Spine Radiosurgery

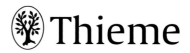

Spine Radiosurgery

Peter C. Gerszten, MD, MPH, FACS
Departments of Neurological Surgery and Radiation Oncology
University of Pittsburgh Medical Center
Pittsburgh, Pennsylvania

Samuel Ryu, MD
Director of Radiosurgery
Departments of Radiation Oncology and Neurosurgery
Josephine Ford Cancer Center
Henry Ford Health System
Detroit, Michigan

Thieme
New York • Stuttgart

Thieme Medical Publishers, Inc.
333 Seventh Ave.
New York, NY 10001

Associate Editor: Ivy Ip
Executive Editor: Kalen D. Conerly
Vice President, Production and Electronic Publishing: Anne T. Vinnicombe
Production Editor: Grace R. Caputo, Dovetail Content Solutions
Vice President, International Sales and Marketing: Cornelia Schulze
Chief Financial Officer: Peter van Woerden
President: Brian D. Scanlan
Compositor: Macmillan Solutions
Printer: Everbest Printing Co.

Library of Congress Cataloging-in-Publication Data
Spine radiosurgery / [edited by] Peter C. Gerszten, Samuel Ryu.
      p. ; cm.
      Includes bibliographical references and index.
      ISBN 978-1-58890-509-3 (alk. paper)
    1. Spinal cord—Tumors. 2. Radiosurgery. I. Gerszten, Peter C. II. Ryu,
Samuel.
      [DNLM: 1. Spinal Cord Neoplasms—surgery. 2. Radiosurgery—methods. WL
400 S75945 2008]
      RD673.S65 2008
      617.4'82059—dc22
                                        2008017405

Important note: Medical knowledge is ever-changing. As new research and clinical experience broaden our knowledge, changes in treatment and drug therapy may be required. The authors and editors of the material herein have consulted sources believed to be reliable in their efforts to provide information that is complete and in accord with the standards accepted at the time of publication. However, in view of the possibility of human error by the authors, editors, or publisher of the work herein or changes in medical knowledge, neither the authors, editors, nor publisher, nor any other party who has been involved in the preparation of this work, warrants that the information contained herein is in every respect accurate or complete, and they are not responsible for any errors or omissions or for the results obtained from use of such information. Readers are encouraged to confirm the information contained herein with other sources. For example, readers are advised to check the product information sheet included in the package of each drug they plan to administer to be certain that the information contained in this publication is accurate and that changes have not been made in the recommended dose or in the contraindications for administration. This recommendation is of particular importance in connection with new or infrequently used drugs.

Some of the product names, patents, and registered designs referred to in this book are in fact registered trademarks or proprietary names even though specific reference to this fact is not always made in the text. Therefore, the appearance of a name without designation as proprietary is not to be construed as a representation by the publisher that it is in the public domain.

Printed in China

5 4 3 2 1

ISBN 978-1-58890-509-3

To my teachers, colleagues, parents, wife, and children for their continuous encouragement and their support of my work.

Peter C. Gerszten

To my parents, who received radiosurgery treatment; to my wife and children for their loving encouragement; and to my teachers, who gave insight of research.

Samuel Ryu

Contents

Contents

Preface

The current trend in modern cancer treatment is for more focused and more targeted therapy. Targeted therapy is not limited to the biological approach. In the 1950s, brain radiosurgery was developed in which large doses of precisely directed focused radiation created lesions in white matter tracts of nuclei. The biologic effect of radiosurgery was almost like the result of a surgical procedure even though traditional surgical instruments were not used. The revolution in medical imaging in the 1970s (computed tomography) and early 1980s (magnetic resonance imaging) provided increasingly sophisticated diagnostic tools for target definition and radiosurgery planning. The development of radiation intensity modulation in the 1990s, with elegant methods of pencil beam and multileaf collimators, coupled with the progress of computer science, made the use of radiosurgery possible outside the brain.

Working independently, we conceived a vision of applying stereotactic radiosurgery for the treatment of spinal tumors. We each risked failures while seeking clinical success for our patients. We finally met in 2003, each bringing with us our own experiences of spine radiosurgery. At that time, we did not realize that this would open an exciting new chapter in the field of spinal oncology. We had many common thoughts and shared our visions for the future progress of spine radiosurgery.

Stereotactic radiosurgery is a demanding discipline that combines knowledge of radiation biology and physics, medical imaging, and radiotherapeutic and neurosurgical practice with oncologic decision making. Therefore, the practice of radiosurgery is the utmost example of the close collaboration of multidisciplinary endeavor that adds a new dimension to the treatment of both benign and malignant disorders. For the safe and effective practice of radiosurgery, physicians involved in the practice of radiosurgery must be qualified to recommend other standard or alternative treatments, whether neurosurgical or radiotherapeutic. The application of radiosurgery demands rigid criteria for selecting individual patients to be treated, with the understanding of the natural course of spine tumors. The practice of spine radiosurgery certainly requires a thorough knowledge of neuroanatomy and neurophysiopathology and an understanding of the radiobiologic effects on therapeutic gain and potential acute and long-term risks, as well as radiosurgery physics and techniques. As the first book dedicated to spine radiosurgery, this volume was conceived as a major resource to consolidate information on the techniques, clinical indications and outcomes, and complications of spine radiosurgery.

We thank the many contributors to this book. They were chosen carefully because of their innovative individual contributions as pioneers in this field. Finally, we are deeply indebted to the patients who bravely agreed to undergo spine radiosurgery during its earliest days of development. It is our sincerest hope that the origin and our vision of spine radiosurgery will positively contribute to the progress of modern medicine and benefit patients.

Introduction I

Stereotactic radiosurgery (SRS) was the brain child of the innovative Swedish pioneer Lars Leksell. He coined the term in 1951 after first combining a prototype intracranial guiding device with an orthovoltage dental x-ray unit that could be swept in arcs over a patient's head. His goal was to provide closed skull irradiation of a tiny intracranial target, the gasserian ganglion, during treatment of patients with intractable trigeminal neuralgia. The results, after more than 30 years, were startling and long-lasting. Leksell collaborated with the Swedish radiobiologist Bore Larsson, who ran the proton beam unit at the University of Uppsala (The Gustav Werner Institute). They expanded their concept of using protons cross-fired on the target employing a specially constructed guiding device with a proton generator attached to a huge arc. Numerous experiments were performed on radiobiological models, including goats that lived peacefully on Larsson's nearby farm, until nature presented the opportunity for an eventual postmortem examination.

Professor Leksell found that discrete lesions could be created in animal models. He began to apply this concept to the construction of a human stereotactic radiosurgical device, eventually called *strålkniven,* or "radiation knife." As the source of the photon beams was found to be best using cobalt 60, the name eventually evolved to Gamma Knife, which became the first successful unit to be applied in the hospital environment. Leksell had hoped to use linear accelerators, but the wobble of the gantry in these early generation units of the 1960s gave him pause. He elected to use 179 sealed sources mounted in a hemispheric array in a specially sealed two-ton unit.

The field of SRS had been born, nurtured, and expanded. During the 1980s, new units were placed in various sites outside Sweden, and applications continued to expand. It first seemed likely that the advantage of radiosurgery—that is, closed skull destruction of an intracranial target using ionizing beams of radiation that could be focused through the intact scalp, skull, and brain—would be restricted to the brain. During this same interval, the revolution in neurodiagnostic imaging brought about first by computed tomography in the 1970s and then by magnetic resonance imaging in the 1980s prompted early and graphic recognition of intracranial and eventually spine and body targets. The revolution in diagnostic imaging drove a concomitant revolution in therapies. Radiosurgery, the older sister of microsurgery, stayed in the background until selected sites began to request the technology, apply it in a wide spectrum of brain disease, and eventually test the concept that it could be performed for targets other than in the brain and skull.

Such an application required the reassessment of the potential role of linear accelerator-created photon irradiation. Linear accelerator manufacturers began collaboration not only with radiation oncology partners, their traditional source of inspiration, but also with surgeons and medical physicists who wanted to apply principles of radiosurgery to both the spine and other body targets. Pioneers such as Alan Hamilton in Tucson, Arizona, and Ingomar Lax in Stockholm, Sweden, developed body stereotactic guiding devices that could be coupled with linear accelerators to deliver radiation in a single session. Many problems had to be solved, including complex attachment of the body-guiding device so that rigid fixation was ensured. In addition, the potential movement of the target within the body during the cardiac and respiratory cycles defied easy solutions. Finally, the selection of appropriate candidates for radiosurgical intervention was paramount. It was logical to apply the SRS principle to spinal targets, both malignant and benign tumors, because of the need for noninvasive treatments for patients with metastatic invasive cancer. In addition, dose-sparing strategies were needed to maintain function of critical surrounding structures such as the spinal cord, while optimizing the therapeutic benefit of mass lesion to control tumor growth and to obtain pain relief.

In this book, the reader will learn much about the current status of spinal radiosurgery from pioneers who helped to demonstrate its worth. Currently, there are many vendors who have adapted their technology or even created new technologies to assist the radiosurgical team in the accurate therapeutic delivery of radiation, usually in a single session (radiosurgery) or, on occasion, using multiple procedures (staged radiosurgery). Usage of single or staged procedures has more to do with the ability of the technology to provide high conformality (three-dimensional volume shaping of the therapeutic target dose to the lesion itself) and high selectivity (rigid dose fall-off in adjacent tissues). For technologies that have high conformality and high selectivity, radiosurgery may be the optimal management, especially for smaller volume targets. For larger lesions, or for targets in which the technological conformality and selectivity is not as good, staged radiosurgical procedures may maintain therapeutic efficacy, while minimizing radiation risk to surrounding tissues. At present, the explosion of knowledge and application related to these technologies provides evidence for enhanced patient outcomes in properly selected patients. SRS is an accepted alternative to traditional surgical or even fractionated radiation therapy. Radiosurgery has not followed the usual course of new technological discoveries, that is, a blip of initial interest followed by an explosion of applications, which is in turn followed by a sobering assessment of the risks and benefits. Instead, there has been a steady and significant growth in the application of radiosurgical principles over the past 55 years.

It cannot be overemphasized that for a center to embark on radiosurgical approaches, a team effort is required. The team consists of surgeons, radiation oncologists, and medical physicists who bring their particular knowledge base to a new paradigm of multidisciplinary cooperation and collaboration. To be effective, the team must realize that what is important is keeping the best interests of patients at heart, not who is the leader or who takes the credit. With this approach, the future will see a widening application of radiosurgery in the field of cancers involving the lungs, extremities, spine, and abdominal cavity.

L. Dade Lunsford, MD
Pittsburgh, Pennsylvania

Introduction II

Decades ago, traditional practitioners of radiotherapy developed the concept of fractionation to enhance the therapeutic ratio. Early in the 20th century, it was already well recognized that the sensitivity of different tissues was unique and dependent on fraction size as well as total dose. The classic teaching in radiobiology illustrates this concept with the oft-quoted story about irradiating ram testicles: whereas a single large fraction resulted in both severe skin toxicity and azoospermia, delivering the same total dose in a fractionated approach resulted in azoospermia with skin sparing, illustrating the greater sensitivity of spermatogenesis to radiation compared with skin, and also demonstrating how fractionation could be used to spare skin.[1] Early pioneering work in France by Bacllese et al established the principles of fractionating radiotherapy in the management of neoplastic disease, setting the basis for current fractionation schedules. In the 1980s, radiobiological research proposed the linear-quadratic model, which was initially simply and practically interpreted to imply that there are two broad categories of tissues: those with "high" α/β ratios (generally 10 or so, and including most "rapidly proliferating" tissues, such as skin, mucosa, bone marrow, and, presumably, most malignancies) and those with "low" α/β ratios (generally 2–3, and including most "late-reacting" tissues, such as lung, brain, liver, and kidneys).[2] At the same time, the concept of "half-life" of repair gained currency, with the expectation, albeit very general and simplified, that most tumors had long or longer half-lives of repair of radiation injury in contrast to most normal tissues, which had shorter (e.g., 1.5–2 hours) half-lives of repair.[3] The extension of this concept was the underpinning for hyperfractionation with interfraction intervals of 6 to 8 hours (with a range of 4–12 hours), assuming that most repairable injury to normal tissues had been completed between radiation fractions delivered 6 to 8 hours apart, but the tumor was still more susceptible as little repair had occurred in it. With the availability of actual data, we now know that the situation is far more complex. For example, the most common cancer in men, prostate cancer, most likely has a very low α/β ratio, perhaps even lower than that for normal tissues.[4] Additionally, a superior understanding of half-lives of repair supports considerable heterogeneity based on the specific tissue.

Whereas traditional radiotherapy has diligently pursued the fractionation paradigm, it has long been known, almost from the time of the Curies, that a single exposure to a large dose of radiation can have significant tissue-ablative/destructive capability. Lars Leksell, the pioneering Swedish neurosurgeon, capitalized on this by applying multiple noncoplanar beams to a small intracranial target with the express purpose of achieving tissue ablation.[5] However, competing modalities for neuroablation, such as cryosurgery and radiofrequency ablation, could also achieve similar results, and radiosurgery, the application of multiple radiation beams to a tiny intracranial target (to a high single fraction dose), found its niche in treating intracranial neoplasms (both benign and malignant), among other applications. Since its origin in the 1960s and widespread application since the 1980s, radiosurgery has remained confined to the cranium.[6]

This book deals with the extracranial use of radiosurgery. Currently, extracranial radiosurgery is primarily used for small targets in the lung, liver, and spine. The biology of extracranial application of radiosurgical principles is indeed very complex, and the technology necessary for this is only just emerging.[7] This book is logically divided into sections that permit one to understand the necessary biology and technology prior to reviewing actual clinical applications. It is in fact the clinical observations that are driving this "revolution." An excellent example of this is the recognition that conventional radiotherapy produces very low local control rates of early-stage lung cancer, but extracranial radiosurgery can yield about 80% local control. Clearly, such a dramatic difference in outcome is made possible simply through the phenomenon of escalating dose sufficiently, but a key consideration here is limiting the dose to normal tissues. To achieve this, major advances in patient immobilization have been made and married to technologies for precise delivery and, more importantly, verification of delivery. Both intensity-modulated and image-guided radiation therapy have made this possible. These advances in treatment delivery and verification, image guidance, patient immobilization, and dosimetric precision make possible the application of the principle of radiosurgery to spinal targets. Clinically, we are in an early, exploratory phase, and the need of the hour is carefully crafted and completed clinical trials to produce level 1 evidence.

Minesh P. Mehta, MD
Madison, Wisconsin

References

1. Hall EJ. Radiobiology for the Radiologist. Philadelphia: Lippincott-Raven; 1994:212.
2. Fowler JF. The linear quadratic formula and progress in fractionated radiotherapy. Br J Radiol 1989;62:679–694.
3. Peters LJ, Withers HR, Thames HD. Radiobiological basis for multiple daily fractionation. In: Kaercher KH, Kogenlink HD, Reinartz G, eds. Progress in Radio-oncology II. New York: Raven Press; 1982:317–323.
4. Bentzen SM, Ritter M. The α/β ratio for prostate cancer: what is it, really? Radiother Oncol 2005;76:1–3.
5. Leksell L. Cerebral radiosurgery I: gammathalamotomy in two cases of intractable pain. Acta Chir Scand 1968;134:585–595.
6. Mehta MP. The physical, biologic and clinical basis of radiosurgery. Curr Probl Cancer 1995;19:265–329.
7. Fowler JF, Tomé WA, Fenwick J, Mehta MP. Stereotactic body radiotherapy: a challenge to conventional radiation oncology. Int J Radiat Oncol Biol Phys 2004;60:1241–1256.

Contributors

John R. Adler, Jr., MD
Professor
Department of Neurosurgery
Stanford University School of Medicine
Stanford, California

Joseph Anderson, MD
Department of Medical Oncology
Henry Ford Health System
Detroit, Michigan

Mark H. Bilsky, MD
Associate Member
Department of Neurosurgery
Memorial Sloan-Kettering Cancer Center, and
Associate Professor
Department of Neurological Surgery
Weill Cornell University Medical Center
New York, New York

Stephen Brown, PhD
Staff Scientist and Associate Professor
Department of Radiation Oncology
Henry Ford Health System and Wayne State School of Medicine
Detroit, Michigan

Steven A. Burton, MD
Associate Professor
Department of Radiation Oncology
University of Pittsburgh Medical Center
Pittsburgh, Pennsylvania

Eric Lin Chang, MD
Associate Professor
Radiation Oncology Unit
The University of Texas M.D. Anderson Cancer Center
Houston, Texas

Steven D. Chang, MD
Associate Professor
Department of Neurosurgery
Stanford University School of Medicine
Stanford, California

Boyle C. Cheng, PhD
Assistant Professor
Department of Neurological Surgery
University of Pittsburgh Medical Center
Pittsburgh, Pennsylvania

Antonio A. F. De Salles, MD, PhD
Professor of Neurosurgery
Stereotactic Surgery Section
Division of Neurosurgery
UCLA Medical Center
Los Angeles, California

Robert L. Dodd, MD, PhD
Assistant Professor
Department of Neurosurgery
Stanford University School of Medicine
Stanford, California

Kathleen M. Faber, RTT
Senior Research Scientist
Department of Radiation Oncology
Henry Ford Health System
Detroit, Michigan

Gregory J. Gagnon, MD
Associate Professor of Radiation Oncology
Department of Radiation Medicine
Georgetown University Hospital
Washington, DC

Marilyn J. G. Gates, MD
Assistant Professor
Department of Neurosurgery
Assistant Program Director, USUHS
Director, Elder Spine Surgical Program
Co-director, Complex Spine
Henry Ford Health System
Detroit, Michigan

Peter C. Gerszten, MD, MPH, FACS
Departments of Neurological Surgery and Radiation
    Oncology
University of Pittsburgh Medical Center
Pittsburgh, Pennsylvania

Iris C. Gibbs, MD
Associate Professor
Department of Radiation Oncology
Stanford University School of Medicine
Stanford, California

Steven L. Hancock, MD
Professor
Department of Radiation Oncology
Stanford University School of Medicine
Stanford Cancer Center
Stanford, California

Fraser C. Henderson, MD
Director, Spine Tumor Center
Co-director, Radiosurgery
Georgetown University Hospital
Washington, DC

Jian-Yue Jin, PhD, DABR
Senior Staff Physicist
Department of Radiation Oncology
Henry Ford Health System
Detroit, Michigan

Jae Ho Kim, MD, PhD
Professor
Department of Radiation Oncology
Henry Ford Health System
Detroit, Michigan

John P. Kirkpatrick, MD, PhD
Assistant Professor
Department of Radiation Oncology
Duke University Medical Center
Durham, North Carolina

Ian Y. Lee, MD
Resident
Department of Neurosurgery
Henry Ford Health System
Detroit, Michigan

Simon S. Lo, MD
Associate Professor of Radiation Medicine and
    Neurosurgery
Department of Radiation Medicine
Arthur G. James Cancer Hospital
Ohio State University Medical Center
Columbus, Ohio

D. Michael Lovelock, PhD
Associate Attending Physicist
Physics Department
Memorial Sloan-Kettering Cancer Center
New York, New York

L. Dade Lunsford, MD
Professor
Department of Neurological Surgery
University of Pittsburgh Medical Center
Pittsburgh, Pennsylvania

Laura A. Massanisso, BSN
Registered Nurse
Department of Radiation Oncology
Henry Ford Health System
Detroit, Michigan

Paul M. Medin, PhD
Associate Professor
Department of Radiation Oncology
University of Nebraska Medical Center
Omaha, Nebraska

Minesh P. Mehta, MD
Professor
Department of Human Oncology
University of Wisconsin School of Medicine and Public
    Health
Madison, Wisconsin

Martin J. Murphy, PhD
Associate Professor
Department of Radiation Oncology
Virginia Commonwealth University
Richmond, Virginia

Cihat Ozhasoglu, PhD
Assistant Professor
Department of Radiation Oncology
University of Pittsburgh Medical Center
Pittsburgh, Pennsylvania

Jack P. Rock, MD
Senior Staff and Residency Program Director
Department of Neurosurgery
Henry Ford Health System
Detroit, Michigan

Samuel Ryu, MD
Director of Radiosurgery
Departments of Radiation Oncology and Neurosurgery
Josephine Ford Cancer Center
Henry Ford Health System
Detroit, Michigan

Arjun Sahgal, MD
Department of Radiation Oncology
Sunnybrook Health Sciences Centre
University of Toronto
Toronto, Ontario, Canada

Timothy D. Solberg, PhD
Professor
Department of Radiation Oncology
University of Texas Southwestern Medical Center
Dallas, Texas

Albert J. van der Kogel, PhD
Professor of Clinical Radiobiology
Department of Radiation Oncology
Nijmegen, The Netherlands

Zhiheng Wang, PhD
Assistant Professor
Department of Radiation Oncology
Duke University Medical Center
Durham, North Carolina

William C. Welch, MD, FACS, FICS
Professor
Department of Neurosurgery
University of Pennsylvania and
    The Pennsylvania Neurologic Institute
Pennsylvania Hospital
Philadelphia, Pennsylvania

C. Shun Wong, MD, FRCPC
Chief, Department of Radiation Oncology
Head, Radiation Treatment Program
Sunnybrook and Women's College Health Sciences Centre,
and
Professor and Vice-Chair
Department of Radiation Oncology
University of Toronto
Toronto, Ontario, Canada

Q. Jackie Wu, PhD
Assistant Professor
Department of Radiation Oncology
Duke University Medical Center
Durham, North Carolina

Yoshiya Yamada, MD
Assistant Attending Radiation Oncologist
Department of Radiation Oncology
Memorial Sloan-Kettering Cancer Center
New York, New York

Fang-Fang Yin, PhD
Professor and Director of Radiation Physics
Department of Radiation Oncology
Duke University Medical Center
Durham, North Carolina

I

Radiobiology

1
Radiobiology of Radiosurgery

Jae Ho Kim and Stephen Brown

Radiosurgery was initially introduced as a new therapeutic modality for the noninvasive treatment of small intracranial benign vascular lesions. Subsequently, the technology was applied to the treatment of malignant lesions of the brain, including primary and metastatic tumors. More recently, extracranial radiosurgery has been expanded to treat tumors outside the brain, such as those in the spine, head and neck, lung, abdomen, and pelvis. When target lesions are relatively small (i.e., < 2 cm in diameter), large single doses are used to capitalize on the inherent geometric advantage of radiosurgery to limit normal tissue radiation exposure. Target volumes for extracranial radiosurgery often are larger than 2 cm in diameter, resulting in a reduction in the inherent geometric advantage. Like conventional radiotherapy, normal tissue tolerance limits the maximum dose and volume of large single-dose radiosurgery. In an attempt to improve the therapeutic ratio and increase the normal tissue tolerance, delivery of radiosurgery in multiple fractions separated in time may improve efficacy by decreasing late effects of critical normal structures while maintaining superior radiation dose distribution within the tumor tissue. This chapter is primarily devoted to the cellular and molecular processes involved in the killing of tumor and adjacent critical normal tissues after either single or fractionated high-dose radiation.

◆ Tumor Cell Killing after Single High Dose of Radiation

Mammalian cells die through different molecular and cellular mechanisms following exposure of cells to ionizing radiation.[1,2] Depending on cell types, irradiated cells undergo (1) reproductive death (mitotic catastrophic death), (2) apoptosis (usually in interphase cell death), or (3) terminal growth inhibition (metabolic death). Reproductive cell death (sometimes called mitotic cell death) becomes the predominant mode of cellular loss in most human tumors (other than lymphoid and germinal tumors) following x-irradiation. The reproductive capacity of tumor cells is quantified using a cell survival curve, a clonogenic assay of single cells' capacity to undergo multiple replications. Apoptosis is an important mode of cell death in normal tissues and in some tumors, particularly during the acute phase of radiation response. Stem cells of self-renewal normal tissues such as hematopoetic and intestinal crypt cells undergo apoptosis following a moderate dose of radiation exposure. Apoptosis occurs within a few hours to days and can be detected using an array of assays, including observing deoxyribonucleic acid (DNA) laddering on a Western blot; antibody detection in situ or with flow cytometry using any of various DNA fragment labels, such as TUNEL (terminal uridine deoxynucleotidyl transferase mediated dUTP [2'-deoxyuridine 5'-triphosphate] nick end labeling) and Annexin V; and caspase kits, such as caspase 3. In contrast to the significance of apoptosis to the manifestation of the acute phase of tissue response to radiation, the late phase is a result of terminal or permanent growth inhibition of either self-renewing or differentiating and metabolically active cells.

◆ Cell Survival Curves of Established Human Tumor Cells in Culture

Are cell survival curves of human tumor cells in culture relevant to the radiobiology of single high-dose radiosurgery? Tumor physiology is usually more complex than simple in vitro models can reasonably characterize. Nonetheless, some human metastatic lesions in the brain or other organs are well circumscribed without significant infiltration into the adjacent normal tissues and with tumor vasculature less developed than the primary tumors arising in the brain or other organs from which they derive. In fact, cell culture models such as single plated monolayer cells and multicellular spheroids have considerable value in modeling pertinent radiobiological parameters important to the tumor control probability in a wide range of tumors, even though they are not perfect representations of human tumors.

A standard in vitro assay of a cell's capacity to reproduce is a clonogenic assay that results in a cell survival curve. Classical cell survival curves are obtained following the growth of single cells maintained in culture media exposed to graded single doses of radiation. Clonogenic assays represent the reproductive capacity of single tumor cells. To produce a cluster of progeny, called a "colony," from single plated cells, human tumor cells excised from the patient are propagated for many generations under optimal tissue culture conditions and allowed to form a colony from single plated cells. However, if single cells from the biopsy or pathology specimens do not form a colony from plated cells, other methods are used, such as short-term growth delay using a colorimetric assay (e.g., MTT [3-(4,5-dimethylthiazol-2-yl)-2,5-diphenyltetrazolium bromide] assay), although quantitative measurement of cell killing of more than 2 logs is problematic. Radiobiological studies with established human tumor cell lines have provided several useful biological determinants influencing the tumor response and tumor control rate of in vivo tumor system.

Two mathematical constructs widely used to model the relationship between cell survival and radiation dose are the single-hit, multitarget (SHMT) and the linear-quadratic models (also called the alpha/beta [α/β] model). The model characterizes the shape of the best-fit curve using two of three related parameters, Do, Dq, and N, which are related by $\ln N = Dq/Do$. Do is a measure of the slope of the log-linear plot of cell survival and radiation dose that reflects the intrinsic radiation sensitivity of the cells. Dq is almost a threshold dose, below which radiation purportedly has no effect, and is a measure of the breadth of the low-dose shoulder region that reflects the cells' capacity to repair radiation damage. N, the extrapolation number, is a measure of the number of targets in the cell and also reflects the cells capacity for repair. The SHMT model describes the relationship between the radiation dose, d, and the surviving fraction of cells, $SF = S(d)/So$, where $S(d)$ is the number of cells that survive a dose of radiation, d, and So is the initial number of cells, $SF = 1 - [1 - \exp(-d/Do)]^N$.

The linear-quadratic model characterizes the best-fit relationship between SF and d using two parameters, α and β, $SF = \exp(-\alpha d - \beta d^2)$. Cell death that is "linearly" proportional to dose (on a semi-logarithmic plot of SF vs d) has been interpreted to be a result of double-strand DNA breaks because such aberrations are lethal and may be caused by the same particle (i.e., photon). Consequently, an increase in dose "linearly" decreases surviving fraction. Cell death that is "quadratically" proportional to dose (on a semi-logarithmic plot of SF vs d) has been interpreted to be a result of single-strand DNA breaks because two such aberrations in close proximity are lethal (more probable at high doses). Consequently, an increase in dose "quadratically" decreases surviving fraction, and the quadratic mode of cell killing dominates at high doses. Interestingly, the ratio of α over β has found utility in characterizing the response of tissues as either acutely responding, those having large magnitudes of the order of 10, and late responding, those having smaller magnitudes of the order of 2.

Radiation survival curves of most human tumor cells other than lymphoma or germinal tumors are well fit by the SHMT model with a shoulder region at low doses, and at higher doses the survival curve decreases exponentially with dose. It is interesting to note that most of the heterogeneity of cellular response to radiation is seen at the low-dose region (maximum variation is 10- or 20-fold), but at the higher dose region, that is, doses higher than 8 to 10 Gy, the differences among cell lines become smaller (maximum variation is 2-fold). This is an important consideration in the difference between the radiobiology of conventional radiation therapy and the radiobiology of radiosurgery. For example, in the conventional 2 Gy dose fractionation radiotherapy, the total cell kill will be determined with the surviving fraction at the 2 Gy level and magnified to 30 or 35 times, depending on the total dose of radiotherapy, whereas in single-dose radiosurgery, the surviving fraction is mostly determined at the high-dose fraction region. Hence, variation in the total surviving fraction from cell line to cell line may be less with radiosurgery. In fractionated radiotherapy, radiobiological parameters such as repair capacity from the sublethal injury and the rate of reoxygenation after each dose fraction are important determinants to the eventual radiocurability of large solid tumors. On the other hand, important radiobiological determinants in radiosurgery are tumor clonogen numbers and intrinsic radiosensitivity of tumor cells. These two parameters are readily calculated from the cell survival curves.

Figure 1.1 shows representative survival curves having different N and Do. It is readily apparent from **Fig. 1.1** that the higher the single dose, the more tumor cells killed and that the magnitude of cell kill depends on the intrinsic radio-

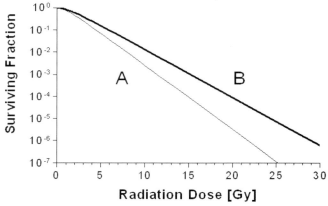

Figure 1.1 At radiosurgery doses, the relationship between surviving fraction and radiation dose is affected most profoundly by the intrinsic cellular radiosensitivity, Do, which is the radiation dose necessary to reduce surviving fraction by 37%, and also by the number of targets, N. Do is the reciprocal of the steepness of the straight-line portion of the curve (the smaller the Do, the more sensitive the cells). N is related to the cells' capacity to accumulate sublethal damage. The two cell lines shown are illustrative of sensitive cells characterized by $Do = 1.5$ and $N = 2$ (line A) and resistant cells characterized by $Do = 2.0$ and $N = 4$ (line B). The population of sensitive cells is 4 times more likely to be killed at a low dose, such as 5 Gy, than a population of resistant cells with approximately equal contributions from Do and N. In contrast, at a high dose, such as 30 Gy, the sensitive cells are 300 times more sensitive, with most of the difference in sensitivity resulting from the difference in Do.

Table 1.1 Characterization of Survival Curves with Varying Sensitivity and Repair Capacity

Dose (Gy)	Surviving Fraction			
	Sensitive Cells ($Do = 1.5$) Smaller Repair ($N = 2$)	Sensitive Cells ($Do = 1.5$) Larger Repair ($N = 4$)	Resistant Cells ($Do = 2.0$) Smaller Repair ($N = 2$)	Resistant Cells ($Do = 2.0$) Larger Repair ($N = 4$)
0	1.0	1.0	1.0	1.0
5	0.070	0.14	0.16	0.29
10	0.0025	0.0051	0.013	0.026
15	9.1×10^{-5}	0.00018	0.0011	0.0022
20	3.2×10^{-6}	6.5×10^{-6}	9.1×10^{-5}	0.00018
30	4.1×10^{-9}	8.2×10^{-9}	6.1×10^{-7}	1.2×10^{-6}
40	5.2×10^{-12}	1.0×10^{-11}	4.1×10^{-9}	8.2×10^{-9}

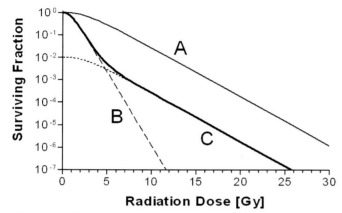

Figure 1.2 The relationship between surviving fraction and radiation dose is critically dependent on the oxygen status of the cells because hypoxic cells are up to three times more resistant ($3 \times Do$) than well-oxygenated cells. (A) Surviving fraction as a function of radiation dose of a hypoxic cell population. (B) Surviving fraction as a function of radiation dose of a uniformly well-oxygenated cell population. (C) Surviving fraction as a function of radiation dose of a population of cells that are 99% well-oxygenated and sensitive to radiation and 1% hypoxic and resistant to radiation. At doses greater than 6 Gy, cellular survival is dictated by the response of the hypoxic cells.

sensitivity of cells. **Table 1.1** shows the surviving fraction of irradiated tumor cells following single doses of radiation. For example, the surviving fraction of cells will be reduced by nearly 6 logs of cell kill at a dose of 20 Gy for cells having Do of 1.50 Gy and $N = 2$, whereas the surviving fraction will be reduced by approximately 4 logs of cell kill for cells exposed to the same dose having Do of 2.00 Gy and $N = 4$. On the other hand, when a tumor cell population contains a small fraction of hypoxic cells (e.g., 1%), the cell survival curve shows a biphasic response (**Fig. 1.2**). Hypoxic tumor cells are about three times more resistant, that is, $3 \times Do$, than oxic cells. **Table 1.2** shows the expected surviving fraction of irradiated tumor cells following single doses of radiation, containing 1% and 10% hypoxic fraction.

◆ In vivo Murine Tumor Control Rate following a Single High Dose of Radiation

Studies of a range of cell lines derived from murine or human tumors have shown a wide variation in the tumor control rates following a single fraction dose of radiation. The most commonly used estimate of the tumor control rate of transplantable murine tumors and human tumor xenografts is the measured radiation dose required to produce tumor control in half of a group of tumors (TCD$_{50}$). A typical determina-

Table 1.2 The Effect of Hypoxia on Cellular Survival

Dose (Gy)	Surviving Fraction			
	No Hypoxia ($Do = 1.0$, $N = 2$)	1% Hypoxia (Do$_{hypoxia}$ = $3 \times Do$, $N = 2$)	10% Hypoxia (Do$_{hypoxia}$ = $3 \times Do$, $N = 2$)	100% Hypoxia (Do$_{hypoxia}$ = $3 \times Do$, $N = 2$)
0	1.0	1.0	1.0	1.0
5	0.013	0.017	0.046	0.34
10	9.1×10^{-5}	0.00079	0.0071	0.070
15	6.1×10^{-7}	0.00013	0.0013	0.013
20	4.1×10^{-9}	2.5×10^{-5}	0.00025	0.0025
30	1.9×10^{-13}	9.1×10^{-7}	9.1×10^{-6}	9.1×10^{-5}
40		3.2×10^{-8}	3.2×10^{-7}	3.2×10^{-6}

tion of TCD involves locally irradiating transplanted tumors growing in syngeneic mice when the tumors reach a certain predefined volume (e.g., 100 mm^3) using a generous region of adjacent normal tissues in the field and usually graded single doses of radiation. The proportion of tumors that are locally controlled within 90 or 120 days after irradiation is plotted as a function of dose, and TCD_{50} is the dose at which 50% of the tumors are free of local tumor at the defined time after irradiation.

The range of 50% tumor control doses (TCD_{50}) for both murine and human tumor xenograft varies widely by a factor of 2 or 3, when tumors are irradiated under normal blood flow conditions. The TCD_{50} range is, approximately, 30 to 70 Gy. The large variation in the TCD_{50} is mostly due to three radiobiologic parameters — intrinsic radiosensitivity, clonogenic fraction, and tumor hypoxia of individual transplantable tumors.[3] Most transplantable tumors implanted into subcutaneous or intramuscular site contain a substantial fraction of hypoxic tumors, which would account for high TCD_{50} values. In the absence of tumor hypoxia, tumor clonogens become a significant determinant of tumor curability after single-dose irradiation.

In addition to the foregoing two radiobiological parameters — that is, clonogen and intrinsic radiosensitivity of tumor cells — a question of relevance is the importance of radiation-induced apoptosis on the tumor cure rates of apoptosis-susceptible versus resistant tumors. Dewey et al discussed the contribution of radiation-induced apoptosis with respect to single high dose versus fractionated radiotherapy.[4] The effect of apoptosis-susceptible tumors (e.g., 20–40% induced apoptosis) after multiple clinically relevant doses of 2 Gy fractions would be very significant to total cell killing, assuming that irradiated tumor cells would be recruited into an apoptosis-susceptible fraction after each dose of radiation. This additional killing from apoptosis could result in a 20% cure rate without apoptosis and increasing to a 50 to 65% cure rate with apoptosis. On the other hand, the contribution of apoptosis following a single high dose of radiation (e.g., TCD_{50}-values) would be minimal, because the maximal effect of cell kill by apoptosis would be less than 1 log cell kill (e.g., 50% induced apoptosis).

However, radiation-induced endothelial apoptosis in the irradiated microvasculature is considered to be an obligatory process in achieving tumor cure in some tumors. Garcia-Barros et al have shown this process by using genetic knockout systems to demonstrate the involvement of the endothelia.[5] They implanted nonimmunogenic transplantable tumors into mice that had radioresistant endothelia because of deficiencies in acid sphingomyelinase. Tumors implanted into these mice were more resistant to radiation than tumors implanted into wild-type acid sphingomyelinase positive mice, which have radiosensitive endothelia.[6] It is interesting to note that tumor response to radiation regulated by endothelial cell apoptosis is seen at the single dose of less than 10 Gy, whereas at higher doses of 18 to 20 Gy, death of tumor cells becomes independent of the endothelial apoptosis.

◆ Molecular Events following a Single High Dose of Radiation

Although radiation can cause molecular damage to any molecule in a cell, damage to DNA and nucleoprotein is most critical to the survival of the cell. Ionizing radiation can cause DNA strand breakage or distortion of the DNA nucleoprotein conformation, events that would trigger the expression of cellular stress response signals. The initial molecular events include rapid upregulation of gene transcription for inflammatory cytokines,[7] angiogenic factors,[8] secondary transcriptional activators,[9] and gene products involved in the repair of damaged DNA. Prominent among the initial upregulation of gene transcription is early growth response protein gene families (*EGR1*). In particular, the functional role of *EGR1* in radiation-induced signaling is crucial because the promoter of *EGR1* contains radiation-inducible DNA sequences.[10] Gene targets mediated by *EGR1* in response to radiation include tumor necrosis factor-alpha (TNF-α), protein 53 (p53), retinoblastoma (Rb), and Bcl-2-associated X protein (Bax), all of which are effectors of apoptosis. It has been shown that activation of both *EGR1* and TNF-α gene is radiation dose dependent.[11] Thus, a high single dose of radiation (e.g., > 10

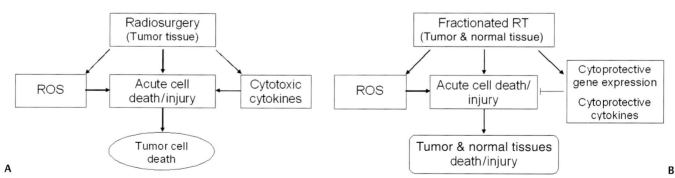

Figure 1.3 The molecular events after fractionated radiotherapy (RT) and radiosurgery (RS) are dictated by the radiation dose used and the tissue volume irradiated. Both the normal tissue response **(A)** and that of the malignant tissue **(B)** contribute to the resulting molecular events. ROS, reactive oxygen species.

Gy) would confer more efficient radiation-inductive signaling cascade through early genes such as *EGR1*.

Radiation-induced stress responses at the molecular level elicit very different responses depending on the level of radiation doses. The diversity of responses with cytoprotective and cytotoxic signals vary widely between the normal tissues and tumor tissues (**Fig. 1.3**). Radiation induces activation of plasma membrane receptors. These activation signals, depending on the radiation dose and the nature of receptors activated, are transmitted through preexisting signal transduction pathways. Cytoprotective responses include members of mitogen-activated protein kinase (MAPK) families, PI3K (phosphoinositide-3 kinase), AKT, STAT3 (signal transducer and activator of transcription 3), nitric oxide synthase, and NF-κ (nuclear factor-κ).[12–15] These pathways engage inhibition of proapoptotic BAD ($Bcl-X_L$/Bcl-2–associated death promoter), increase the ratio of Bcl-2/Bax, and upregulate DNA repair enzymes.[16] Cytotoxic response pathways include activation of death receptors and ceramide pathway.[17] Another part of the early response involves the induction of sets of secreted molecules, such as pro-inflammatory cytokines, proteases, and antiproteases. The larger the volume of normal tissue being irradiated, the more induction of proinflammatory cytokines. Basic fibroblast growth factor (bFGF) can protect apoptosis of endothelial cells by an autocrine pathway. Secretion of vascular endothelial growth factor (VEGF) would make endothelial cells radioresistant. Proinflammatory cytokines play an important role in the development of late effects of normal tissues.

◆ Radiobiology of Fractionated Radiosurgery

Geometric superiority of radiosurgery for the treatment of a small target volume becomes less evident when the target field increases. More normal tissue is necessarily irradiated as the tumor volume increases even if the tumor margin remains the same. For example, the volume of a 1 mm margin of a 1 cm diameter spherical tumor is 0.4 cm^3, whereas the volume of a 1 mm margin of a 3 cm diameter spherical tumor is 3.0 cm^3. **Figure 1.4** illustrates the increased area of normal tissue that is irradiated when larger fields and margins are used. Normal tissue tolerance limits the dose and volume of large single-dose fraction radiosurgery. Consequently, as with conventional fractionated radiotherapy, large tumors represent a treatment challenge limited by the dose that surrounding normal tissues can tolerate.

With the advent of a relocatable frame, it has become possible to exploit the radiobiological advantages of fractionation with the possibility of improving the therapeutic ratio, as compared with single-fraction radiosurgery. If fractionated radiosurgery is to be used, the question arises as to how many fractions to use and what the optimum overall time frame would be. Fractionated schemes that have been used in the clinic for radiosurgery vary from conventional daily fractionation to various types of hypofractionation.

As with conventional fractionated radiotherapy, fractionated radiosurgery would provide several potential ra-

diobiological advantages over single-fraction radiosurgery, although tumor cell killing efficiency may be less with fractionated radiosurgery. These biological factors include reoxygenation of tumors containing a radioresistant hypoxic fraction (the larger the tumor, the more likely it is to have a hypoxic fraction), recruitment of noncycling plateau phase tumor cells into the more radiosensitive cycling phase, and differential repair and recovery of tumor and normal tissues from sublethal and potentially lethal damage.

Because the normal tissue tolerance is directly related to the volume and dose of tissues being irradiated, the smaller incremental exposure of the normal tissue would be advantageous. The dose volume histogram would be a useful guide in estimating the volume of normal tissues being exposed. Kim et al addressed the issue of response of tumor and late-responding normal tissue of critical intracranial structures to both single-dose and fractionated radiosurgery.[18] As expected, single-dose radiosurgery was found to be more effective in curing small intracranial tumors (9L gliosarcoma) than large tumors. They further tested the validity of the linear-quadratic isoeffect formula for the normal tissue injury using the optic neuropathy as an end point. The sparing effect of fractionated radiosurgery is greater for late-responding tissues, relative to the rapidly proliferating tumor tissues. However, it is not clear whether conventional dose fractionated radiotherapy (e.g., 2 Gy × 30) would be able to achieve a similar tumor control rate with hypofractionated radiosurgery (e.g., 14 Gy × 3).

Intriguing recent experimental evidence from cell culture studies demonstrates that a prior radiation exposure can elicit an inducible-like radioprotective response that is not dependent on the cellular intrinsic radiosensitivity or cell cycle effects.[19] The magnitude of protection is not small; cell killing can vary by 2 logs of cell kill in response to a high single exposure depending on whether the cells were primed (i.e., exposed to prior radiation) or not. Notwithstanding the need for confirmatory studies, these results give theoretical support to the use of single high-dose radiosurgery in favor of fractionated radiotherapy. A complete understanding of the radiobiology of radiosurgery will allow for improvements in routine clinical radiation therapy.

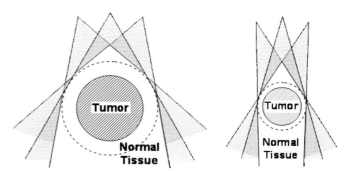

Figure 1.4 Radiobiological parameters are affected by cellular factors differently under conditions of fractionated radiotherapy and single-dose radiosurgery. The radiobiological response of normal tissue depends on the volume of irradiation, which in turn is a function of the field size and margins used.

◆ Conclusion

In summary, as with all radiation therapy, the response of adjacent irradiated normal tissue impacts tumor curability by limiting radiation doses obtainable. For large tumors, normal tissue volume irradiated is substantially larger than for small tumors. Fractionated radiosurgery is one approach to spare normal tissue while maintaining tumor response. The radiobiological response of normal tissue depends on the volume irradiated, the radiation dose, the number of fractions, and the dose per fraction. Our understanding of the radiobiology of both normal tissue and tumor affects the success of radiosurgery.

References

1. Hall EJ. Radiobiology for the Radiologist. 5th ed. Philadelphia: Lippincott Williams & Wilkins; 2000.
2. Tannock IF, Hill RP, Bristow RC, Harrington L. The Basic Science of Oncology. 4th ed. New York: McGraw-Hill; 2005.
3. Gerweck LE, Zaidi ST, Zietman A. Multivariate determinants of radiocurability. 1: Prediction of single fraction tumor control doses. Int J Radiat Oncol Biol Phys 1994;29(1):57–66.
4. Dewey WC, Ling CC, Meyn RE. Radiation-induced apoptosis: relevance to radiotherapy. Int J Radiat Oncol Biol Phys 1995;33:781–796.
5. Garcia-Barros M, Kolesnick R, Fuks Z, et al. Tumor response to radiotherapy regulated by endothelial cell apoptosis. Science 2003;300:1155–1159.
6. Paris F, Fuks Z, Kang A, et al. Endothelial apoptosis as the primary lesion initiating intestinal radiation damage in mice. Science 2001;293:293–297.
7. Hallahan DE, Haimovitz-Friedman A, Kufe DW, et al. The role of cytokines in radiation oncology. Important Adv Oncol 1993;71–80.
8. Gorski DH, Beckett NT, Jaskowiak DP, et al. Blockade of vascular endothelial growth factor stress response increases the antitumor effects of ionizing radiation. Cancer Res 1999;59:3374–3378.
9. Dalton TP, Shertzer HG, Puge A. Regulation of gene expression by reactive oxygen. Annu Rev Pharmacol Toxicol 1999;39:67–101.
10. Datta R, Rubin E, Sukhatme V, et al. Ionizing radiation activates transcription of the EGR1 gene via CarG elements. Proc Natl Acad Sci U S A 1992;89:10149–10153.
11. Weichselbaum RR, Kufe DW, Hellman S, et al. Radiation-induced tumor necrosis factor-alpha expression: clinical application of transcriptional and physical targeting of gene therapy. Lancet Oncol 2002;3:665–671.
12. Kavanagh BD, Lin PS, Chen P, et al. Radiation-induced enhanced proliferation of human squamous cancer cells in vitro: a release from inhibition by epidermal growth factor. Clin Cancer Res 1995;1:1557–1562.
13. Schmidt-Ullrich RK, Dent P, Grant S, et al. Signal transduction and cellular radiation responses. Radiat Res 2000;153:245–257.
14. Dent P, Reardon DB, Park JS, et al. Radiation-induced release of TGF-alpha activates the epidermal growth factor receptor and mitogen-activated protein kinase pathway in carcinoma cells, leading to increased proliferation and protection from radiation-induced cell death. Mol Biol Cell 1999;10:2493–2506.
15. Bromberg JF, Horvath CM, Besser D, et al. Stat3 activation is required for cellular transformation by V-SRC. Mol Cell Biol 1998;18:2553–2558.
16. Iliakis G, Wang Y, Guan J, et al. DNA damage checkpoint control in cells exposed to ionizing radiation. Oncogene 2003;22:5834–5847.
17. Kolesnick R, Fuks Z. Radiation and ceramide-induced apoptosis. Oncogene 2003;22:5897–5906.
18. Kim JH, Khil MS, Kolozsvary A, et al. Fractionated radiosurgery for 9L gliosarcoma in the rat brain. Int J Radiat Oncol Biol Phys 1999;45:1035–1040.
19. Qutob SS, Multani AS, Pathak S, et al. Fractionated X-radiation treatment can elicit an inducible-like radioprotective response that is not dependent on the intrinsic cellular X-radiation resistance/sensitivity. Radiat Res 2006;166:590–599

2

Spinal Cord Radiobiology

Arjun Sahgal, Albert J. van der Kogel, and C. Shun Wong

Central nervous system (CNS) radiation injury is a major toxicity in radiation therapy (XRT) for tumors located within or near the brain and spinal cord. White matter necrosis, demyelination, and vascular damage (including increased vascular permeability) are prominent histopathologic findings following XRT to the CNS. Treatment-related sequelae such as focal neurological deficits, neurocognitive dysfunction, and myelopathy are of such concern that they severely limit the clinician's ability to deliver curative doses of XRT.

Radiation injury to the CNS is manifested as three distinct clinical entities.[1] During a course of XRT, patients often experience fatigue and an exacerbation of preexisting neurologic symptoms and signs. However, death from brain herniation, especially after a large single dose as delivered during stereotactic radiosurgery, has been reported.[2] These acute CNS radiation injuries (early effects) are generally considered to be secondary to edema and disruption of the blood–brain barrier (BBB).[3,4]

A self-limiting delayed reaction known as Lhermitte syndrome is well recognized after XRT to the spinal cord. It occurs after a latent period of 2 to 4 months and is characterized by paresthesia in the back and extremities upon neck flexion. After cranial XRT, a corresponding syndrome characterized by somnolence has been described (somnolence syndrome).[5] These syndromes typically last for a few months followed by complete clinical recovery. Transient demyelination is believed to be the underlying mechanism of these early delayed reactions (subacute effects).[6] There is, however, no correlation of Lhermitte syndrome with permanent radiation myelopathy.

Late effects are typically irreversible and most devastating, and thus are the most clinically important. Radiation myelopathy is one of the most distressing late complications of radiotherapy. It generally occurs after a latent time of 12 to 14 months, but it has been reported 3 to 4 years after XRT.[7,8] Clinical symptoms and signs of radiation myelopathy vary depending on the level of injury; they can occur in various combinations of motor and sensory deficits and at different rates of progression. Moreover, myelopathy can be fatal if the damage occurs at the upper cervical level.[9]

Initial signs of radiation-induced myelopathy may be nonspecific and often include a diminished temperature sensation, diminished sense of proprioception, muscle weakness (typically beginning in the legs), and clumsiness. Changes in gait, incontinence, Brown-Séquard syndrome, spasticity, paresis, plegia, hyperreflexia, and the Babinski sign are examples of more characteristic symptoms and signs that develop as the injury manifests.

◆ Structure of the Spinal Cord

Anatomy

The spinal cord is an elongated cylindrical structure and an extension of the brain. In the adult mammal, the spinal cord extends from the superior border of the atlas (foramen magnum) to the lumbar vertebrae. In the human adult, the spinal cord typically ends at the junction between the first and second lumbar vertebrae (L1–L2) and is typically 45 cm in length.[10] The spinal cord is bathed in cerebrospinal fluid (CSF) and enclosed by the dura, arachnoid, and pia mater, which are separated by the subdural and subarachnoid spaces.

A spinal cord segment provides the attachment of the rootlets of a pair of spinal nerves. From both sides of a segment of cord, dorsal and ventral roots traverse the dura and unite close to their intervertebral foramina to form mixed spinal nerves.[10,11] Nerve roots of the lumbar and sacral segments of the cord form a bundle of roots (known as the cauda equina) as they descend to their respective intervertebral foramina. In total there are 31 pairs of spinal nerves (i.e., segments).[10,11]

The spinal cord lies inside the spinal column, which is made up of 33 vertebrae in the human. Five vertebrae are fused together to form the sacrum, and four small vertebrae are fused together to form the coccyx. The spine is typically divided into four sections (excluding the coccyx): the cervical (C1–C7), thoracic (T1–T12), lumbar (L1–L5), and sacral (S1–S5) vertebrae.[10,11] Between the vertebral bodies (except C1 and C2) are disks that serve as the supporting structure for the spine. Ligaments attached to the vertebrae also serve as supporting structures.

The transverse diameter of the cord gradually tapers craniocaudally except at the level of two enlargements. The cervical enlargement (C3–T2) is the source of large spinal nerves innervating the upper limbs, and the lumbar enlargement (L1–S3) is the source of large spinal nerves supplying the lower limbs.[10,11]

On transverse section of the cord, the basic structural organization consists of central gray matter and outer white matter. Ascending tracts of sensory fibers and descending motor tracts are the main components of the white matter that are organized into funiculi (white columns) and grouped into dorsal, lateral, and ventral funiculi. Gray matter contains the neuronal cell bodies, and on transverse section it resembles the letter H with ventral and dorsal horns. The more prominent ventral horns contain cell bodies of the large lower motor neurons, and the dorsal horns contain the cell bodies of second-order sensory neurons involved in pain and temperature sensation. Details of specific cell columns and tracts are not the focus of this chapter and can be obtained from neuroanatomy textbooks.

Cell Types

The major cell types in the spinal cord, similar to those in the brain, are neurons, glia, and vascular endothelial cells.

Neurons are of neuroectodermal origin and, despite great variation in size and shape, consist of a cell body (containing the nucleus and surrounding cytoplasm known as the perikaryon), a short number of dendrites, and a long, single, straight axon. The receptive parts of the neuron are the dendrites, and the axon transmits the impulse to its terminal branches.

Glial cells are also of neuroectodermal origin and are generally divided into oligodendrocytes, astrocytes, and microglia. Oligodendrocytes are responsible for myelination of axons and dendrites in the CNS.[12] The process of myelination allows propagation of nerve impulses or action potentials. Myelin sheaths are formed by the wrapping of oligodendrocyte cytoplasmic processes around the axon and are interrupted by the nodes of Ranvier, which serve to enhance propagation of action potentials. One oligodendrocyte can myelinate segments of several adjacent axons via its processes.

Astrocytes are irregularly shaped glial cells with a large number of branched processes. Many of these processes end in terminal expansions upon the basement membrane of capillaries known as perivascular feet. Astrocytes participate in neuronal growth and development, as well as in the transmission of the neuronal signals.[13] They also play a key role in the formation and maintenance of the BBB and, in the spinal cord, the blood–spinal cord barrier (BSCB).[14]

Microglia are small cells that, upon activation in response to tissue damage, transform into phagocytic cells. They are thought to be part of the monocyte–macrophage defense system in the brain and spinal cord.[15]

Vascular endothelial cells in the spinal cord are responsible for the BSCB. Similar to the BBB, the BSCB severely restricts the passage into the spinal cord of most proteins, hydrophilic molecules, and ions in the circulation. In addition to the spe-cialized endothelium of the spinal cord, other components of BSCB include the basement membrane, astrocytes, and pericytes in immediate proximity. The unusual impermeability of CNS capillaries is attributed to tight junctions between endothelial cells and a paucity of endothelial vesicular transport. These features are the basis for the characteristic resistance to para- and transcellular transport, respectively.[16,17]

It is now recognized that neural progenitors and neural stem cells persist in the adult CNS.[18,19] Although these cells are generally believed to reside in certain areas of the brain, they can be isolated from the adult spinal cord.[19] The role of these cells in the radiation response of the CNS, including the spinal cord, is beginning to emerge, as discussed later. Recent studies have highlighted the importance of interactions of endothelial cells, glia neurons, and neural progenitors in the normal and diseased CNS.[20,21] An understanding of how these interactions are disturbed and disrupted in spinal cord radiation injury could lead to the development of novel neuroprotective strategies.

◆ General Radiobiological Concepts Pertinent to the Spinal Cord

XRT for patient therapy is ionizing, meaning that its photons, upon interaction with matter, contain sufficient energy to release an electron orbiting around the nucleus of an atom or molecule. XRT can cause any damage to any molecule in a cell, but damage to deoxyribonucleic acid (DNA) is most crucial in causing cell lethality. Damage to DNA can occur directly through the free electrons themselves or indirectly through free radicals generated from these electrons.[22]

Cellular damage following XRT may lead to cell-cycle arrest, mitosis-linked death, or apoptotic cell death.[23] The probability of cell survival after a single dose of XRT is a function of absorbed dose and is measured as energy per unit mass of tissue in gray units (Gy). In cells cultured in vitro following XRT, the capability of a single cell to grow and form a large colony is typically used as a measure of reproductive integrity. The formation of these colonies provides the basis for quantitative assays that can be used to describe the survival of cells after XRT. Whereas differentiated cells such as neurons, astrocytes, and oligodendrocytes in the CNS do not form colonies, neural stem cells and progenitors can be cultured in vitro and form colonies under specific growth conditions. These assays have been used to characterize the clonogenic survival of neural progenitors isolated from the spinal cord after in vivo XRT.[24,25]

Many different mathematical models have been used to describe cell survival after XRT. One that is widely used in the clinic is the linear-quadratic model,[26] and it can be used to describe the fractionation sensitivity of tissues after XRT.[27,28] Late-responding normal tissues such as the spinal cord have low values of the alpha to beta (α/β) coefficient based on the linear-quadratic model. This is indicative of tissues where significant sparing can be achieved with fractionation. Values of α/β for the spinal cord ranged from 1.5 to 3.0 Gy.[29,30] The concepts of cell survival curves and fractionation are discussed in Chapter 1. It should be pointed out these mathematical models, including the linear-quadratic model, are likely to be overly simplistic and flawed, given what is currently known about the molecular responses of cells and tissues after XRT.

A functional assay that has been used extensively to assess the radiation response of the spinal cord is paralysis.[30,31] The assumption is that the defined level of functional deficit (paralysis) corresponds to a decrease in the number of surviving target cells in the spinal cord. In rats, the ED_{50} (the estimated isoeffective dose for induction of paralysis in 50% of animals) for forelimb paralysis due to white matter necrosis was 19 Gy following single doses to the cervical spinal cord and went up to 87 Gy for 40 daily fractions.[30] Therefore, the total dose to cause necrosis of the spinal cord is much lower for a single dose of radiosurgery as compared with conventional fractionation.

When it comes to sparing of the spinal cord, it must be emphasized that there are no radiobiological advantages of single high doses as compared with fractionated regimens for malignant tumors. With a single high-dose treatment for a given rate of tumor cure, or control, the risk of myelopathy is much greater as compared with fractionated regimens. Therefore, a narrower therapeutic ratio must be respected, as the risk of late effects increases with increasing dose per fraction. Technology has evolved such that single high-dose treatments can be delivered safely and precisely with the

aim of equivalent or even better tumor control, as compared with fractionated regimens, while minimizing dose delivered to organs at risk. The net result is a shorter overall patient treatment time, and therefore improved patient convenience while maintaining a sufficient therapeutic ratio.

Many proteins and complex signaling cascades are involved in the general molecular response to XRT.[22,23] These molecular events are described in several textbooks on radiobiology.[22,23,26] The cellular and molecular details to follow in this chapter will be specific to spinal cord radiation.

Histopathogic Features of Spinal Cord Injury

As spinal cord injury (myelopathy) is objectively detectable by the onset of paralysis, radiation-induced cord injury has been studied in greater detail in animal models than has brain injury. Much of what is known about the radiation responses of the CNS has been based on radiobiological studies of the spinal cord. Most studies of spinal cord radiation responses were performed in rodent species, particularly in rats, using single doses. These studies are thus particularly relevant to spine radiosurgery.

In rat spinal cord, forelimb paralysis is observed at 4 to 5 months after single doses exceeding 20 Gy.[30] In these animals, the most important and predominant histopathologic change is necrosis confined to white matter (**Fig. 2.1A,B**).

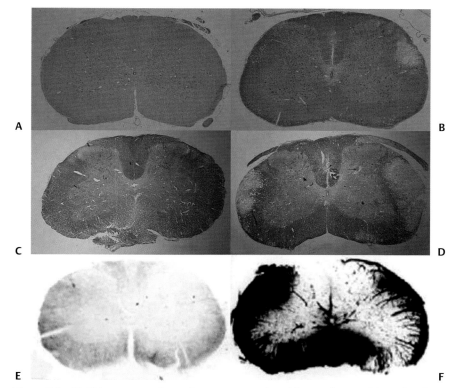

Figure 2.1 **(A,B)** Low-power views of transverse sections of control **(A)** and irradiated **(B)** cervical rat spinal cord on routine hematoxylin and eosin staining. **(B)** In animals that developed forelimb paralysis at 20 weeks, there is evidence for necrosis confined to white matter after a myelopathic dose of 25 Gy. **(C,D)** Nonirradiated spinal cord shows no evidence of demyelination upon luxol blue staining for myelin **(C)**, whereas demyelination is evident in lateral white matter at 20 weeks after 22 Gy **(D)**. **(E)** Using horseradish peroxidase as a vascular tracer, control nonirradiated spinal cord shows no extravasation of the tracer. **(F)** The transverse section of the cervical spinal cord at 17 weeks after 25 Gy shows reaction product of horseradish peroxidase in almost all of the white matter. Disruption of the blood–spinal cord barrier invariably precedes histologic evidence of demyelination and necrosis.

Histologically, these changes consist of randomly distributed areas of cell loss, necrotic debris, swollen axons, and focal to extensive demyelination and necrosis (**Fig. 2.1C,D**). A scant mononuclear infiltrate is occasionally seen.[30]

There are no specific vascular changes observed for radiation myelopathy. In rat spinal cord, the vascular changes are generally not prominent, although foci of fibrinoid degeneration of vascular walls are sometimes observed. In other mammalian species, vascular changes that have been described include telangiectasia, perivascular fibrosis and inflammation, hyaline degeneration and thickening, edema and fibrin exudation, stagnation and leakage of erythrocytes, and thrombosis with vessel obliteration and hemorrhage.[32,33] Perhaps the most consistent vascular abnormality is the disruption of the BSCB. In rat spinal cord, gross histopathologic changes were invariably preceded by a generalized disruption in vascular permeability in white matter (**Fig. 2.1E,F**).[34]

Studies that described histopathological changes at lower doses, or doses below the threshold of paralysis, have not been reported as often. Similarly, few studies have tracked the histopathologic changes during the latent time prior to the onset of paralysis. In rat spinal cord following doses of only 5 to 10 Gy, paranodal demyelination, nodal widening, and wallerian-type degeneration of fibers in white matter has been described as early as 2 weeks postradiation.[35,36] However, in the 5 to 10 Gy dose range, remyelination was observed at 3 months post-XRT. This observation has led investigators to conclude that early delayed effects (Lhermitte syndrome) are related to demyelination that could occur at doses below the threshold for tissue necrosis.

In rhesus monkeys that underwent XRT to the cord but did not develop myelopathy by 2 years, the lesions consisted of single or multiple small mineralized foci in nonmotor tracts, astrocytes that were increased in size and often adjacent to foci of malacia, and microglial cells surrounding flecks of mineral.[37] In addition, vasculopathy of hyaline degeneration was frequently observed as both an independent process and in close association with lesions of the neurophil (brain tissue that lies between cell bodies).

Histopathologic description of human myelopathy is typically based on case reports or small series where autopsy materials were available. In an analysis of these reports, there were lesions that involved only white matter parenchyma with minor vascular changes, lesions that were mainly vascular, and lesions that demonstrated characteristics of both white matter parenchyma and vascular damage.[38] Human studies are limited due to many unknown patient, tumor, treatment, and other confounding factors that may influence the development of damage. In addition, the damage reported typically represented patients with the most severe damage, such that histologic or autopsy materials were available for examination.

Cellular and Molecular Mechanisms in Spinal Cord Myelopathy

For decades, largely based on extrapolation of histopathologic changes described above, the debate on the pathogenesis of spinal cord myelopathy after ionizing radiation was focused on the role of the oligodendrocyte versus the vascular endothelial cell. The support for the "glial hypothesis" stems from the observation of demyelination and lesions confined to white matter, whereas the "vascular hypothesis" stems from the observation of disruption of the BSCB that precedes or is associated with white matter lesions and other vascular changes observed. With recent advances in neurobiology, it is now recognized that spinal cord injury is unlikely to be related only to clonogenic cell death of one or two target cell types.

Whereas at the clinical and histopathologic level, there is a latent period of months to years prior to the onset of myelopathy, at the cellular and molecular level, there is no evidence of a latent time. The development of spinal cord damage is currently best viewed as a damage continuum culminating in tissue necrosis with clinical myelopathy. In terms of mode of cell death in the CNS after XRT, certain glial, neuronal, and endothelial cells in the CNS also undergo apoptosis within hours after XRT. However, the clinical relevance of this mode of cell death remains unclear.[4,39-43] Furthermore, there is also a component of secondary injury and cell death that may be mediated by microenvironmental alterations such as hypoxia/ischemia and neuroinflammation.[44-48] **Figure 2.2** illustrates a model of the molecular and cellular responses in the irradiated spinal cord. Insight into potentially reversible components of damage may offer neuroprotective avenues against radiation injury.

Gene Induction and Oxidative Stress

Ionizing radiation produces a variety of DNA and other cellular lesions that elicit a stress response. Altered gene profiles represent one characteristic feature of this response. In the rodent CNS, increased expression of proinflammatory and other genes has been demonstrated within hours following XRT.[49-52] These include genes of transcription factors such as nuclear factor-kappa B (NF-κB), cytokines such as tumor necrosis factor-alpha (TNF-α) and interleukin-1 beta (IL-1β), basic fibroblast growth factor (bFGF), adhesion molecules such as intercellular adhesion molecule-1 (ICAM-1), and selectins.

NF-κB is important in the regulation of cytokine expression, including expression of TNF-α and IL-1β, both of which have been implicated in the development of demyelination.[53] The expression of TNF-α is associated with edema observed after ischemic and hypoxic injury,[54] and is also a key regulator of ICAM-1. ICAM-1 is associated with BBB disruption in a variety of injuries,[55] and increased ICAM-1 expression has been observed in rat spinal cord within 24 hours after XRT.[56-58] Increased neurologic abnormalities and extensive demyelination were observed in *TNFRp75*-deficient mice after cranial irradiation as compared with *TNFRp55*-deficient and control mice. These findings implicate a role for TNF-α in radiation-induced demyelination.[59]

Similar to other CNS injury models, a state of oxidative stress is associated with an increase in reactive oxygen species (ROS). Levels of malonaldehyde (MDA), an end product of lipid peroxidation, were found elevated in the mouse hippocampus at 1 week after a dose of 10 Gy, and cells immu-

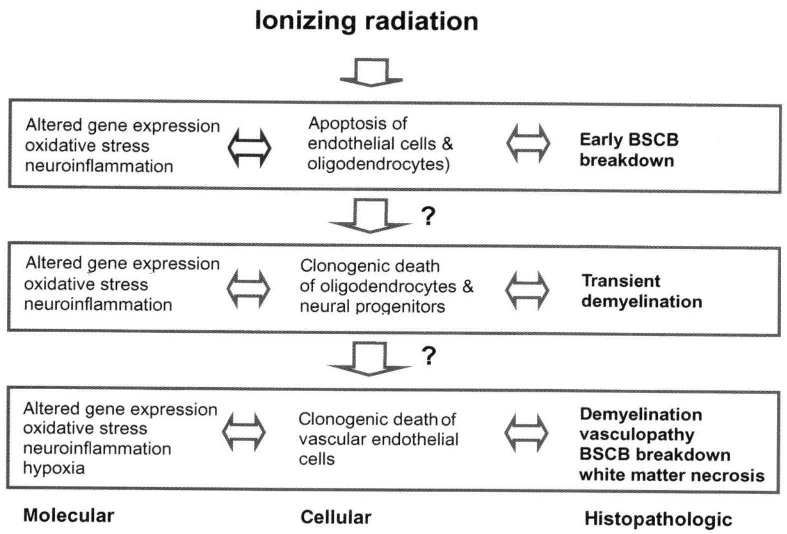

Ionizing radiation

Figure 2.2 A model of the molecular and cellular responses of the irradiated spinal cord. Whereas at the histopathologic level injury to the spinal cord after irradiation may be distinct entities, at the cellular and molecular level, the response is best viewed as a continuous and interacting process in which altered gene expression, neuroinflammation, and oxidative stress all contribute to cell kill induced by irradiation. BSCB, blood–spinal cord barrier.

noreactive for MDA were observed in the dentate gyrus at 24 hours.[60] It has been suggested that the ROS responses may be tied to p53-dependent regulation of cell cycle control and stress-activated pathways. Oxidative stress and ROS are associated with activation of heme oxygenase 1 (Hmox 1), a stress protein,[61] and a dose-dependent increase in Hmox1 gene expression has been observed in rat spinal cord after XRT.[62] Oxidative stress and increases in ROS are likely to interact with radiation-induced altered gene profiles and to participate in responses to XRT of the CNS.

Recently, microarrays have allowed for the study of global gene expression in rodent CNS after XRT. These studies showed very complex patterns of gene expression profiles in mouse brain after XRT, and these expression profiles appeared to be dose- and time-dependent after cranial XRT.[63,64] When expression profiles in the irradiated mouse kidney were compared with those in the irradiated brain, striking differences were observed. These observations are consistent with the notion that cellular and tissue response to XRT is complex and critically dependent on cell and tissue types.[65] Microarray analysis may allow the identification of novel genes that may play a role in CNS radiation injury.

Oligodendrocytes, Oligodendroglial Progenitors, and Demyelination

It is now recognized that clonogenic cell death is not the only mode of cell death in the CNS after XRT.[4,39–43] Following single doses, an apoptotic response occurs within hours in rodent spinal cord and is not observed by 24 hours. The apoptotic cells that have been best characterized in the spinal cord are oligodendrocytes.[39,40,66] Some of the apoptotic cells have the phenotype of oligodendroglial progenitors.[67]

In the irradiated spinal cord, following an apoptotic response of oligodendrocytes peaking at approximately 8 hours, a reduction of oligodendrocytes was observed at 24 hours.[39,66] After XRT of the rat cervical spinal cord with 15 or 23 Gy, the oligodendroglial progenitor cell (OPC) pool was reduced to < 0.1% of its normal population at 2 to 4 weeks. This was followed by a dose-dependent recovery reaching a maximum of 40 to 80% of control values at 3 months.[68] This recovery was preceded by proliferation of OPCs. Early proliferation of OPCs, however, was not impaired in the irradiated spinal cord of p53-knockout mice. Given the dependence of radiation-induced apoptosis of oligodendroglial cells on p53, this suggests that the early proliferation of oligodendroglial progenitors observed may not be linked directly to apoptosis of oligodendrocytes.[67]

In rat spinal cord, several early events such as oligodendroglial apoptosis, reduced oligodendroglial density, and changes in oligodendroglial gene expression were observed after a myelopathic dose of 22 Gy. Similar changes occurred after a much lower dose of 8 Gy. In addition, only after a myelopathic dose was there a secondary decline of OPCs, with subsequent demyelination, observed between 4 and 5 months. These findings suggest that these early cellular and molecular events affecting the oligodendroglial populations are unlikely to be directly associated with late demyelination observed after XRT.[66]

OPCs are bipotential glial (O-2A) progenitors that can also differentiate into astrocytes, depending on the in vitro growth condition.[69] The radiosensitivity, repair, and regeneration of OPCs in rat spinal cord have been characterized using an in vivo–in vitro clonogenic assay of these cells.[24,70–72] This assay was used in a study of boron neutron capture therapy (BNCT) to rat spinal cord to determine the role of OPCs versus vascular damage in white matter injury. Results of this study will be discussed later.

Role of Neural Stem Cells and Neural Progenitors

In the brain, cells that are susceptible to radiation-induced apoptosis are largely concentrated in the subependymal zone of the lateral ventricles and the subgranular layer of the dentate gyrus.[43,73] These apoptotic cells are of particular interest, as neural progenitors and stem cells reside in the adult subependymal zone and dentate gyrus.[74,75] Similar to the apoptotic response of oligodendrocytes, radiation-induced apoptosis of subventricular cells is p53 dependent and is virtually absent in transgenic mice knockout of the *p53* gene.[41]

Neural stem cells with multipotential and self-renewing properties are present in adult spinal cord. They can be isolated and form neurospheres in vitro.[19] Similar to the studies in OPCs,[24,70–72] the radiation response of these neural progenitors has been described recently using in vitro neurosphere assay following in vivo irradiation of the rat spinal cord.[25,76] This in vivo–in vitro assay can be used to describe the repair and repopulation of these neural stem cells/progenitors after irradiation.

Recent studies suggest that cranial XRT was associated with inhibition of neurogenesis.[45,46,77] In rat brain after a single XRT dose of 10 Gy, there was ablation of neurogenesis in the hippocampal dentate gyrus, an area where there is ongoing generation of new neurons, and it was observed that neural stem cells/progenitors instead differentiated into glial cells. Furthermore, the inhibition of neurogenesis was accompanied by disruption of the microvascular angiogenesis associated with neurogenesis, and an increase in the number and activation status of microglia was observed.[78] The deficit in neurogenesis after XRT is postulated to reflect alterations in the neural stem cell niche that regulates progenitor cell fate. These findings highlight the role of the microenvironment, in particular the presence of neuroinflammation, in mediating the damage response.

Although the presence of newly generated neurons may be necessary for intact hippocampal function, other factors, including an enriched environment and exercise, are associated with enhanced neurogenesis.[79,80] Thus, the causal role of inhibition of hippocampal neurogenesis to the impairment of learning and memory function observed after XRT remains unproven. To what extent these neural stem cells and neuroprogenitors participate in the radiation injury response in spinal cord remains to be investigated.

Endothelial Cell Apoptosis and Early BSCB Disruption

Endothelial cells in the CNS also undergo early apoptosis.[4,42] In rat brain, there was a 15% decrease in the number of endothelial cells at 24 hours following a single dose of 25 Gy.[81] A dose-dependent loss of endothelial cells at 24 hours was also observed in rat spinal cord after XRT.[82] These findings are consistent with the observation of a peak of endothelial apoptosis at 8 to 12 hours in the rodent CNS post-XRT.[42] Importantly, whereas oligodendrocyte apoptosis after XRT is p53 dependent,[41] endothelial cell apoptosis is not p53 dependent. Radiation-induced endothelial cell apoptosis is mediated by the second messenger ceramide, which is generated from sphingomyelin following activation of sphingomyelinases.[83] Thus, consistent with the notion that radiation-induced endothelial apoptosis is mediated by the acid sphingomyelinase (*ASMase*) pathway, endothelial apoptosis after XRT was reduced in the brain and spinal cord of ASMase-knockout mice.[4,42]

Following a single dose of 50 Gy (ED$_{50}$ for white matter necrosis) to the spinal cord, endothelial density was reduced by almost 50%, and there was evidence for disruption of the BSCB in *ASMase* wild-type mice but not in *ASMase*-knockout animals.[4] Both *p53* wild-type and knockout mice exhibited a similar reduction in endothelial cell numbers, as well as BSCB disruption after spinal cord XRT. These data suggest that apoptosis of endothelial cells initiates acute BBB disruption in the CNS after XRT. Whether early endothelial cell apoptosis mediates tissue injury that appears months later remains to be investigated.

Late BSCB Disruption

A consistent and prominent feature of spinal cord damage after XRT is disruption of the BSCB. Barrier disruption is well documented at both early and late intervals after CNS XRT, and is likely to play an important role in both acute and late radiation toxicities.[34,84–86]

Microvessels constitute about 95% of the blood–tissue interface. Evidence for microvascular injury, as critical to the pathogenesis of radiation myelopathy, was described by a series of experiments using BNCT to irradiate the rat spinal cord. BNCT involves the systemic delivery of a boron compound followed by irradiation with low-energy neutrons. The capture of neutrons by the boron releases α particles and lithium ions with a short range of approximately 10 μm. Therefore, only cells within the immediate vicinity are irradiated. Using the boron compound borocaptate sodium (BSH), which does not cross the BSCB and is thus confined to the microcirculation, BNCT was found to result in myelopathy with white matter necrosis and similar histological changes at doses equivalent to those following photon XRT.[87]

A subsequent study compared the in vitro clonogenic survival of OPC or O-2A cells after in vivo BNCT irradiation of rat spinal cord with capture agents that did or did not cross the BSCB.[88] When the radiation dose was primarily delivered in the vascular endothelium, there was significantly higher survival of OPC compared with photons only, despite the fact that all treatments resulted in an equal incidence of white matter necrosis. These results serve to highlight the critical role of the vasculature rather than OPC survival in mediating white matter injury after XRT.

Hypoxia and Microenvironmental Disruption

Although vascular injury, including BBB disruption, implicates vascular endothelial cells as an important target of CNS radiation injury, recent studies suggest that complex interactions involving endothelial cell death, altered gene expression, neuroinflammation, and microenvironmental changes contribute to the development of damage.[62,82]

Hypoxia develops where oxygen supply from the vasculature is compromised because of deficient vascularization or local microcirculation disturbances, such as in ischemic or traumatic injury. Hypoxia causes a wide range of responses at both the systemic and cellular level, and may regulate many physiological and pathological processes. Hypoxia is an important inducer for vascular endothelial growth factor (VEGF), also known as vascular permeability factor, which is known to mediate increased permeability in a wide range of tissues, including the CNS.[89] In the neonatal rat spinal cord, induced VEGF expression was observed within days and persisted for 2 weeks after a very high dose of XRT (55 Gy).[90] In rats that develop paralysis associated with necrosis of the white matter within 20 weeks after single doses of 20 to 25 Gy, an increase in the number of VEGF-expressing cells was observed in white matter beginning at 16 weeks. The increase in the number of VEGF-expressing cells demonstrated a dose-dependent response above 17 Gy. The majority of these cells were astrocytes.[91]

When hypoxia in rat spinal cord was assessed using a hypoxic marker, ^{125}I-iodoazomycin arabinoside (IAZA), there was a dose- (17–22 Gy) and time-dependent (16–20 weeks after 22 Gy) increase in ^{125}I-IAZA in the irradiated spinal cord. A similar pattern of dose- and time-dependent increase in immunoreactivity of 2-(2-nitro-1H-imidazol-1-l)-N-(2,2,3,3,3-pentafluoropropyl) acetamide (EF5), another nitroimidazole hypoxic marker, was observed in white matter. This dose-dependent increase in hypoxia correlated temporally and spatially with a dose-dependent increase in BSCB permeability and expression of VEGF,[44] hypoxia-inducible factor-1 alpha (HIF-1α), and glucose transporter-1 (Glut-1) in white matter of the spinal cord (**Fig. 2.3**).[47] The response of *VEGF-lacZ* (beta galactosidase) knock-in transgenic mice with increased or decreased functional VEGF expression to spinal cord XRT was assessed following XRT to the thoracolumbar spinal cord. Protection and a longer latent time to development of hindlimb weakness and paralysis was observed in transgenic mice with reduced VEGF, as compared with wild-type mice and transgenic mice with increased VEGF.[47] These results provided evidence for a causal role of VEGF in the development of radiation myelopathy.

The underlying mechanisms of VEGF-mediated increase in vascular permeability are unclear. There is evidence that VEGF-mediated vascular permeability changes do not require receptor binding.[92] In radiation-induced late BBB disruption, VEGF upregulation was not associated with evidence for increased or even detectable VEGF receptor expression.[47] The integrity of the BBB is dependent on tight junctions, and possibly adherens junctions, between endothelial cells.[93] VEGF may alter the expression and distribution of tight junction proteins such as occludin and zonula occludens-1 in brain endothelial cells.[94] However, in a morphometric study using the electron microscope, no disruption or expansion of microvessel tight junction contacts was detected in the irradiated rat spinal cord.[34] A different study also demonstrated no apparent change in the distribution or amount of immunoreactivity of occludin and zonula occludens-1 in rat spinal cord after myelopathic radiation doses.[58]

Increased ICAM-1 expression is associated with a diversity of CNS injury models where BBB disruption is present,[95-98] including radiation injury.[47,99] VEGF increases the expression of ICAM-1 in the CNS, as well as in cultured brain microvascular endothelial cells.[89,100,101] In rat spinal cord, the time course, dose response, and spatial distribution of increased ICAM-1 expression paralleled the observations of BSCB disruption and albumin leakage.[58] ICAM-1-mediated leukocyte binding, cytoskeletal rearrangements, and signaling to tight junctions may all contribute to barrier disruption.[102,103] Given the central role of ICAM-1 in the inflammatory status of endothelial cells, these findings are also consistent with the role of "inflammation" in propagating the CNS damage after XRT.

Other mechanisms, such as the generation of free radicals under hypoxic conditions,[104,105] may also contribute to the

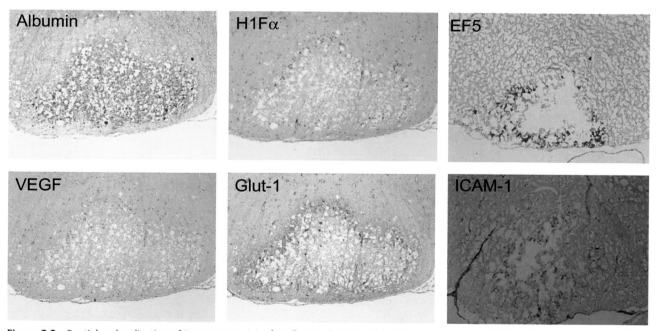

Figure 2.3 Spatial co-localization of immunoreactivity for albumin, hypoxia-inducible factor-1 alpha (HIF-1α), the hypoxia marker EF5, vascular endothelial growth factor (VEGF), glucose transporter-1 (Glut-1), and intercellular adhesion molecule-1 (ICAM-1) in adjacent transverse rat spinal cord sections. Rats received 22 Gy to the cervical spinal cord and were sacrificed at 20 weeks.

damage development. Hmox 1, a stress protein, is induced by hypoxia through HIF-1α.[106] Upregulation of Hmox 1 in the rat spinal cord at 5 and 6 months after 26 Gy has been reported as evidence for oxidative stress.[62] Because ROS are implicated in several degenerative and injurious processes in the CNS,[107] this observation also suggests a central role of hypoxia in mediating secondary damage in radiation myelopathy.

In summary, **Fig. 2.2** illustrates a model in which gene expression and microenvironmental changes affect cell fate and cell interactions and contribute to tissue injury. For white matter injury, clonogenic death of endothelial cells following XRT may initiate the breakdown of the BSCB, leading to ischemia, hypoxia, and neuroinflammation. Hypoxia induces HIF1-mediated increases in VEGF and other cytokine expression, such as ICAM-1 and TNF-α. This secondary damage cascade leads to a further increase in vascular permeability, demyelination, and ultimately tissue necrosis.

Regional Differences in Cord Radiation Sensitivity

In rat spinal cord following XRT, a predominance of dorsal tract lesions in high cervical segments, ventrolateral at mid-cervical levels, and a shift to dorsal lesions in the upper thoracic cord (with greater variability) have been observed.[108–112] Despite these differences in distribution of lesions, there was no evidence for a regional difference in radiosensitivity. Similar data in rhesus monkeys also suggest no difference in radiation sensitivity between the cervical and thoracic cord.[37]

In rodents, the lumbar/lumbosacral and cauda equina pathology is markedly different than that for the cervical or thoracic region, and a gradual diminishing severity of cord damage is observed. Below L1–L2, damage to the cauda equina was predominantly nerve root necrosis.[111] Similar patterns of radiation response have been reported in both mouse and guinea pig spinal cords.[113–117] Taken together, there is little evidence to support the existence of a significant difference in regional radiosensitivity of the human spinal cord[38] that should affect clinical practice, including spine radiosurgery.

◆ Fractionation, Volume, and Overall Treatment Time

Fractionation

The recognition of a high fractionation sensitivity of the CNS is largely based on extensive rodent studies, particularly in rat spinal cord, whose threshold for induction of paralysis is about 20 to 22 Gy after a single dose.[30,36] The benefits of fractionation for late normal tissue have been studied extensively and widely accepted in the practice of radiation oncology (see Chapter 1).

These fractionation studies also led to the investigation of altered fractionation studies where the dose per fraction was reduced, and more than a single fraction was given daily, in an attempt to improve the therapeutic ratio. For the spinal cord, it was hypothesized that the use of multiple small fractions per day will increase tolerance, but this proved not to be the case.[118,119] Subsequently, several extensive experiments

involving rat cervical cord were performed to determine the kinetics of sublethal repair in spinal cord. Although the results varied from study to study in terms of mathematical models that best described the repair kinetics, the consistent observation is the lack of complete repair when more than a single fraction was given daily.[120–122] Thus, for altered fractionation studies, it is generally recommended that a reduction of the interfraction interval to 6 to 8 hours is associated with a small but nonetheless significant reduction in spinal cord dose tolerance of 10 to 15%.[29] This may not be clinically applicable to single-dose spine radiosurgery, but it has important implications if multiple fractions per day protocols are contemplated. In summary, the risk of spinal cord injury increases with increasing dose per fraction, total radiation dose, and, in the case of multiple daily fractions, shortened interfraction time intervals.

Volume Effect and Cord Tolerance

As mentioned previously, the tolerance of normal tissues to radiation is unlikely to be dependent solely on the number and radiosensitivity of one or two target cell types. However, the ability of the clonogenic/target cells to maintain a sufficient number of mature cells suitably structured to maintain organ function may still be important. One model that was advanced in the 1980s described functional subunits (FSUs), defined as discrete anatomically delineated structures whose relationship to tissue function is clear.[28] Thus, tissue survival may depend on FSU organization and the proportion of FSU necessary for adequate organ function. However, none of the mathematical models that incorporate parameters for serial and parallel behavior have shown a good fit for the cord as a serial organ.[123,124]

In rhesus monkeys, when lengths of cord of 4, 8, and 16 cm were treated to a total dose of 70.4 Gy in 2.2 Gy per fraction,[37] a volume effect was not apparent. However, there was the suggestion of volume dependence, but only when the data were extrapolated to higher doses and shorter cord lengths than those used in the experiment. In irradiated pig spinal cord, no significant volume effect was apparent, and similar ED$_{50}$ values of 27.0, 27.7, and 28.3 Gy were obtained for irradiated cord lengths of 2.5, 5.0 and 10.0 cm, respectively.[125] However, a significant volume effect was found in beagle dogs irradiated with 4 Gy fractions to 4 and 20 cm lengths of the thoracic spinal cord. The ED$_{50}$ was 56.9 Gy for 20 cm versus 68.8 Gy for 4 cm fields.[126]

In an early study in rat spinal cord,[127] it was suggested that the effect of volume was complex and might differ depending on the histologic end point examined. A greater volume effect was observed using white matter lesions compared with using vascular lesions as end points. Some of the limitations of early experiments, such as dosimetric uncertainties and dose inhomogeneity, were addressed recently in a series of experiments using high precision proton beams to irradiate very short lengths of rat spinal cord.[128]

Four different lengths of the rat spinal cord (2, 4, 8, and 20 mm) were irradiated with single fractions of protons (150–190 MeV) using paralysis as the functional end point. A marginal increase in tolerance was observed when the irradiated rat cord length was decreased from 20 mm (ED_{50} = 20.4 Gy) to 8 mm (ED_{50} = 24.9 Gy), whereas a large increase in tolerance was observed when the length was further reduced to 4 mm (ED_{50} = 53.7 Gy) and 2 mm (ED_{50} = 87.8 Gy).[129] It was concluded that for small field lengths, there is an important volume effect. Furthermore, none of the models for normal tissue–complication probability provided an adequate fit of the dose–volume data.

Inhomogeneous Dose Distributions

These investigators also addressed the significance of partial volume irradiation and inhomogeneous dose distributions to the cord using a "bath and shower" proton radiation approach. The bath represents low doses to a large volume, whereas the shower represents high doses to a small volume. The effect was compared with homogeneous irradiation of the spinal cord to the same volume. The results indicated that the high ED_{50} values of a small region of 4 mm decreases significantly when the adjacent tissue is irradiated with a subthreshold dose (bath) as low as 4 Gy.[130] Furthermore, the effect of a low bath dose appeared to be highest for a shower field of 2 mm, less for 4 mm, and absent for 8 mm (**Fig. 2.4**).

When an asymmetrical dose distribution was arranged by irradiation of 12 mm (bath) of spinal cord with a dose of 4 Gy, and irradiating only the caudal 2 mm (shower) of the 12 mm bath with variable single doses, the addition of a 4 Gy bath to only one side of a 2 mm field still showed a large effect.[131] Thus, not only is the integral irradiated volume a determining factor for cord tolerance, but the shape of the dose distribution is of great importance. Interestingly, the low bath doses did not result in any apparent histologic damage.

Therefore, the integrity of surrounding tissue around an area of high dose damage may influence repair, and may be disabled by doses, which on its own would not cause functional deficit.

In another study using grazing proton beams to irradiate the lateral or central parts of the rat cervical spinal cord, a greater sensitivity of the white matter in the lateral cord was observed as compared with the central white and gray matter.[132] The observed difference in radiosensitivity is postulated based on regional sensitivities within the white matter rather than a volume effect. Similar to many previous studies, the gray matter was found to be radioresistant with little or no histopathogic abnormalities observed even after very high doses (**Fig. 2.4**).

Although the underlying mechanisms of the volume effects remain speculative, these observations have important clinical relevance to modern radiotherapy specifically, in the interpretation of complex treatment plans and normal tissue–complication probability in intensity-modulated radiation therapy (IMRT). Whereas models for normal tissue–complication probability might be valid in describing the dose–volume effect of spinal cord in routine or standard external beam XRT, serious and significant deviations exist where there is inhomogeneous dose distribution and very small volumes. For example, with planned radiosurgery of spine lesions, inhomogeneity is expected in the dose distribution, as the complexity of the optimization problem increases with proximity of the target to the cord. In evaluating the treatment plan, the dose variation within the tumor volume must be observed and be acceptable. Furthermore, the location of hot spots (volume outside the planned target volume that receives a dose > 100% of the prescribed dose and exceeds a minimum diameter of

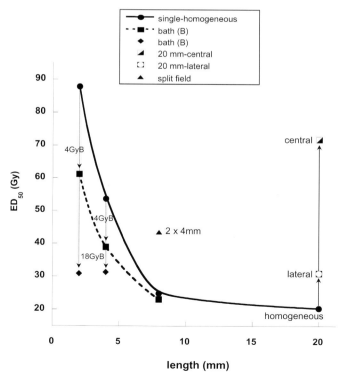

Figure 2.4 Dose–volume relationships in the rat spinal cord: the impact of inhomogeneous dose distributions. The ED_{50} values for paresis are due to white matter necrosis versus the length of the cervical cord irradiated with high-energy protons. A 4 or 18 Gy bath dose significantly decreased the ED_{50} values of a 2 or 4 mm midcervical segment. Irradiation of the lateral side of the full length of the cervical cord showed a relatively modest increase of the ED_{50} by ~10 Gy but a very large increase to an ED_{50} of 70 Gy when irradiating predominantly the central gray and white matter.

1.5 mm) must be observed to ensure they do not lie within organs at risk. To illustrate: the dose volume histogram of spinal cord may indicate that 99% of the cord is receiving < 50 Gy (within tolerance), but 1% (or even a single 2 mm voxel) is receiving 65 Gy. The significance of such a small volume receiving 65 Gy is not known. Based on recent experimental data that showed a steep rise in ED_{50} with small volumes of cord irradiated, it may be acceptable to allow for higher maximum point doses. Similarly, where there are overlapping fields over the cord, a high dose may be tolerable provided that the region of overlap is small. Currently, there are no human data that parallel these recent rodent experiments on volume effects; therefore, one must be cautious in extrapolating these experimental data to the clinic.

Furthermore, for spine radiosurgery, multiple beams, segments, and intensity-modulated delivery, characteristic of IMRT, result in an increase in the integral dose within the patient. Higher integral doses have the potential of resulting in larger volumes of the cord receiving a low (below threshold) dose, as compared with a straight anteroposterior parallel-opposed field with defined beam edges. The clinical impact may be individualization of radiosurgery cord tolerance dose by accounting for the volume of cord exposed to a low dose (i.e., the bath), when considering the clinical acceptability of the location and volume of doses traditionally thought unacceptable.

Overall Treatment Time and Re-irradiation Tolerance

Retreatment potential to the cord is particularly relevant and important for radiosurgery for spine metastases. When other treatment options are not feasible, radiosurgery, due to the technical precision, is a potential application for previously irradiated patients. By applying the necessary dose constraints to account for the dose previously delivered to the cord, IMRT planning may result in safe re-irradiation treatment plans.

For rapidly proliferating tissues, these generally recover from initial treatments and will tolerate almost full retreatment doses.[133–137] Extensive investigations have been conducted on rat spinal cord to characterize cord retreatment potential. These experiments were designed with a framework of varying the initial doses delivered to the cord (therefore, the percent of remaining retreatment tolerance), the subsequent retreatment doses and dose fractionation schedules to the cord (to characterize the tolerance and fractionation sensitivity of retreatment), and the time intervals between the initial and subsequent dose to determine the sensitivity of the effect of recovery time.

Several general conclusions can be made based on these important rodent studies. The most important and consistent observation is the presence of time-dependent long-term recovery of damage in rat spinal cord after an interval of 6 to 8 weeks. Other observations include:

1. Shortened latency times to paralysis with increasing doses of re-irradiation
2. Shortened latency times to paralysis with increasing size or total doses of the initial treatment
3. A significant increase in retreatment tolerance with increasing times between initial treatment and re-irradiation

4. Influence of size of initial doses or injury on extent of recovery
5. Lack of a difference in subsequent fractionation sensitivity with retreatment
6. Recovery never being complete, regardless of time intervals or size of initial injury[30,121,138–140]

Recovery of occult radiation injury was also observed in a series of experiments in rhesus monkeys. These experiments consisted of initial radiation to the cord of 44 Gy in 2.2 Gy/day fractions[141,142] (~60% of the biologic effective dose [BED] for the ED_{50} [76 Gy in 2.2 Gy/day]) followed by increasing re-irradiation doses at 2 years (cumulative doses ranging from 83.6–110.0 Gy), and experiments where the time interval to retreatment varied, as did the re-irradiation dose, depending on that interval (1–3 years and cumulative dose 101.2–110.0 Gy, respectively). These experiments indicate substantial (~75% at 2 years) recovery from the initial 44 Gy, as well as a dose response relationship with subsequent re-irradiation. Furthermore, with increasing time to re-irradiation recovery, estimates also increased with significant recovery within the first year and additional recovery between years 1 and 3. Therefore, a large capacity to recover from occult cord radiation injury has been shown in the primate spinal cord. Because human myelopathy has been observed after many years, caution was raised, as the follow-up was limited to 2.0 to 2.5 years post–re-irradiation.

Human clinical data also suggest a capacity for long-term recovery from occult radiation injury; however, data are very limited. In a series of 35 patients who developed permanent radiation myelopathy at the Princess Margaret Hospital, Canada, 11 had retreatment to the spinal cord.[7] Consistent with experimental data, latent times for myelopathy following a single course of treatment (mean of 19 months) were significantly longer than those after re-irradiation (mean of 11 months).

In an analysis of all published clinical data on spinal cord retreatment, dose-fractionation and other prescription information was available in a total of 40 patients.[143] Assuming an α/β ratio of 2 Gy for the cervical and thoracic cord (37 of 40 patients) and 4 Gy for the lumbar cord (3/40 patients treated to the lumbar cord alone), the cumulative BEDs ranged from 108 to 205 Gy_2 and the median dose was 135 Gy_2. Two risk factors for retreatment myelopathy were identified: a dose of at least 102 Gy_2 (9/40) for one of the radiation courses and an interval of less than 2 months between radiation courses (2/40). In the absence of these risk factors, no myelopathy was observed in 19 patients treated to ≤ 135.5 Gy_2, 7 patients treated to 136 to 150 Gy_2, or 3 patients treated to > 150 Gy_2.

Prospective data are currently being collected for retreatment of the spinal cord in an international randomized trial for re-irradiation of painful bone metastases (protocol CAN-NCIC-SC.20).[144] Patients with spine metastases previously treated with a single fraction of 6, 7, or 8 Gy, or fractionated treatment of 18 Gy in 4, 25 Gy in 6, or 20 Gy in 5 fractions are eligible for retreatment. Retreatment dose (following a minimum of 4 weeks post-initial radiation) is randomized to a second course of either a single 8 Gy fraction or 20 Gy in 5 fractions (20 Gy in 8 if previously treated with 18 Gy in 4, 24 in 6, or 20 Gy in 5 fractions) (personal communication, Dr.

Edward Chow, Toronto Sunnybrook Health Sciences Centre, University of Toronto). These regimens were based on a spinal cord tolerance of a BED of 100 to 120 Gy_2.

The mechanism of time-dependent recovery of radiation tolerance remains unclear. In rat spinal cord, an irradiated 7 mm region of thoracic spinal cord was repopulated completely by OPCs from adjacent unirradiated tissue within 6 weeks after a single dose of 40 Gy.[145] Restoration of the density of progenitor cells was observed similar to that of normal tissue, and it was not associated with a loss in secondary progenitor cells within the adjacent tissue. Given that the microenvironment can affect cell fate determination of progenitors, it is unlikely that the ability to migrate alone is sufficient for recovery of function.[131]

◆ Conclusion

Recent advances in neurobiology have challenged many dogmas but have helped in advancing much of our knowledge regarding the cellular and molecular basis of radiation response of the spinal cord. As new technological developments in radiation oncology are pushing the limits of radiation planning and delivery, the influence of inhomogeneous dose distributions, integral doses, and regional sensitivity on cord tolerance becomes clinically relevant. In spine radiosurgery protocols, factors that influence retreatment tolerance of the cord need to be identified and addressed. Novel experimental design and animal models will be required to determine the molecular and cellular basis of spinal cord injury pertinent to spine radiosurgery and to answer important clinical questions related to the tolerance of spinal cord in spine radiosurgery.

References

1. Schultheiss TE, Kun LE, Ang KK, Stephens LC. Radiation response of the central nervous system. Int J Radiat Oncol Biol Phys 1995;31(5):1093–1112.
2. Engenhart R, Kimmig BN, Hover KH, et al. Stereotactic single high dose radiation therapy of benign intracranial meningiomas. Int J Radiat Oncol Biol Phys 1990;19(4):1021–1026.
3. Moore AH, Olschowka JA, Williams JP, Paige SL, O'Banion MK. Radiation-induced edema is dependent on cyclooxygenase 2 activity in mouse brain. Radiat Res 2004;161(2):153–160.
4. Li YQ, Chen P, Haimovitz-Friedman A, Reilly RM, Wong CS. Endothelial apoptosis initiates acute blood-brain barrier disruption after ionizing radiation. Cancer Res 2003;63(18):5950–5956.
5. Freeman JE, Johnston PG, Voke JM. Somnolence after prophylactic cranial irradiation in children with acute lymphoblastic leukaemia. BMJ 1973;4(891):523–525.
6. Delattre JY, Rosenblum MK, Thaler HT, Mandell L, Shapiro WR, Posner JB. A model of radiation myelopathy in the rat: pathology, regional capillary permeability changes and treatment with dexamethasone. Brain 1988;111(Pt 6):1319–1336.
7. Wong CS, Van Dyk J, Milosevic M, Laperriere NJ. Radiation myelopathy following single courses of radiotherapy and retreatment. Int J Radiat Oncol Biol Phys 1994;30(3):575–581.
8. Schultheiss TE, Higgins EM, El-Mahdi AM. The latent period in clinical radiation myelopathy. Int J Radiat Oncol Biol Phys 1984;10(7):1109–1115.
9. Schultheiss TE, Stephens LC, Peters LJ. Survival in radiation myelopathy. Int J Radiat Oncol Biol Phys 1986;12(10):1765–1769.
10. Gray H. Anatomy of the Human Body. Philadelphia: Lea & Febiger, 1918/2000.
11. Moore K, Dalley A. Clinically Oriented Anatomy. 4th ed. Philadelphia: Williams and Wilkins; 1999.
12. Sherman DL, Brophy PJ. Mechanisms of axon ensheathment and myelin growth. Nat Rev Neurosci 2005;6(9):683–690.
13. Vernadakis A. Neuron-glia interrelations. Int Rev Neurobiol 1988;30:149–224.
14. Abbott NJ, Ronnback L, Hansson E. Astrocyte-endothelial interactions at the blood–brain barrier. Nat Rev Neurosci 2006;7(1):41–53.
15. Kim SU, de Vellis J. Microglia in health and disease. J Neurosci Res 2005;81(3):302–313.
16. Goldstein GW. Endothelial cell-astrocyte interactions: a cellular model of the blood–brain barrier. Ann N Y Acad Sci 1988;529:31–39.
17. Rubin LL, Staddon JM. The cell biology of the blood–brain barrier. Annu Rev Neurosci 1999;22:11–28.
18. Sanai N, Tramontin AD, Quinones-Hinojosa A, et al. Unique astrocyte ribbon in adult human brain contains neural stem cells but lacks chain migration. Nature 2004;427(6976):740–744.
19. Weiss S, Dunne C, Hewson J, et al. Multipotent CNS stem cells are present in the adult mammalian spinal cord and ventricular neuroaxis. J Neurosci 1996;16(23):7599–7609.
20. Alvarez-Buylla A, Lim DA. For the long run: maintaining germinal niches in the adult brain. Neuron 2004;41(5):683–686.
21. Shen Q, Goderie SK, Jin L, et al. Endothelial cells stimulate self-renewal and expand neurogenesis of neural stem cells. Science 2004;304(5675):1338–1340.
22. Tannock I, Hill R, Bristow R, Harrington L. The Basic Science of Oncology. 4th ed. New York: McGraw-Hill; 2005.
23. Faulhaber O, Bristow R. Basis of cell kill following clinical radiotherapy. In: Sluyser M, ed. Application of Apoptosis to Cancer Treatment. New York: Kluwer-Springer Press; 2005:293–320.
24. van der Maazen RW, Verhagen I, van der Kogel AJ. An in vitro clonogenic assay to assess radiation damage in rat CNS glial progenitor cells. Int J Radiat Biol 1990;58(5):835–844.
25. Lu F, Wong CS. A clonogenic survival assay of neural stem cells in rat spinal cord after exposure to ionizing radiation. Radiat Res 2005;163(1):63–71.
26. Hall EJ. Radiobiology for the Radiologist. 5th ed. Philadelphia: Lippincott Williams & Wilkins; 2000.
27. Thames HD Jr, Withers HR, Peters LJ, Fletcher GH. Changes in early and late radiation responses with altered dose fractionation: implications for dose-survival relationships. Int J Radiat Oncol Biol Phys 1982;8(2):219–226.
28. Withers HR, Taylor JM, Maciejewski B. Treatment volume and tissue tolerance. Int J Radiat Oncol Biol Phys 1988;14(4):751–759.
29. Ang KK. Radiation injury to the central nervous system: clinical features and prevention. In: Meyer JL, ed. Radiation Injury: Advances in Management and Prevention. Vol 32. Basel: Karger; 1999:145–154.
30. Wong CS, Minkin S, Hill RP. Linear-quadratic model underestimates sparing effect of small doses per fraction in rat spinal cord. Radiother Oncol 1992;23(3):176–184.
31. van der Kogel AJ, Barendsen GW. Late effects of spinal cord irradiation with 300 kV X rays and 15 MeV neutrons. Br J Radiol 1974;47(559):393–398.
32. Schultheiss TE, Stephens LC. Invited review: permanent radiation myelopathy. Br J Radiol 1992;65(777):737–753.
33. Okada S, Okeda R. Pathology of radiation myelopathy. Neuropathology 2001;21(4):247–265.
34. Stewart PA, Vinters HV, Wong CS. Blood–spinal cord barrier function and morphometry after single doses of x-rays in rat spinal cord. Int J Radiat Oncol Biol Phys 1995;32(3):703–711.
35. Mastaglia FL, McDonald WI, Watson JV, Yogendran K. Effects of x-radiation on the spinal cord: an experimental study of the morphological changes in central nerve fibres. Brain 1976;99(1):101–122.
36. van der Kogel AJ. Central nervous system radiation injury in small animal models. In: Gutin PH, Leibel SA, Sheline GE, eds. Radiation Injury to the Nervous System. New York: Raven Press; 1991:91–111.
37. Schultheiss TE, Stephens LC, Ang KK, Price RE, Peters LJ. Volume effects in rhesus monkey spinal cord. Int J Radiat Oncol Biol Phys 1994;29(1):67–72.
38. Schultheiss TE, Stephens LC, Maor MH. Analysis of the histopathology of radiation myelopathy. Int J Radiat Oncol Biol Phys 1988;14(1):27–32.

39. Li YQ, Jay V, Wong CS. Oligodendrocytes in the adult rat spinal cord undergo radiation-induced apoptosis. Cancer Res 1996;56(23):5417–5422.

40. Li YQ, Guo YP, Jay V, Stewart PA, Wong CS. Time course of radiation-induced apoptosis in the adult rat spinal cord. Radiother Oncol 1996;39(1):35–42.

41. Chow BM, Li YQ, Wong CS. Radiation-induced apoptosis in the adult central nervous system is p53-dependent. Cell Death Differ 2000;7(8):712–720.

42. Pena LA, Fuks Z, Kolesnick RN. Radiation-induced apoptosis of endothelial cells in the murine central nervous system: protection by fibroblast growth factor and sphingomyelinase deficiency. Cancer Res 2000;60(2):321–327.

43. Mizumatsu S, Monje ML, Morhardt DR, Rola R, Palmer TD, Fike JR. Extreme sensitivity of adult neurogenesis to low doses of X-irradiation. Cancer Res 2003;63(14):4021–4027.

44. Li YQ, Ballinger JR, Nordal RA, Su ZF, Wong CS. Hypoxia in radiation-induced blood–spinal cord barrier breakdown. Cancer Res 2001;61(8):3348–3354.

45. Monje ML, Mizumatsu S, Fike JR, Palmer TD. Irradiation induces neural precursor-cell dysfunction. Nat Med 2002;8(9):955–962.

46. Monje ML, Toda H, Palmer TD. Inflammatory blockade restores adult hippocampal neurogenesis. Science 2003;302(5651):1760–1765.

47. Nordal RA, Nagy A, Pintilie M, Wong CS. Hypoxia and hypoxia-inducible factor-1 target genes in central nervous system radiation injury: a role for vascular endothelial growth factor. Clin Cancer Res 2004;10(10):3342–3353.

48. Nordal RA, Wong CS. Intercellular adhesion molecule-1 and blood–spinal cord barrier disruption in central nervous system radiation injury. J Neuropathol Exp Neurol 2004;63(5):474–483.

49. Hong JH, Chiang CS, Campbell IL, Sun JR, Withers HR, McBride WH. Induction of acute phase gene expression by brain irradiation. Int J Radiat Oncol Biol Phys 1995;33(3):619–626.

50. Chiang CS, Hong JH, Stalder A, Sun JR, Withers HR, McBride WH. Delayed molecular responses to brain irradiation. Int J Radiat Biol 1997;72(1):45–53.

51. Raju U, Gumin GJ, Tofilon PJ. Radiation-induced transcription factor activation in the rat cerebral cortex. Int J Radiat Biol 2000;76(8):1045–1053.

52. Kyrkanides S, Moore AH, Olschowka JA, et al. Cyclooxygenase-2 modulates brain inflammation-related gene expression in central nervous system radiation injury. Brain Res Mol Brain Res 2002;104(2):159–169.

53. Palma JP, Kwon D, Clipstone NA, Kim BS. Infection with Theiler's murine encephalomyelitis virus directly induces proinflammatory cytokines in primary astrocytes via NF-kappa B activation: potential role for the initiation of demyelinating disease. J Virol 2003;77(11):6322–6331.

54. Meistrell ME III, Botchkina GI, Wang H, et al. Tumor necrosis factor is a brain damaging cytokine in cerebral ischemia. Shock 1997;8(5):341–348.

55. Dobbie MS, Hurst RD, Klein NJ, Surtees RA. Upregulation of intercellular adhesion molecule-1 expression on human endothelial cells by tumour necrosis factor-alpha in an in vitro model of the blood–brain barrier. Brain Res 1999;830(2):330–336.

56. Olschowka JA, Kyrkanides S, Harvey BK, et al. ICAM-1 induction in the mouse CNS following irradiation. Brain Behav Immun 1997;11(4):273–285.

57. Gaber MW, Sabek OM, Fukatsu K, Wilcox HG, Kiani MF, Merchant TE. Differences in ICAM-1 and TNF-alpha expression between large single fraction and fractionated irradiation in mouse brain. Int J Radiat Biol 2003;79(5):359–366.

58. Nordal RA, Wong CS. Intercellular adhesion molecule-1 and blood–spinal cord barrier disruption in central nervous system radiation injury. J Neuropathol Exp Neurol 2004;63(5):474–483.

59. Daigle JL, Hong JH, Chiang CS, McBride WH. The role of tumor necrosis factor signaling pathways in the response of murine brain to irradiation. Cancer Res 2001;61(24):8859–8865.

60. Limoli CL, Giedzinski E, Rola R, Otsuka S, Palmer TD, Fike JR. Radiation response of neural precursor cells: linking cellular sensitivity to cell cycle checkpoints, apoptosis and oxidative stress. Radiat Res 2004;161(1):17–27.

61. Foresti R, Goatly H, Green CJ, Motterlini R. Role of heme oxygenase-1 in hypoxia-reoxygenation: requirement of substrate heme to promote cardioprotection. Am J Physiol Heart Circ Physiol 2001;281(5):H1976–H1984.

62. Tofilon PJ, Fike JR. The radioresponse of the central nervous system: a dynamic process. Radiat Res 2000;153(4):357–370.

63. Yin E, Nelson DO, Coleman MA, Peterson LE, Wyrobek AJ. Gene expression changes in mouse brain after exposure to low-dose ionizing radiation. Int J Radiat Biol 2003;79(10):759–775.

64. Mahmoud-Ahmed AS, Atkinson S, Wong CS. Early gene expression profile in mouse brain after exposure to ionizing radiation. Radiat Res 2006;165(2):142–154.

65. Zhao W, Chuang EY, Mishra M, et al. Distinct effects of ionizing radiation on in vivo murine kidney and brain normal tissue gene expression. Clin Cancer Res 2006;12(12):3823–3830.

66. Atkinson S, Li YQ, Wong CS. Changes in oligodendrocytes and myelin gene expression after radiation in the rodent spinal cord. Int J Radiat Oncol Biol Phys 2003;57(4):1093–1100.

67. Atkinson SL, Li YQ, Wong CS. Apoptosis and proliferation of oligodendrocyte progenitor cells in the irradiated rodent spinal cord. Int J Radiat Oncol Biol Phys 2005;62(2):535–544.

68. Chari DM, Huang WL, Blakemore WF. Dysfunctional oligodendrocyte progenitor cell (OPC) populations may inhibit repopulation of OPC depleted tissue. J Neurosci Res 2003;73(6):787–793.

69. Raff MC, Lillien LE. Differentiation of a bipotential glial progenitor cell: what controls the timing and the choice of developmental pathway? J Cell Sci Suppl 1988;10:77–83.

70. van der Maazen RW, Kleiboer BJ, Verhagen I, van der Kogel AJ. Repair capacity of adult rat glial progenitor cells determined by an in vitro clonogenic assay after in vitro or in vivo fractionated irradiation. Int J Radiat Biol 1993;63(5):661–666.

71. van der Maazen RW, Verhagen I, Kleiboer BJ, van der Kogel AJ. Radiosensitivity of glial progenitor cells of the perinatal and adult rat optic nerve studied by an in vitro clonogenic assay. Radiother Oncol 1991;20(4):258–264.

72. van der Maazen RW, Kleiboer BJ, Verhagen I, van der Kogel AJ. Irradiation in vitro discriminates between different O-2A progenitor cell subpopulations in the perinatal central nervous system of rats. Radiat Res 1991;128(1):64–72.

73. Otsuka S, Coderre JA, Micca PL, et al. Depletion of neural precursor cells after local brain irradiation is due to radiation dose to the parenchyma, not the vasculature. Radiat Res 2006;165(5):582–591.

74. Doetsch F, Caille I, Lim DA, Garcia-Verdugo JM, Alvarez-Buylla A. Subventricular zone astrocytes are neural stem cells in the adult mammalian brain. Cell 1999;97(6):703–716.

75. Morshead CM, van der Kooy D. Disguising adult neural stem cells. Curr Opin Neurobiol 2004;14(1):125–131.

76. van der Maazen RW, Verhagen I, Kleiboer BJ, van der Kogel AJ. Repopulation of O-2A progenitor cells after irradiation of the adult rat optic nerve analyzed by an in vitro clonogenic assay. Radiat Res 1992;132(1):82–86.

77. Madsen TM, Kristjansen PE, Bolwig TG, Wortwein G. Arrested neuronal proliferation and impaired hippocampal function following fractionated brain irradiation in the adult rat. Neuroscience 2003;119(3):635–642.

78. Monje ML, Palmer T. Radiation injury and neurogenesis. Curr Opin Neurol 2003;16(2):129–134.

79. van Praag H, Christie BR, Sejnowski TJ, Gage FH. Running enhances neurogenesis, learning, and long-term potentiation in mice. Proc Natl Acad Sci U S A 1999;96(23):13427–13431.

80. Kempermann G, Kuhn HG, Gage FH. More hippocampal neurons in adult mice living in an enriched environment. Nature 1997;386(6624):493–495.

81. Ljubimova NV, Levitman MK, Plotnikova ED, Eidus L. Endothelial cell population dynamics in rat brain after local irradiation. Br J Radiol 1991;64(766):934–940.

82. Li YQ, Chen P, Jain V, Reilly RM, Wong CS. Early radiation-induced endothelial cell loss and blood–spinal cord barrier breakdown in the rat spinal cord. Radiat Res 2004;161(2):143–152.

83. Santana P, Pena LA, Haimovitz-Friedman A, et al. Acid sphingomyelinase-deficient human lymphoblasts and mice are defective in radiation-induced apoptosis. Cell 1996;86(2):189–199.

84. Siegal T, Pfeffer MR. Radiation-induced changes in the profile of spinal cord serotonin, prostaglandin synthesis, and vascular permeability. Int J Radiat Oncol Biol Phys 1995;31(1):57–64.

85. Rubin P, Gash DM, Hansen JT, Nelson DF, Williams JP. Disruption of the blood–brain barrier as the primary effect of CNS irradiation. Radiother Oncol 1994;31(1):51–60.

86. Sheline GE, Wara WM, Smith V. Therapeutic irradiation and brain injury. Int J Radiat Oncol Biol Phys 1980;6(9):1215–1228.

87. Morris GM, Coderre JA, Bywaters A, Whitehouse E, Hopewell JW. Boron neutron capture irradiation of the rat spinal cord: histopathological evidence of a vascular-mediated pathogenesis. Radiat Res 1996;146(3):313–320.

88. Coderre JA, Morris AD, Micca PL, et al. Late effects of radiation on the central nervous system: role of vascular endothelial damage vs glial stem cell survival. Radiat Res 2006;116(3):495–503.

89. Proescholdt MA, Heiss JD, Walbridge S, et al. Vascular endothelial growth factor (VEGF) modulates vascular permeability and inflammation in rat brain. J Neuropathol Exp Neurol 1999;58(6):613–627.

90. Bartholdi D, Rubin BP, Schwab ME. VEGF mRNA induction correlates with changes in the vascular architecture upon spinal cord damage in the rat. Eur J Neurosci 1997;9(12):2549–2560.

91. Tsao MN, Li YQ, Lu G, Xu Y, Wong CS. Upregulation of vascular endothelial growth factor is associated with radiation-induced blood–spinal cord barrier breakdown. J Neuropathol Exp Neurol 1999;58(10):1051–1060.

92. Stacker SA, Vitali A, Caesar C, et al. A mutant form of vascular endothelial growth factor (VEGF) that lacks VEGF receptor-2 activation retains the ability to induce vascular permeability. J Biol Chem 1999;274(49):34884–34892.

93. Rubin LL, Staddon JM. The cell biology of the blood–brain barrier. Annu Rev Neurosci 1999;22:11–28.

94. Wang W, Dentler WL, Borchardt RT. VEGF increases BMEC monolayer permeability by affecting occludin expression and tight junction assembly. Am J Physiol Heart Circ Physiol 2001;280(1):H434–H440.

95. Iwahashi T, Koh CS, Inoue A, Yahikozawa H, Yamazaki M, Yanagisawa N. Characterization of infiltrating mononuclear cells in the spinal cords of Lewis rats with experimental autoimmune encephalomyelitis (EAE) [in Japanese]. Arerugi 1994;43(11):1345–1350.

96. Brown H, Hien TT, Day N, et al. Evidence of blood–brain barrier dysfunction in human cerebral malaria. Neuropathol Appl Neurobiol 1999;25(4):331–340.

97. Engelhardt B, Conley FK, Butcher EC. Cell adhesion molecules on vessels during inflammation in the mouse central nervous system. J Neuroimmunol 1994;51(2):199–208.

98. Quarmby S, Kumar P, Kumar S. Radiation-induced normal tissue injury: role of adhesion molecules in leukocyte-endothelial cell interactions. Int J Cancer 1999;82(3):385–395.

99. Quarmby S, Kumar P, Kumar S. Radiation-induced normal tissue injury: role of adhesion molecules in leukocyte-endothelial cell interactions. Int J Cancer 1999;82(3):385–395.

100. Mayhan WG. VEGF increases permeability of the blood–brain barrier via a nitric oxide synthase/cGMP-dependent pathway. Am J Physiol 1999;276(5 Pt 1):C1148–C1153.

101. Radisavljevic Z, Avraham H, Avraham S. Vascular endothelial growth factor up-regulates ICAM-1 expression via the phosphatidylinositol 3 OH-kinase/AKT/nitric oxide pathway and modulates migration of brain microvascular endothelial cells. J Biol Chem 2000;275(27):20770–20774.

102. Miyamoto K, Khosrof S, Bursell SE, et al. Vascular endothelial growth factor (VEGF)-induced retinal vascular permeability is mediated by intercellular adhesion molecule-1 (ICAM-1). Am J Pathol 2000;156(5):1733–1739.

103. Greenwood J, Etienne-Manneville S, Adamson P, Couraud PO. Lymphocyte migration into the central nervous system: implication of ICAM-1 signalling at the blood-brain barrier. Vascul Pharmacol 2002;38(6):315–322.

104. Beal MF. Aging, energy, and oxidative stress in neurodegenerative diseases. Ann Neurol 1995;38(3):357–366.

105. Bindokas VP, Jordan J, Lee CC, Miller RJ. Superoxide production in rat hippocampal neurons: selective imaging with hydroethidine. J Neurosci 1996;16(4):1324–1336.

106. Lee PJ, Jiang BH, Chin BY, et al. Hypoxia-inducible factor-1 mediates transcriptional activation of the heme oxygenase-1 gene in response to hypoxia. J Biol Chem 1997;272(9):5375–5381.

107. Smith KJ, Kapoor R, Felts PA. Demyelination: the role of reactive oxygen and nitrogen species. Brain Pathol 1999;9(1):69–92.

108. Bradley WG, Fewings JD, Cumming WJ, Harrison RM. Delayed myeloradiculopathy produced by spinal X-irradiation in the rat. J Neurol Sci 1977;31(1):63–82.

109. van der Kogel AJ. Radiation-induced nerve root degeneration and hypertrophic neuropathy in the lumbosacral spinal cord of rats: the relation with changes in aging rats. Acta Neuropathol (Berl) 1977;39(2):139–145.

110. van der Kogel AJ. Radiation tolerance of the rat spinal cord: time–dose relationships. Radiology 1977;122(2):505–509.

111. van der Kogel AJ. Late effects of radiation on the spinal cord–dose effect relationships and pathogenesis. Radiobiol Inst Org Health Res 1979.

112. van der Kogel AJ. Mechanisms of late radiation injury in the spinal cord. In: Meyn R, Withers H, eds. Radiation biology in Cancer Research. New York: Raven Press; 1980:461–470.

113. Goffinet DR, Marsa GW, Brown JM. The effects of single and multifraction radiation courses on the mouse spinal cord. Radiology 1976;119(3):709–713.

114. Travis EL, Parkins CS, Holmes SJ, Down JD. Effect of misonidazole on radiation injury to mouse spinal cord. Br J Cancer 1982;45(3):469–473.

115. Habermalz HJ, Valley B, Habermalz E. Radiation myelopathy of the mouse spinal cord–isoeffect correlations after fractionated radiation. Strahlenther Onkol 1987;163(9):626–632.

116. Knowles JF. The effects of single dose X-irradiation on the guinea-pig spinal cord. Int J Radiat Biol Relat Stud Phys Chem Med 1981;40(3):265–275.

117. Knowles JF. The radiosensitivity of the guinea-pig spinal cord to X-rays: the effect of retreatment at one year and the effect of age at the time of irradiation. Int J Radiat Biol Relat Stud Phys Chem Med 1983;44(5):433–442.

118. Saunders MI, Dische S, Hong A, et al. Continuous hyperfractionated accelerated radiotherapy in locally advanced carcinoma of the head and neck region. Int J Radiat Oncol Biol Phys 1989;17(6):1287–1293.

119. Wong CS, Van Dyk J, Simpson WJ. Myelopathy following hyperfractionated accelerated radiotherapy for anaplastic thyroid carcinoma. Radiother Oncol 1991;20(1):3–9.

120. Landuyt W, Fowler J, Ruifrok A, Stuben G, van der Kogel A, van der Schueren E. Kinetics of repair in the spinal cord of the rat. Radiother Oncol 1997;45(1):55–62.

121. Ruifrok AC, Kleiboer BJ, van der Kogel AJ. Reirradiation tolerance of the immature rat spinal cord. Radiother Oncol 1992;23(4):249–256.

122. Kim JJ, Hao Y, Jang D, Wong CS. Lack of influence of sequence of top-up doses on repair kinetics in rat spinal cord. Radiother Oncol 1997;43(2):211–217.

123. Philippens ME, Pop LA, Visser AG, Schellekens SA, van der Kogel AJ. Dose-volume effects in rat thoracolumbar spinal cord: an evaluation of NTCP models. Int J Radiat Oncol Biol Phys 2004;60(2):578–590.

124. van Luijk P, Bijl HP, Konings AW, van der Kogel AJ, Schippers JM. Data on dose-volume effects in the rat spinal cord do not support existing NTCP models. Int J Radiat Oncol Biol Phys 2005;61(3):892–900.

125. van den Aardweg GJ, Hopewell JW, Whitehouse EM. The radiation response of the cervical spinal cord of the pig: effects of changing the irradiated volume. Int J Radiat Oncol Biol Phys 1995;31(1):51–55.

126. Powers BE, Thames HD, Gillette SM, Smith C, Beck ER, Gillette EL. Volume effects in the irradiated canine spinal cord: do they exist when the probability of injury is low? Radiother Oncol 1998;46(3):297–306.

127. Hopewell JW, Morris AD, Dixon-Brown A. The influence of field size on the late tolerance of the rat spinal cord to single doses of X rays. Br J Radiol 1987;60(719):1099–1108.

128. van Luijk P, Bijl HP, Coppes RP, et al. Techniques for precision irradiation of the lateral half of the rat cervical spinal cord using 150 MeV protons [corrected]. Phys Med Biol 2001;46(11):2857–2871.

129. Bijl HP, van Luijk P, Coppes RP, Schippers JM, Konings AW, van der Kogel AJ. Dose-volume effects in the rat cervical spinal cord after proton irradiation. Int J Radiat Oncol Biol Phys 2002;52(1):205–211.

130. Bijl HP, van Luijk P, Coppes RP, Schippers JM, Konings AW, van der Kogel AJ. Unexpected changes of rat cervical spinal cord tolerance caused by inhomogeneous dose distributions. Int J Radiat Oncol Biol Phys 2003;57(1):274–281.

131. Bijl HP, van Luijk P, Coppes RP, Schippers JM, Konings AW, van der Kogel AJ. Influence of adjacent low-dose fields on tolerance to high doses of protons in rat cervical spinal cord. Int J Radiat Oncol Biol Phys 2006;64(4):1204–1210.

132. Bijl HP, van Luijk P, Coppes RP, Schippers JM, Konings AW, van der Kogel AJ. Regional differences in radiosensitivity across the rat cervical spinal cord. Int J Radiat Oncol Biol Phys 2005;61(2):543–551.

133. Brown JM, Probert JC. Early and late radiation changes following a second course of irradiation. Radiology 1975;115(3):711–716.

134. Carpenter SG, Raju MR. Residual radiation damage in the mouse foot after exposure to heavy particles. Radiology 1981;138(2):483–485.

135. Denekamp J. Residual radiation damage in mouse skin 5 to 8 months after irradiation. Radiology 1975;115(1):191–195.

136. Hendry JH, Rosenberg I, Greene D, Stewart JG. Re-irradiation of rat tails to necrosis at six months after treatment with a "tolerance" dose of x rays or neutrons. Br J Radiol 1977;50(596):567–572.

137. Terry NH, Tucker SL, Travis EL. Time course of loss of residual radiation damage in murine skin assessed by retreatment. Int J Radiat Biol 1989;55(2):271–283.

138. Ruifrok AC, Kleiboer BJ, van der Kogel AJ. Radiation tolerance and fractionation sensitivity of the developing rat cervical spinal cord. Int J Radiat Oncol Biol Phys 1992;24(3):505–510.

139. Wong CS, Poon JK, Hill RP. Re-irradiation tolerance in the rat spinal cord: influence of level of initial damage. Radiother Oncol 1993;26(2):132–138.

140. Wong CS, Hao Y. Long-term recovery kinetics of radiation damage in rat spinal cord. Int J Radiat Oncol Biol Phys 1997;37(1):171–179.

141. Ang KK, Jiang GL, Feng Y, Stephens LC, Tucker SL, Price RE. Extent and kinetics of recovery of occult spinal cord injury. Int J Radiat Oncol Biol Phys 2001;50(4):1013–1020.

142. Ang KK, Price RE, Stephens LC, et al. The tolerance of primate spinal cord to re-irradiation. Int J Radiat Oncol Biol Phys 1993;25(3):459–464.

143. Nieder C, Grosu AL, Andratschke NH, Molls M. Proposal of human spinal cord reirradiation dose based on collection of data from 40 patients. Int J Radiat Oncol Biol Phys 2005;61(3):851–855.

144. Chow E. Protocol CAN-NCIC-SC20. Available at: http://www.cancer.gov/search/ViewClinicalTrials.aspx?cdrid=357423&protocolsearchid=2504181&versionfiltered=healthprofessional.

145. Chari DM, Blakemore WF. Efficient recolonisation of progenitor-depleted areas of the CNS by adult oligodendrocyte progenitor cells. Glia 2002;37(4):307–313.

3

Clinical Spinal Cord Tolerance to Radiosurgery

Simon S. Lo and Eric Lin Chang

Stereotactic spine radiosurgery and stereotactic spine radiation therapy are advanced radiation therapy techniques that enable focused delivery of radiation treatments to spinal lesions while sparing the spinal cord. A very steep radiation dose fall-off beyond the target volume is a prerequisite for a stereotactic radiation delivery system. Because of this favorable dosimetric characteristic, it is possible to treat spinal lesions with a few fractions or only one fraction of a high dose of radiation and to more safely give a higher radiation dose than could be given by conventional radiotherapy techniques. It is also possible to re-irradiate spinal lesions that have previously been irradiated by avoiding the spinal cord as much as possible. Radiation-induced myelopathy is one of the most feared complications associated with radiation therapy. Although there has been ample experience with using conventional external beam irradiation to treat spinal tumors, as well as growing experience with stereotactic techniques, the true spinal cord tolerance to radiation has not been clearly defined due to conservative dose constraints placed on the spinal cord. Although very limited clinical data exist on the spinal cord's tolerance to re-irradiation, practitioners of stereotactic body radiation therapy often encounter this situation. This chapter examines clinical spinal cord tolerance in the context of radiobiology, historical literature on conventional radiation therapy, and recent reports in the literature on stereotactic radiation for spinal tumors.

◆ Overview of Mechanisms of Radiation-Induced Myelopathy

Demyelination and necrosis of the spinal cord, both being manifestations of white matter injury, are the main morphologic features of radiation-induced myelopathy, although they are not pathognomonic of radiation injury.[1] Apart from the white matter changes, vasculopathies and glial reaction can also be seen in radiation-induced myelopathy.[1] Injury of the microvasculature has been implicated as a mecha-

nism of myelopathy, but there are circumstances in which white matter necrosis occurs without accompanied vascular changes in the previously irradiated areas. Glial reaction has been observed in other demyelinating conditions not related to radiation injury, and it is believed it may have some role in radiation myelopathy. There is some suggestion that the cytokine network in the central nervous system may also have a role in radiation myelopathy.[1]

◆ Radiobiology of Spinal Cord Tolerance

The use of intensity-modulated radiation therapy (IMRT) can create highly conformal dose distributions for spinal tumors with steep dose gradients that spare the spinal cord (**Fig. 3.1**). The use of stereotactic radiation techniques enables delivery of IMRT with millimeter precision. The combination of these techniques translates into high-dose, highly conformal irradiation that can be delivered with much greater safety than previously possible. From a radiobiological standpoint, this means that an increased therapeutic ratio is created with greater separation between the normal tissue complication curve for the spinal cord and the tumor control probability curve for the spinal tumor. The spinal cord, a late responding tissue, is highly sensitive to fraction size, as shown in **Fig. 3.2**, and is therefore best treated with relatively small fraction sizes when using conventional radiation therapy. Whereas hypofractionated stereotactic radiation uses larger fraction sizes, the steep dose gradients associated with IMRT previously described permit one to keep the actual fraction size seen by the spinal cord relatively small, so that late effects are minimized. It should be emphasized that conventional radiation therapy is very useful and should be considered the first line of radiation treatment for radiosensitive lesions of the spine such as breast cancer, plasmacytoma, lymphoma, and germ cell tumors, where the tumor control curve lies to the left of the normal tissue complication curve (**Fig. 3.3A**). However, for recurrent spinal tumors previously irradiated,

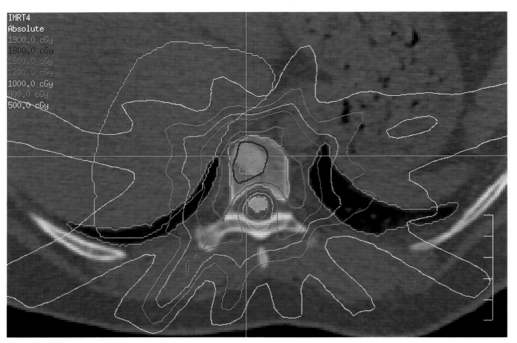

Figure 3.1 Intensity-modulated radiation therapy plan for stereotactic spine radiosurgery delivering 16 Gy to the entire T9 vertebral body and 18 Gy to the gross tumor volume; the spinal cord dose was limited to < 10 Gy.

as well as radioresistant tumors such as renal cell carcinoma, melanoma, and sarcomas, the tumor control curve lies to the right of the normal tissue complication curve (**Fig. 3.3B**). In these cases, conventional irradiation is often inadequate, as tumoricidal doses cannot be given without exceeding spinal cord tolerance. One must then resort to stereotactic spine radiation techniques to improve the therapeutic window that will allow higher doses to be given to the tumor while sparing the spinal cord. The large dose per fraction used in

hypofractionated radiation therapy or single-session radiosurgery may help overcome radioresistant tumors, which are late responding tissues, by "getting over the shoulder," going from dose point A to dose point B, resulting in greater log cell kill (**Fig. 3.4**).

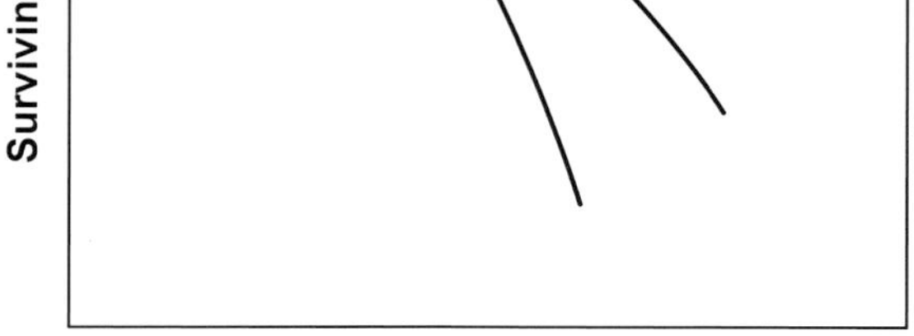

The studies reported to date on stereotactic irradiation of spinal tumors in general show that these techniques are safe (**Table 3.1**). The problem for one trying to determine spinal cord tolerance is that the field has done such a good job of minimizing spinal cord complications, that the incidence of such occurrences is too low to make any determinations on what is the upper bound of a safe dose. For instance, in our review of 13 studies on stereotactic spine irradiation involving 459 patients, only Dodd et al[41] reported any neurologic complication. The tumor control curve and normal tissue complication curve can be combined into an uncomplicated local cure curve (**Fig. 3.5**). Although it is clear that practitioners are operating along this curve with almost no complication somewhere between dose A and dose B, it is not clear what the optimum dose B is because the upper limit has not yet been defined. From our own data at M. D. Anderson Cancer Center in Houston, Texas, it appears that giving spinal tumors 27 Gy in three fractions or 30 Gy in five fractions while limiting the spinal cord to < 10 Gy is relatively safe. However, this spinal cord constraint may be overly conservative. How much to relax this constraint is currently unknown. For single-session stereotactic radiation series reported by others, it appears that limiting the surface dose of the spinal cord to 10, 12, and perhaps even 14 Gy appears safe, although patient numbers are still limited and follow-up is relatively short. Further experience with larger numbers of patients and longer follow-up will be needed. It is currently unclear

Figure 3.2 Normal tissue effect of smaller versus larger fractions of radiation therapy on early and late responding tissues.
(Adapted from Hall EJ, ed. Radiobiology for the Radiologist. 5th ed. Philadelphia: Lippincott Williams & Wilkins; 2000:401, with permission.)

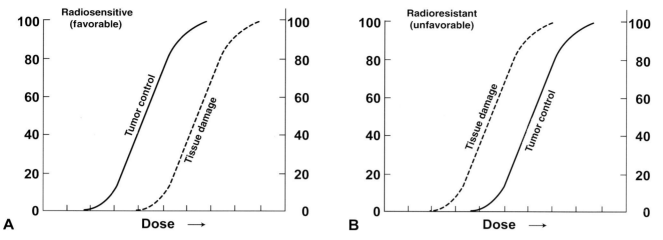

Figure 3.3 Tumor control probability and incidence of tissue damage as a function of dose for radiosensitive (A) and radioresistant (B) tumors. (Reprinted from Rubin P. Clinical Oncology: A Multidisciplinary Approach for Physicians and Students. 7th ed. Philadelphia: Elsevier; 1993, with permission.)

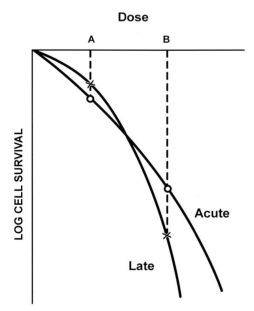

Figure 3.4 Compared with small fraction sizes (dose A) used in conventional radiation therapy, greater fraction sizes (dose B) used in hypofractionated radiation therapy may help overcome radioresistance in tumors with low α/β, which behave like late responding tissues. (Adapted from Fowler JR, Fractionation and therapeutic gain. In: Stell GG, Adams GE, Peckham MJ, eds. The Biological Basis for Radiotherapy. Philadelphia: Elsevier; 1983:181–194,with permission.)

and remains to be seen how much higher a surface dose the spinal cord will tolerate in a single fraction.

◆ Spinal Cord and Cauda Equina Tolerance

Spinal Cord Tolerance to Conventionally Fractionated Radiation Therapy

Traditionally, the spinal cord tolerance is generally accepted to be between 45 and 50 Gy in conventional fractionation. Emami et al estimated the TD 5/5 (the radiation dose at which there is a 5% risk of radiation myelopathy at 5 years from radiation therapy) for irradiation of 5, 10, and 20 cm of spinal cord in conventional fractionation to be 50, 50, and 47 Gy, respectively.[2] However, this estimate was based on data that went back as far as the 1940s. Data in the literature suggest that the spinal cord tolerance to conventional radiation should be higher than the estimated level of 45 to 50 Gy (**Table 3.2**). Marcus and Million reviewed the 1112 evaluable patients treated with radiation therapy for head and neck cancer.[3] These patients received > 30 Gy to > 2 cm of spinal cord and were followed for at least 1 year. The incidence of myelitis was 0.18%. The risk of radiation-induced myelitis was 0/124 at 30.0 to 39.99 Gy, 0/442 at 40.0 to 44.99 Gy, 2/471 at 45.0 to 49.99 Gy, and 0/75 at a cord dose of 50 Gy or higher.[3] One can conclude from these data that the spinal cord tolerance has not been reached with these doses. McCunniff and Liang examined the rate of myelitis in 144 patients who received 56 Gy or higher to a portion of the cervical spinal cord during head and neck radiation therapy.[4] Most of the patients received ≥ 60 Gy to the cervical spinal cord in 1.33 to 2.0 Gy fractions. Among the 53 patients (approximately half of them received 60 Gy or higher to the spinal cord) who had at least 2 years of follow-up, only 1 of them developed spinal cord injury 20 months after treatment.[4] The investigators at Princess Margaret Hospital, Toronto, did not observe any cases of radiation-induced myelopathy in patients who

Table 3.1 Summary of the Spinal Cord/Cauda Equina Toxicity from Different Stereotactic Spine Radiosurgery and Stereotactic Spine Radiotherapy Series

Series	n (pt/l/lpxrt)	Tumor Rose, range (Gy)	No. of Fractions	Median Cord/ CE Dose, range (Gy)	Median Follow-up, range (Months)	Neurologic Complications, n (%)
Stereotactic Spine Radiosurgery Series						
Hamilton et al[26]	9/9/9	8 (8–10)	1	Cord: 1.79 (0.52–3.2)	NA	0 (0)
Ryu et al[27]	10/10/10	6 (6–8)	1	Cord: > 4 (NA)	6 (3–12)	0 (0)
Ryu et al[28]	49/61/0	NA (10–16)	1	Cord: NA	NA (6–24)	0 (0)
Ryu et al[29]	18/18/5	11.4 (6–14)	1	Neural elements: NA (5.28–12.32)	7 (4–36)	0 (0)
Gerszten et al[35]	50/68/48	19 (15–22.5)	1	Cord: 10 (6.5–13.0) CE: 10.5 (1–17)	16 (6–48)	0 (0)
Gerszten et al[36]	48/60/42	20 (17.5–25.0)	1	Cord: 9.68 (2.42–14.02) CE: 9.15 (0.51–14.31)	37 (14–48)	0 (0)
Gerszten et al[37]	28/36/23	21.7 (17.5–25.0)	1	Cord: 8.6 (1.3–13.1) CE: 9 (1.1–13.3)	13 (3–43)	0 (0)
Gerszten et al[33]	115/125/78	14 (12–20)	1	Spinal canal: > 8 (NA)*	18 (9–30)	0 (0)
Gerszten et al[34]	15/15/3	16 (12–20)	1	Spinal canal: > 8 (NA)	12 (NA)	0 (0)
Dodd et al[41]	19/NA/NA	NA (16–30)†	1	Cord: > 10 (maximum dose)	23 (6–73)‡	0 (0)
Stereotactic Spine Radiotherapy Series						
Chang et al[38]	15/15/5	30 (20–30)	5	Cord: 10 (NA)	9 (6–16)	0 (0)
Bilsky et al[39]	16/16/10	PTs: NA (59.4–70.8) SSTs: NA (20–50) MTs: 20 (20–55.8)	PTs: NA (33–38) SSTs: NA(5–15) MTs: 5 (4–31)	PTs: NA (14.3–52.5) SSTs: NA (2.6–4.2) MTs: 6 Gy (3.6–25.5)	12 (2–23)	0 (0)
Yamada et al[40]	35/35/24	PTs: 70 (59.4–70.2) MTs: 20 (20–30)	PTs: 35 (33–39) MTs: 5	PTs: 68% (14–75%) MTs: 34% (13–60%)	11 (1–42)	0 (0)
Dodd et al[41]	32/NA/NA	NA (16–30)†	2–5	Cord: NA (NA)	23 (6–73)‡	1 (3%)§

Abbreviations: CE, cauda equina; l, lesions; lpxrt, lesions with prior external beam radiation therapy; MTs, metastatic tumors; n, number; NA, not available, pt, patients; PTs, primary tumors; SSTs, superior sulcus tumors.
* Maximum dose to the spinal canal was 13 Gy.
† This was the range of the total prescribed radiation dose delivered in one to five fractions in the whole series of 51 patients (only 19 patients received all of the radiation dose in one session).
‡ These follow-up times were for the entire group of 51 patients in the series treated with single or multiple sessions of CyberKnife-based stereotactic irradiation.
§ This patient received > 8 Gy per fraction × 3.

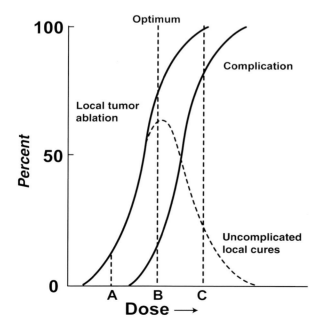

Figure 3.5 Dose A results in low probability of tumor control and low complication rate. Dose B (optimum dose) achieves high probability of tumor control and low complication rate. Dose C results in a high probability of tumor control and high complication rate. The dashed curve represents the probability of uncomplicated local cures. (Adapted from Mendelsohn ML. The biology of dose-limiting tissues. In: Time and Dose Relationships in Radiation Biology as Applied to Radiotherapy. Brookhaven National Laboratory [BNL] Report 5023 [C-57]. Upton, NY: Brookhaven National Laboratory; 1969:154–173, with permission.)

Table 3.2 Summary of Studies on Spinal Cord Tolerance to Conventionally Fractionated Radiation Therapy

Series	n	Radiation Dose (Gy)	No. of Patients with Myelopathy/Percentage
Marcus & Million[3]	124	30.0–39.99	0/0
	442	40.0–44.99	0/0
	471	45.0–49.99	2/0.4
	75	≥ 50	0/0
McCunniff & Liang[4]	56	≥ 56	1/1.7
Jeremic et al[6]	72*	≥ 55 (one third of patients received > 60)	4/5.6
Lindstadt et al[7]	14	66–78†	0/0
Marucci et al[8]	85	Surface: 55–58 CGE Center: 67–70 CGE	Grade 1–2: 15.3% Grade 3: 4.7%

* All patients had follow-up of at least 2 years.
† In 1.0 Gy twice per day fractionation.
Abbreviations: CGE, cobalt gray equivalent; *n*, number of patients.

received 50 Gy to the spinal cord if conventional fractionation (1.8–2.0 Gy) was used.[5] Schultheiss et al estimated the TD 5/5 to be between 57 and 61 Gy and the TD 50/5 to be between 68 and 73 Gy in conventional fractionation.[1] Jeremic and colleagues examined the incidence of radiation-induced myelopathy in the cervical spinal cord at doses of ≥ 55 Gy.[6] Seventy-two of 176 patients had follow-up longer than 2 years. One third (26 patients) of those patients received a dose of > 60 Gy with fraction sizes of 1.57 to 1.7 Gy. Four (5.6%) patients developed permanent radiation myelitis.[6] In adult patients with diffuse pontine glioma, hyperfractionated regimens delivering a total dose of > 70 Gy have been used without any incidence of myelitis.[7] This suggests that smaller fraction sizes may increase spinal cord tolerance to radiation as predicted by the linear-quadratic model of radiation response, although only a small segment of cervical spinal cord received the prescribed dose. In a study of combined proton-photon radiation therapy, the dose constraints to the surface of the cervical spinal cord and the center of the cervical spinal cord were 67 to 70 and 55 to 58 cobalt gray equivalent (CGE), respectively. The spinal cord toxicity was graded using the European Organization for Research and Treatment of Cancer (EORTC) and Radiation Therapy Oncology Group (RTOG) late effects scoring system. With a median follow-up of 41.3 months, 15.3 and 4.7% of the patients developed grade 1 to 2 and grade 3 toxicity, respectively.[8]

Spinal Cord Tolerance to Hypofractionated Radiation Therapy

Hypofractionated radiation therapy is usually given in a palliative setting. Because of the different fraction sizes used, it is difficult to make comparisons between studies. Macbeth et al from the Medical Research Council estimated the risk of myelopathy in patients treated with different hypofractionated regimens for lung cancer.[9] Those regimens were 8.5 Gy × 2 (*n* = 524), 4.5 Gy × 6 (*n* = 47), 5 Gy × 6 (*n* = 36), 3 Gy × 10 (*n* = 88), 3 Gy × 12 (*n* = 126), and 3 Gy × 13 (*n* = 153). The corresponding rates of myelopathy were 3/524 (0.6%), 0, 0, 0, 0, and 2/153 (1.3%), respectively.[9] For the three patients who developed radiation myelopathy after 8.5 Gy × 2 fractions, the time of onset ranged from 8 to 42 months

after radiation therapy compared with an onset time of 8 to 10 months for the two patients who developed radiation myelopathy after 39 Gy in 13 fractions.[9] Because all the patients were treated with two-dimensional techniques in the study, the spinal cord doses stated were approximate. The authors may have underestimated the actual dose delivered to the spinal cord because it might be 5% greater than the prescribed dose as a result of tissue lateral effect and sloping chest.[9] Assuming that the alpha/beta (α/β) value is 2 Gy (as suggested by the authors) and taking into account the 5% hot spot, the estimated equivalent biological total doses given as 2 Gy fractions were 48.8, 47.7, 57.1, 40.6, 48.7, and 52.7 Gy, respectively.[7] No radiation-induced myelopathy was observed in patients who received 45 Gy in 15 fractions (3 Gy per fraction) in two studies.[10,11]

In a randomized trial comparing short-course versus split-course radiation therapy in metastatic spinal cord compression, approximately half of the patients (*n* = 142) received 16 Gy in two fractions for spinal cord compression.[12] With a median follow-up of 33 months, none of those patients were scored to have late toxicity, although 10 of the 93 patients (10.8%) who were ambulatory before treatment lost the ability to walk after treatment.[12] In a Dutch trial, the palliative regimens of 30 Gy in 10 fractions and 16 Gy in 2 fractions were compared in patients with advanced non–small cell lung cancer. No myelopathy was observed in both arms.[13] Radiation-induced myelopathy has been observed in patients treated with various hypofractionated regimens to the spinal cord in other series.[14–18] In patients treated to a dose of 40 Gy in 10 fractions to the spinal cord, the reported rate of radiation-induced myelopathy ranged from 0 to 13.3% in different series.[14–17,19] Dische et al reported a radiation myelopathy rate of 11.4% when the spinal cord dose exceeded 33.5 Gy (in six fractions).[18] There were other studies showing significant incidence of radiation myelopathy after a combination of various fraction sizes.[1] Because of the use of various fraction sizes in those studies, it is difficult to draw any useful conclusion regarding dose–response rates for radiation-induced myelopathy. **Table 3.3** summarizes the incidence of radiation-induced myelopathy reported in selected studies of patients treated to the spinal cord using hypofractionated regimens.

Table 3.3 Summary of the Incidence of Radiation-Induced Myelopathy Reported in Selected Studies of Patients Treated to the Spinal Cord Utilizing Hypofractionated Regimens

Series	n	Radiation Dose	No. of Patients with Myelopathy/Percentage
Macbeth et al[9]	524	8.5 Gy × 2	3/0.6
	47	4.5 Gy × 6	0/0
	36	5 Gy × 6	0/0
	88	3 Gy × 10	0/0
	126	3 Gy × 12	0/0
	153	3 Gy × 13	2/1.3
Choi et al[10]	16	3 Gy × 15	0/0
Hazra et al[11]	75	3 Gy × 15	0/0
Maranzano et al[12]	142	8 Gy × 2	0/0
Kramer et al[13]	149	8 Gy × 2	0/0
Madden et al[14]	43	4 Gy × 10	1/2.3
Miller et al[15]	97	4 Gy × 10	4/4.1
Fitzgerald et al[16]	45	4 Gy × 10	6/13.3
Abramson & Cavanaugh[17]	103	4 Gy × 10	4/3.9
Dische et al[18]	71	33.5 Gy in 6 fractions	8/11.3
Guthrie et al[19]	42	4 Gy × 10	0/0

Abbreviation: n, number of patients.

Spinal Cord Tolerance to a Single Dose of Radiation

Data on spinal cord tolerance to a single dose of radiation therapy are limited. Macbeth et al examined the rates of radiation-induced myelopathy in patients treated with various hypofractionated regimens for lung cancer, including those patients who received a single dose of 10 Gy.[9] None of the 114 patients treated with a single dose of 10 Gy developed myelopathy.[9] The risk of radiation-induced myelopathy was estimated to be zero in patients treated with a single dose of 10 Gy by 2 years. As suggested by the authors, some patients might have received a radiation dose to the spinal cord 5% higher than the prescribed dose in the study. Rades et al treated patients with spinal cord compression to a single dose of 10 Gy with no myelopathy observed.[20,21] The RTOG conducted a randomized trial comparing a single dose of 8 Gy and 30 Gy in 10 fractions for palliation of osseous metastases, including spinal metastases. Four hundred fifty-five patients were treated with the single-dose regimen to various osseous sites, including the spine, with no incidence of radiation-induced myelopathy.[22]

Spinal Cord Tolerance to Re-irradiation

Because of the conservative spinal cord dose constraints adopted by most radiation oncologists, it had been a very uncommon practice to re-irradiate the spine until recently, when the image-guided stereotactic radiation delivery system for the spine became available. As a result, the data on re-irradiation of the spinal cord are very limited. In a retrospective review of 62 patients with metastatic spinal cord compression who received spinal re-irradiation after initial primary spinal radiation therapy to a dose of either 8 Gy in one fraction or 20 Gy in five fractions, Rades et al reported no incidence of radiation myelitis after re-irradiation of the spine to a dose of either 8 Gy in one fraction, 15 Gy in five fractions, or 20 Gy in five fractions after a median follow-up (after re-irradiation) of 8 months (range 2–42 months).[23] The cumulative biologically effective dose (BED) was 80 to 100 Gy_2. The authors concluded that the risk of radiation myelopathy should be low if the cumulative BED is ≤ 100 Gy_2. Nieder et al reviewed data in the literature on 40 patients who underwent re-irradiation to the spinal cord and estimated the risk of myelopathy to be small after ≤ 135.5 Gy_2 when the interval is not shorter than 6 months and the dose of each course is ≤ 98 Gy_2.[24] However, due to the relatively small number of patients in these studies and the retrospective nature and relatively short follow-up periods of these studies, these datasets should be interpreted with caution.

Anatomical Considerations and Dose-Volume Effect

It has long been suggested that the radiation tolerance is different for different regions of the spinal cord.[1] However, data in the literature did not seem to support this theory. In an extensive literature review, Schultheiss et al did not find any definite evidence of difference in radiation tolerance for spinal cord in the cervical and thoracic levels.[1]

It has been a general belief that the radiation tolerance of the spinal cord is dependent upon the length of the spinal cord irradiated. Emami et al estimated TD 5/5 to be different for different lengths of spinal cord irradiated.[2] However, there are no definite clinical data to support this hypothesis. Primate models have been used to examine the relationship between the volume of spinal cord irradiated and the spinal cord tolerance. It is determined that in the regular treatment setting, it is unlikely that the volume of spinal cord irradiated will have any significant impact on the cord tolerance.[1] The spinal cord tolerance to stereotactic radiation will need to be reassessed for a variety of reasons. The first is

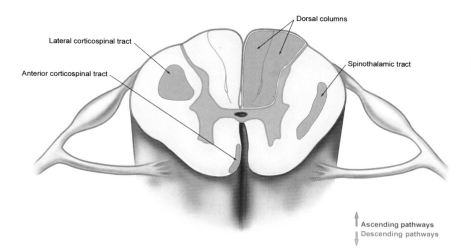

Figure 3.6 Cross-sectional anatomy of the thoracic spinal cord showing spinal cord tracts at differential risk to radiation damage depending on the anatomical location.

that conventional techniques typically irradiated the spinal cord through and through. The dose distribution from IMRT used with stereotactic irradiation typically results in a dose gradient across the spinal cord, so that the surface dose to the spinal cord should be tracked. The anatomy of the spinal cord is such that there may be differential damage to the corticospinal tracts for lesions involving the anterior column of the spine, and there may be differential damage to the dorsal columns in treating lesions involving the posterior elements of the spine (**Fig. 3.6**). One can speculate that there may be partial lesions induced by stereotactic radiation resulting in complications that are less severe than complete cord transection. Although it is true that the spinal cord is a serial structure, there are multiple serial structures or pathways in the spinal cord that could be differentially damaged. The presence of steep dose gradients, recognition of multiple pathways in the spinal cord, and use of hypofractionation or single-session schemes of radiation therapy will require continued reassessment of spinal cord tolerance and its patterns of neurologic sequelae.

◆ Cauda Equina Tolerance

In a seminal publication, Emami et al determined the TD 5/5 to be 60 Gy.[2] A study by Pieters et al examined the cauda equina tolerance to conventional fractionated high-dose radiation therapy to the region from the second lumbar vertebra downward in 53 patients.[25] The median cauda equina dose was 65.8 CGE. With a median follow-up of 87 months, 13 patients developed neurologic toxicity. Approximately half of the patients developed neurologic toxicity 5 years or longer after treatment. The median cauda equina doses were 73.7 CGE in the patients who developed neurologic toxicity and 55.6 CGE in those who did not develop neurologic toxicity.[25] Interestingly, female patients had a higher cauda equina tolerance than male patients. The TD 5/5 and TD 50/5 were 67 and 84 CGE, respectively, for females and 55 and 72 CGE, respectively, for males.[25] The tolerance dose was estimated to be 8 CGE lower 10 years after treatment.

◆ Literature on Stereotactic Spine Irradiation

There are emerging data in the literature on the safety of stereotactic spine radiosurgery and stereotactic spine radiation therapy (**Table 3.1**). Various stereotactic radiation delivery systems have been used. Although favorable outcomes have been reported, it should be noted that the overall follow-up periods are relatively short in most studies. This section focuses on the spinal cord tolerance when stereotactic radiation has been used.

Literature on Stereotactic Spine Radiosurgery

The earliest experience in stereotactic spine radiosurgery came from the University of Arizona.[26] Utilizing an invasive rigid fixation device for immobilization of the spine, Hamilton and colleagues treated nine patients with recurrent spinal tumors with stereotactic radiosurgery. All patients received prior external beam radiation therapy to the same areas. The median radiosurgical dose was 8 Gy (range 8–10 Gy) prescribed at the 80% isodose line. The spinal cord dose ranged from 0.52 to 3.2 Gy (median 1.79 Gy). No neurologic toxicity was observed.[26]

Ryu and colleagues reported the results of a prospective trial in which 10 patients received external beam radiation therapy to 25 Gy in 10 fractions followed by a radiosurgical boost of 6 to 8 Gy. With a mean follow-up of 6 months (range 3–12 months), no acute neurologic toxicity was observed.[27] The median spinal cord dose was higher than 4 Gy. In a subsequent study, Ryu and colleagues treated 49 patients with 61 spinal metastases with no prior external beam radiation therapy with stereotactic spine radiosurgery alone.[28] The prescribed dose was 10 to 16 Gy. The spinal cord dose was not specified in the study. With follow-up times ranging from 6 to 24 months, no neurologic toxicity was reported.[28] In a more recent study, the same group treated 18 patients with spinal tumors with postoperative stereotactic spine radiosurgery.[29] Five of the 18 patients had prior external beam radiation therapy. The marginal radiosurgical dose ranged from 6 to 16 Gy (mean 11.4 Gy) prescribed to the 90% isodose line. The authors reported that significant doses were delivered to the spinal cord and the nerve roots. The volume of irradiated spinal cord and nerve roots receiving 30, 50, and 80% of the total prescribed dose ranged from 0.51 to 11.05 cm³, 0.19 to 6.34 cm³, and 0.06 to 1.73 cm³, respectively.[29] With a median follow-up of 7 months (range 4–36 Gy), no neurologic complications occurred.[29] Ryu et al recently demonstrated a partial volume tolerance of spinal cord after a single dose of radiosurgery in patients with solitary spine metastasis in 230 procedures of 177 patients.[30] The spinal cord volume was defined as 6 mm above and below the radiosurgery target. Average spinal cord volume defined at the treated spinal segment was 5.9 ± 2.2 cc. The average dose to the 10% spinal cord volume was 9.8 ± 1.5 Gy. Among the 86 patients who survived longer than 1 year, there was one case of radiation-induced cord injury 13 months after radiosurgery. There were no other cases of spinal cord sequelae. Based on these findings, partial volume tolerance of the human spinal cord is at least 10 Gy to 10% of the cord volume defined as above.[30]

De Salles and colleagues treated 14 patients with stereotactic spine radiosurgery or stereotactic spine radiation therapy (13 patients were treated with stereotactic spine radiosurgery) for 22 spinal lesions.[31] A mean dose of 12 Gy (range 8–21 Gy) prescribed to the 91% isodose line was given. With a mean follow-up of 6 months (range 1–16 months), no neurologic complications were observed.[31] However, the authors did not specify the spinal cord dose from stereotactic spine radiosurgery. Benzil and colleagues treated 31 patients with 35 spinal tumors treated with stereotactic spine radiosurgery (6–8 Gy) or stereotactic spine radiation therapy (10 Gy in two fractions).[32] The spinal cord doses were not specified. Two patients (6.5%) developed transient radiculitis, and both received a biological equivalent dose of > 60 Gy.[32] The details of the two patients who developed neurologic complications were not provided.

Gerszten and colleagues reported the treatment results utilizing a CyberKnife radiosurgical system for spinal lesions in various studies.[33–37] In one of the studies, 115 patients with 125 spinal lesions (78 lesions had prior external beam radiation therapy) were treated with stereotactic spine radiosurgery to a mean dose of 14 Gy (range 15–20 Gy) at the 80% isodose line.[33] It should be noted that the spinal canal instead of the spinal cord was contoured during treatment planning. The canal volume receiving more than 8 Gy ranged from 0.0 to 1.7 cm³. The maximum spinal canal dose was 13 Gy. With a median follow-up of 18 months (range 9–30 months), there was no neurologic toxicity reported.[33] In another report from Gerszten et al, 15 patients were treated with stereotactic spine radiosurgery for benign spinal tumors.[34] Three patients had prior radiation therapy to the same segment of spine. Again, the spinal canal was contoured for treatment planning purposes. The prescribed dose was 16 Gy (range 12–20 Gy). The spinal canal volume receiving more than 8 Gy was 0.2 cm³ (range 0.0–0.9 cm³). The maximum spinal canal dose was not stated by the authors. With a follow-up of 12 months, no neurologic complications occurred.[34] In other studies from the same institution, the spinal cord (not spinal canal) and the nerve roots were contoured, thus allowing for a more accurate estimation of the radiation dose delivered to the spinal cord and the nerve roots.[35–37] Fifty patients with 68 lesions were treated with stereotactic spine radiosurgery for spinal metastases from breast cancer.[35] Forty-eight lesions had prior external beam radiation therapy. The prescribed dose was 19 Gy (range 15.0–22.5 Gy). The spinal cord and cauda equina doses were 10 Gy (range 6.5–13.0 Gy) and 10.5 Gy (range 1–17 Gy), respectively.[35] With a median follow-up of 16 months, no neurologic toxicity was observed.[35] In another study of stereotactic spine radiosurgery for spinal metastases from renal cell carcinoma, 48 patients with 60 lesions (42 lesions had prior radiation therapy) were treated.[36] The prescribed dose was 20 Gy (range 17.5–25.0 Gy). The spinal cord and cauda equina doses were 9.68 Gy (range 2.42–14.02 Gy) and 9.15 Gy (range 0.51–14.31 Gy).[36] With a median follow-up of 37 months, which was the longest among all the stereotactic spine series, there was no spinal cord toxicity.[36] In the 28 patients with 36 lesions (23 lesions were also irradiated previously) treated with stereotactic spine surgery to a dose of 21.7 Gy (range 17.5–25.0 Gy) for spinal metastases from melanoma, none developed spinal cord toxicity, with a median follow-up of 13 months.[37] The spinal cord and cauda equina doses were 8.6 Gy (range 1.3–13.1 Gy) and 9.15 Gy (range 0.51–14.31 Gy), respectively.

Literature on Stereotactic Spine Radiation Therapy

In a non-dose-escalating stereotactic spine radiation therapy phase I trial, Chang and colleagues treated 15 patients for spinal metastases.[38] Five of them had received 30 to 50 Gy to the same segment of spine previously. A conservative spinal cord dose constraint of 10 Gy in five fractions was used. The prescribed dose to the clinical target volume was 30 Gy in five fractions (6 Gy per fraction). With a median follow-up time of 9 months (range 6–16 months), no neurologic toxicity was observed.[38] Bilsky and colleagues reported their initial experience with stereotactic spine radiation therapy for primary and metastatic spinal tumors at Memorial-Sloan Kettering Cancer Center.[39] Sixteen patients with 16 tumors were treated. Ten patients had prior radiation therapy to the same segment of the spine. A variety of doses were used. For primary tumors, a dose ranging from 59.4 to 70.8 Gy in conventional fractionation was delivered. The spinal cord dose ranged from 14.3 to 52.5 Gy. For metastatic tumors, a dose of 20 Gy (range 20.0–55.8 Gy) was delivered in four or five fractions (range 4–31 fractions). The maximum spinal cord dose was 6 Gy (range 3.6 Gy to 25.5 Gy). With a median follow-up of 12 months, none of the patients developed myelopathy.[39] In a subsequent report including more patients, 35 patients with 35 primary or metastatic spine tumors (24 tumors had prior radiotherapy) were treated with stereotactic spine radiation therapy.[40] For patients with primary tumors, a dose of 70 Gy (range 59.4–70.2 Gy) in 33 to 39 fractions was given. The spinal cord dose was 68% (range 14–75%) of the prescribed dose. For patients with metastatic tumors, the prescribed dose was 20 Gy (range 20–30 Gy) in five fractions. The estimated spinal cord dose was 34% of the prescribed dose (range 13–60%). Again, no spinal toxicity occurred with a median follow-up of

11 months.[40] Dodd and colleagues treated 51 patients with 55 benign spinal tumors with stereotactic spine radiosurgery or stereotactic spine radiation therapy at Stanford University.[41] A total dose of 16 to 30 Gy was delivered in one to five sessions. Thirty-two patients received prior fractionated radiation treatments, but the exact doses were not specified. One patient developed radiation-induced myelopathy 8 months after treatment.[41] The estimated maximum spinal cord dose was > 24 Gy in three fractions.

◆ Conclusion

Data from the external beam radiation therapy studies suggest that the spinal cord may have a higher tolerance to radiation than the traditional dose limit of 45 to 50 Gy (1.8–2.0 Gy equivalent). When hypofractionated regimens are used, the linear-quadratic equivalent dose at 2 Gy has been proposed to predict for neural tissue toxicity, but caution should always be applied when applying models to real-world scenarios. One has to keep in mind, however, that most of the clinical datasets from the external beam radiation therapy studies were based on two-dimensional estimations, and some uncertainty exists. The interpretation of the datasets is further hindered by the fact that most patients in those studies were treated with palliative intent and might not have survived long enough to develop late spinal cord toxicity. Clinical data on spinal cord tolerance upon re-irradiation are scarce.

Data in the literature on stereotactic spine radiosurgery and stereotactic spine radiation therapy suggest that the dose constraints currently used for this procedure are, in general, safe. The upper limit of tolerance for dose escalation is not definitively established because there are insufficient clinical data to make such an inference. For stereotactic spine radiosurgery, Gerszten and colleagues have delivered a clinically significant maximum single dose of 13 to 14 Gy without myelopathy, and the longest median follow-up was 37 months.

The difference between external beam radiation therapy and stereotactic radiation delivery to the spine lies in the fact that in the former scenario, the whole column of the spinal cord receives a dose close to the prescribed dose, whereas in the latter scenario, only a partial circumference of the spinal cord receives a fraction of the prescribed dose. The dose-volume effect does not appear to be clinically significant in regular clinical settings. However, the dose-volume effect that is often referred to is virtually the dose–spinal cord length effect (with the assumption that the whole circumference of the spinal cord is included in the radiation field). The true relationship between the percentage of circumference of the spinal cord irradiated and the maximum spinal cord tolerance to radiation is unclear. Because most spinal cord tolerance studies were done in the conventional radiation therapy era, treating the spinal cord through and through, anatomical analyses are lacking. In the image-guided era of conformal radiotherapy, there is now an opportunity to perform analyses that can pinpoint damage to specific regions of the spinal cord. An example of such a study on the partial volume tolerance of spinal cord after a single dose of radiosurgery in patients with a solitary spine metastasis has now been completed.[30] Although the spinal cord is a serial structure, damage to any long tracts at one level will result in the loss of neurologic function below that level, and the clinical manifestations will depend on what nerve tracts are affected. It should be recalled that the spinal cord is a highly heterogeneous structure where different regions are responsible for different neurologic functions (**Fig. 3.6**). Theoretically, the spatial distribution of the radiation dose to the spinal cord should have clinical relevance, especially in the setting of stereotactic radiation delivery to the spine, because typically only a particular area of the spinal cord is touching the isodose line of the prescribed dose constraint, rather than through-and-through irradiation of the spinal cord. The risk and the nature of the neurologic deficits will depend on what particular nerve tracts receive the maximum dose to the spinal cord.

Unlike in the setting of conventional radiation therapy, the spinal cord instead of the spinal canal should be contoured because the spinal tumor volume is nearly always located immediately adjacent to the spinal cord. Because of the steep dose gradient achieved by stereotactic radiation delivery, it is extremely important to accurately delineate the spinal cord, which is to be contoured as a structure of avoidance. Postsurgical metallic instrumentation can create artifacts on the treatment planning computed tomography. In these cases, myelography should be used to delineate the spinal cord. The effects of prior surgery on spinal cord tolerance are not well determined, although in one study such a relationship was implicated.[8] Further studies are needed to better determine this relationship.

It appears that cauda equina has a higher tolerance to radiation compared with spinal cord. In terms of its tolerance to a single high dose of radiation (radiosurgery), three studies by Gerszten showed zero neurotoxicity after a maximum dose of 13.3 to 17.0 Gy was delivered. It should be noted that the follow-up times of these studies are still relatively short and that longer follow-up is needed to determine the long-term toxicity in relation to the radiation dose delivered.

References

1. Schultheiss TE, Kun LE, Ang KK, Stephens DV. Radiation response of the central nervous system. Int J Radiat Oncol Biol Phys 1995;31:1093–1112.
2. Emami B, Lyman J, Brown A, et al. Tolerance of normal tissue to therapeutic irradiation. Int J Radiat Oncol Biol Phys 1991;21(1):109–122.2032882
3. Marcus RB Jr, Million RR. The incidence of myelitis after irradiation of the cervical spinal cord. Int J Radiat Oncol Biol Phys 1990;19(1):3–8.
4. McCunniff AJ, Liang MJ. Radiation tolerance of the cervical spinal cord. Int J Radiat Oncol Biol Phys 1989;16(3):675–678.
5. Wong CS, Van Dyk J, Milosevic M, Laperriere NJ. Radiation myelopathy following single courses of radiotherapy and retreatment. Int J Radiat Oncol Biol Phys 1994;30(3):575–581.
6. Jeremic B, Djuric L, Mijatovic L. Incidence of radiation myelitis of the cervical spinal cord at doses of 5500 cGy or greater. Cancer 1991;68(10):2138–2141.
7. Lindstadt DE, Edwards MS, Prados M, Larson DA, Wara WM. Hyperfractionated irradiation for adults with brainstem gliomas. Int J Radiat Oncol Biol Phys 1991;20(4):757–760.

8. Marucci L, Niemierko A, Liebsch NJ, Aboubaker F, Liu MC, Munzenrider JE. Spinal cord tolerance to high-dose fractionated 3D conformal proton-photon irradiation as evaluated by equivalent uniform dose and dose volume histogram analysis. Int J Radiat Oncol Biol Phys 2004;59(2):551–555.

9. Macbeth FR, Wheldon TE, Girling DJ, et al. Radiation myelopathy: estimates of risk in 1048 patients in three randomized trials of palliative radiotherapy for non-small cell lung cancer. The Medical Research Council Lung Cancer Working Party. Clin Oncol (R Coll Radiol) 1996;8(3):176–181.

10. Choi NC, Grillo HC, Gardiello M, Scannell JG, Wilkins EW Jr. Basis for new strategies in postoperative radiotherapy of bronchogenic carcinoma. Int J Radiat Oncol Biol Phys 1980;6(1):31–35.

11. Hazra TA, Chandrasekaran MS, Colman M, Prempree T, Inalsignh M. Survival in carcinoma of the lung after a split course of radiotherapy. Br J Radiol 1974;47(560):464–466.

12. Maranzano E, Bellavita R, Rossi R, et al. Short-course versus split-course radiotherapy in metastatic spinal cord compression: results of a phase III, randomized, multicenter trial. J Clin Oncol 2005;23(15):3358–3365.

13. Kramer GW, Wanders SL, Noordijk EM, et al. Results of the Dutch national study of the palliative effect of irradiation using two different treatment schemes for non-small-cell lung cancer. J Clin Oncol 2005;23(13):2962–2970.

14. Madden FJ, English JS, Moore AK, Newton KA. Split course radiation in inoperable carcinoma of the bronchus. Eur J Cancer 1979;15(9):1175–1177.

15. Miller RC, Aristizabal SA, Leith JT, Manning MR. Radiation myelitis following split-course therapy for unresectable lung cancer. Int J Radiat Oncol Biol Phys 1977;2:179.

16. Fitzgerald RH Jr, Marks RD Jr, Wallace KM. Chronic radiation myelitis. Radiology 1982;144(3):609–612.

17. Abramson N, Cavanaugh PJ. Short-course radiation therapy in carcinoma of the lung. A second look. Radiology 1973;108(3):685–687.

18. Dische S, Martin WM, Anderson P. Radiation myelopathy in patients treated for carcinoma of bronchus using a six fraction regime of radiotherapy. Br J Radiol 1981;54(637):29–35.

19. Guthrie RT, Ptacek JJ, Hass AC. Comparative analysis of two regimens of split course radiation in carcinoma of the lung. Am J Roentgenol Radium Ther Nucl Med 1973;117(3):605–608.

20. Rades D, Stalpers LJ, Veninga T, et al. Evaluation of five radiation schedules and prognostic factors for metastatic spinal cord compression. J Clin Oncol 2005;23(15):3366–3375.

21. Rades D, Stalpers LJ, Hulshof MC, Zschenker O, Alberti W, Koning CC. Effectiveness and toxicity of single-fraction radiotherapy with 1 × 8 Gy for metastatic spinal cord compression. Radiother Oncol 2005;75(1):70–73.

22. Hartsell WF, Scott CB, Bruner DW, et al. Randomized trial of short- versus long-course radiotherapy for palliation of painful bone metastases. J Natl Cancer Inst 2005;97(11):798–804.

23. Rades D, Stalpers LJ, Veninga T, Hoskin PJ. Spinal reirradiation after short-course RT for metastatic spinal cord compression. Int J Radiat Oncol Biol Phys 2005;63(3):872–875.

24. Nieder C, Grosu AL, Andratschke NH, Molls M. Proposal of human spinal cord reirradiation dose based on collection of data from 40 patients. Int J Radiat Oncol Biol Phys 2005;61(3):851–855.

25. Pieters RS, Niemierko A, Fullerton BC, Munzenrider JE. Cauda equina tolerance to high-dose fractionated irradiation. Int J Radiat Oncol Biol Phys 2006;64(1):251–257.

26. Hamilton AJ, Lulu BA, Fosmire H, Gossett L. LINAC-based spinal stereotactic radiosurgery. Stereotact Funct Neurosurg 1996;66(1–3):1–9.

27. Ryu S, Fang Yin F, Rock J, et al. Image-guided and intensity-modulated radiosurgery for patients with spinal metastasis. Cancer 2003;97(8):2013–2018.

28. Ryu S, Rock J, Rosenblum M, Kim H. Patterns of failure after single-dose radiosurgery for spinal metastasis. J Neurosurg 2004;101(Suppl 3):402–405.

29. Rock JP, Ryu S, Shukairy MS, et al. Postoperative radiosurgery for malignant spinal tumors. Neurosurgery 2006;58(5):891–898.

30. Ryu S, Jin JJ, Jin RY, et al. Partial volume tolerance of spinal cord and complication of single dose radiosurgery. Cancer 2007;109(3):628–636.

31. De Salles AA, Pedroso AG, Medin P, et al. Spinal lesions treated with Novalis shaped beam intensity-modulated radiosurgery and stereotactic radiotherapy. J Neurosurg 2004;101(Suppl 3):435–440.

32. Benzil DL, Saboori M, Mogilner AY, Rocchio R, Moorthy CR. Safety and efficacy of stereotactic radiosurgery for tumors of the spine. J Neurosurg 2004;101(Suppl 3):413–418.

33. Gerszten PC, Ozhasoglu C, Burton SA, et al. CyberKnife frameless stereotactic radiosurgery for spinal lesions: clinical experience in 125 cases. Neurosurgery 2004;55(1):89–98.

34. Gerszten PC, Ozhasoglu C, Burton SA, et al. CyberKnife frameless single-fraction stereotactic radiosurgery for benign tumors of the spine. Neurosurg Focus 2003;14(5):e16.

35. Gerszten PC, Burton SA, Welch WC, et al. Single-fraction radiosurgery for the treatment of spinal breast metastases. Cancer 2005;104(10):2244–2254.

36. Gerszten PC, Burton SA, Ozhasoglu C, et al. Stereotactic radiosurgery for spinal metastases from renal cell carcinoma. J Neurosurg Spine 2005;3(4):288–295.

37. Gerszten PC, Burton SA, Quinn AE, Agarwala SS, Kirkwood JM. Radiosurgery for the treatment of spinal melanoma metastases. Stereotact Funct Neurosurg 2005;83(5–6):213–221.

38. Chang EL, Shiu AS, Lii MF, et al. Phase I clinical evaluation of near-simultaneous computed tomographic image-guided stereotactic body radiotherapy for spinal metastases. Int J Radiat Oncol Biol Phys 2004;59(5):1288–1294.

39. Bilsky MH, Yamada Y, Yenice KM, et al. Intensity-modulated stereotactic radiotherapy of paraspinal tumors: a preliminary report. Neurosurgery 2004;54(4):823–830.

40. Yamada Y, Lovelock DM, Yenice KM, et al. Multifractionated image-guided and stereotactic intensity-modulated radiotherapy of paraspinal tumors: a preliminary report. Int J Radiat Oncol Biol Phys 2005;62(1):53–61.

41. Dodd RL, Ryu MR, Kamnerdsupaphon P, Gibbs IC, Chang SD Jr, Adler JR Jr. CyberKnife radiosurgery for benign intradural extramedullary spinal tumors. Neurosurgery 2006;58(4):674–685.

Physics and Techniques

4

Patient Immobilization and Movement

Martin J. Murphy and Jian-Yue Jin

Patient immobilization is an important part of the spine radiosurgery procedure and directly influences the accuracy of target localization. Radiosurgical targeting accuracy has traditionally been obtained by rigidly immobilizing the patient in a stereotactic frame that defines a coordinate system for configuring the treatment beams and simultaneously positions the target site at the isocenter of the radiation delivery device. Frame-based treatment in the cranial site can achieve a targeting precision of 1 mm but has three shortcomings: (1) the frame is invasive, (2) fractionation is inhibited, and (3) treatment is restricted to sites amenable to frame fixation.

Hamilton et al were the first to use an invasive spine immobilization frame, which rigidly attached to the spinal processes of a patient in the prone position, for spine radiosurgery.[1] Target accuracy of 2 mm in the transverse plane and < 4 mm in the longitudinal direction was reported. However, due to its highly invasive nature, the technique was not widely adopted. Noninvasive stereotactic body frames had also been developed.[2–4] However, due to the lack of rigid fixation to the vertebral column, the targeting accuracy solely based on the frame was not ideal. Image-guided target localization, in combination with proper patient immobilization, has been developed to overcome these limitations.[4–8] The Novalis (BrainLab AG, Feldkirchen, Germany) and the CyberKnife (Accuray Inc., Sunnyvale, California) systems are currently two dedicated commercial radiosurgical units that have been widely used for image-guided spine radiosurgery. This chapter will discuss patient immobilization and potential motion during treatment specifically for these two units.

◆ CyberKnife

The spine is an example of a site that is difficult to immobilize in a traditional frame and that also benefits from fractionated treatment. It was thus an early candidate for frameless radiosurgery using the CyberKnife.[5,6] When the treatment site is not immobilized with a rigid frame, however, patient movement can occur and potentially affect dose alignment. Therefore, it is important to investigate movement during frameless radiosurgery.

The CyberKnife is a frameless image-guided stereotactic radiosurgery system that uses x-ray radiographic imaging in the treatment room to locate and track the treatment site while controlling the alignment of radiation beams via a robot-mounted linear accelerator.[9] This system is unique in the way it eliminates all three functions of the stereotactic frame: (1) the target reference coordinates provided by the external frame are replaced by reference coordinates in the patient's anatomy; (2) the radiation delivery system has no isocenter but instead moves the beam to the position of the tumor; and (3) a real-time control loop between the imaging and beam delivery systems allows the beam to adapt to changes in the target position, eliminating the need for rigid fixation.

The CyberKnife radiosurgery system is illustrated in **Fig. 4.1**. The system uses a robotic arm to direct the x-ray beam generated by an X-band 6 MV linear accelerator (linac). A pair of orthogonally positioned amorphous silicon diagnostic x-ray cameras is used to image the patient during treatment. The acquired radiographs are automatically registered to digitally reconstructed radiographs (DRRs) derived from the treatment planning computed tomography (CT) study to determine the patient's position. A control loop between the imaging system and the robotic arm allows the pointing of the treatment beam to be adapted automatically to the observed position of the treatment site. This allows the system to monitor and adjust to patient movement during treatment.

The CyberKnife maintains a quasi-continuous record of target position throughout each fraction, thus providing the data needed to assess patient motion during frameless spine radiosurgery. Because the CyberKnife can adapt to intrafraction movement during spine radiosurgery, it is possible to use comparatively nonrestrictive positioning restraints. It

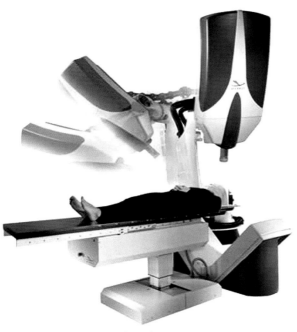

Figure 4.1 The CyberKnife Radiosurgery System. (From Accuray Inc., with permission.)

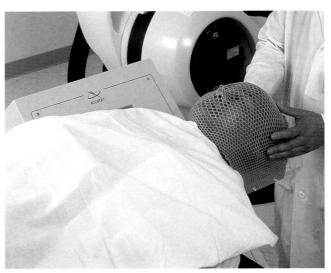

Figure 4.2 Using an Aquaplast mask to limit cervical spine movement.

is important to recognize that the nature of the patient restraint will influence the residual intrafraction motion. CyberKnife treatments to the cervical spine rely on restraint of the head in an Aquaplast mask (Aquaplast Corp., Wyckoff, New Jersey; **Fig. 4.2**), whereas treatments to the thoracic and lumber spine are done while the patient lies supine in a conformable alpha cradle. The face mask constrains motion (but does not rigidly immobilize) in all directions, whereas the alpha cradle supports and stabilizes the patient without constriction. The movement data discussed here were observed for these two restraint methods.

Treatment sites along the cervical spine were located with reference to the nearest vertebral body. The image guidance system acquired orthogonal views of the neck at oblique angles and determined the position of the vertebral landmark by highlighting bony edges and registering them to the corresponding bony structures in the treatment planning CT study. **Figure 4.3** illustrates a cervical spine DRR used for the position determination. Lesions along the thoracic and lumbar spine were also located with reference to the nearby spine, but in these cases the bony structures themselves were difficult to detect in the images, so stainless steel fiducials were implanted percutaneously in the bone for use as targeting landmarks.

Intrafraction movement can consist of moment-by-moment random fluctuations, periodic respiratory movement, and systematic slow drifting in the mean position. The random, periodic, and systematic components will have different effects on the dose distribution.

Image-guided frameless spine radiosurgery begins with orthogonal setup images to establish the initial target posi-

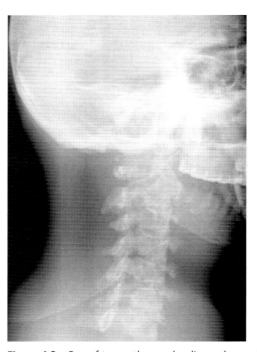

Figure 4.3 One of two orthogonal radiographs used to measure and monitor cervical spine position during a CyberKnife treatment.

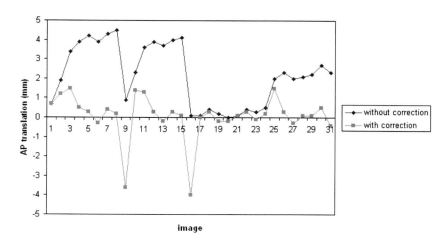

Figure 4.4 An example record of thoracic spine position in the anteroposterior direction at 1-minute intervals during delivery of a CyberKnife treatment. The blue curve measures absolute position relative to the starting setup; the red curve measures the change in position from 1 minute to the next.

tion. It then may or may not involve periodic corrections for movement during the fraction. If targeting is based solely on the initial setup position, the delivered dose distribution will be perturbed by the cumulative random and systematic shifts throughout the fraction. If intrafraction realignment is done, the systematic offset will be removed, and the dose distribution will be perturbed only by the net random fluctuations that occur between position corrections. These two scenarios have different dosimetric consequences.

For spine radiosurgery with the CyberKnife, the target position is observed episodically rather than continuously during treatment. The imaging frequency for each patient is based on a combination of past experience and an assessment of the patient's own particular movement patterns observed during setup and treatment. Typically, the imaging frequency is set at ~1 to 2 frames per minute. If at any time during treatment the patient appears to be moving more frequently than anticipated in the imaging duty cycle, the system can be reprogrammed to increase the frequency of position measurements.

Intrafraction target position and movement data have been collected and analyzed for 17 cervical and 19 thoracic/lumbar sites treated with the CyberKnife.[10,11] The movement data were analyzed in two ways: (1) as net translational offsets from the initial setup position and (2) as fluctuations in position from 1 minute to the next. The net translation from setup is the targeting error that perturbs the dose when periodic realignments are not employed during the fraction, and the periodic fluctuations represent the targeting perturbation when realignment is employed (because each new image acquisition effectively represents a new reference setup position).

Figure 4.4 is an example of the anteroposterior (AP) position record for one patient, showing the combined random and systematic movement relative to the initial setup position (in blue) and relative to the most recent previous intrafraction measurement of position (in red). This patient showed a mean systematic drift of 2.2 mm in the AP direction.

When all of the patient position records for spine treatment were analyzed, there was no evidence of respiratory movement of the spine itself at a level of 1 mm for patients treated in the supine position.[10] No data were obtained for treatments in the prone position.

Figure 4.5 shows the frequency distribution of intrafraction movements away from the initial setup position (in blue) and the net fluctuations from one position measurement to the next (in red) observed for the 36 patients in the database. Net systematic drift away from the setup position was detected in about 20% of the patients. By retargeting the beam after each intrafraction position measurement, the random radial misalignment was reduced by a factor of approximately 2.0 to a mean magnitude of 0.8 mm, and the systematic misalignment due to drift was reduced to zero.

These measurements indicate that, on average, the Aquaplast mask and the alpha cradle can limit patient movement to 1 to 3 mm without relying on severe constriction. The alpha cradle in particular exploits gravity to limit patient movement, in that the patient must make an active effort to shift position.

Although most patient records showed an approximately gaussian distribution of large and small fluctuations during treatment, a small number of patients accounted for a disproportionate number of large (> 2 mm) fluctuations. Therefore, each patient should be monitored closely (especially during the first part of the treatment fraction) to observe the frequency and magnitude of motion. If it significantly exceeds the usual experience, steps should be taken to restrain the patient, increase the frequency of positioning corrections, or, in extreme cases, stop the treatment. Conversely, if motion is minimal and appears random, the frequency of positioning checks (and thus the treatment time) can be reduced. This underscores the value of repeatedly measuring the target position rather than relying on an initial setup position.

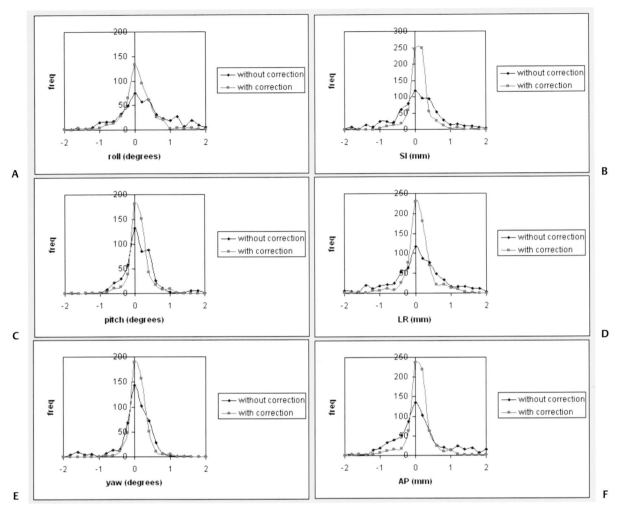

Figure 4.5 The frequency of position changes of a given magnitude observed during a CyberKnife treatment. The blue curve represents changes away from the initial setup position; the red curve represents changes from the most recently measured prior position.

◆ Novalis System

Immobilization Procedure

Patient immobilization can be achieved with different methods. Here, a method with the double-vacuum sandwiched BodyFix system (Medical Intelligence GmbH, Schwabmünchen, Germany) is described. It consists of a sealed vacuum cushion (blue bag), a clear plastic foil wrapping on a patient's lower part of the body up to the thorax, a vacuum pump, and accessory parts such as hoses connecting the wrapping foil and the vacuum cushion to the pump, as shown in **Fig. 4.6.** The blue bag is filled with radiotranslucent polystyrene microspheres, with a valve that allows the air to be pumped into or out of the bag. The following steps are performed for the patient immobilization procedure:

1. The blue bag is placed on the simulation couch, with the microspheres uniformly distributed inside the bag. The

air inside the bag is pumped out slightly until the cushion starts to flatten out but still feel soft (**Fig. 4.6A**). The patient is placed on top of the cushion in the supine position with two hands on the sides.
2. Air is then pumped back into the bag until it is inflated and the microspheres can move freely. The patient, the bag, and the microspheres are maneuvered appropriately to have the best comfortable position for the patient and to have enough microspheres build up support in the crucial areas.
3. The air is removed until a slight vacuum is developed but the microspheres can still move freely. Pumping is stopped, and the microspheres are rearranged to build adequate rims around the body, the shoulder, and the extremities. The air is then pumped out again until a firm mold of the body is formed.
4. The patient is wrapped with plastic foil. Air is pumped between the foil and the patient through a perforated hose placed across the wrapped area under the foil so

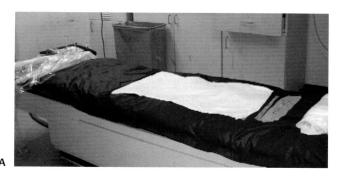

A

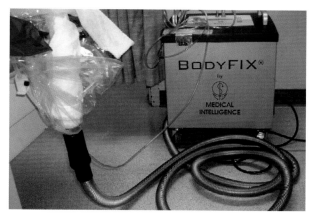

B

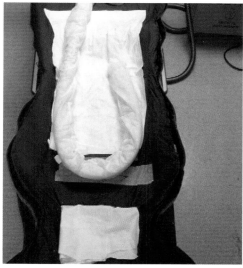

C

Figure 4.6 Immobilization procedure using the BodyFix device. **(A)** The blue bag is placed on the simulation couch top before a patient is placed on it. The air inside the bag is pumped out slightly until the cushion starts to flatten out but still feels soft. **(B)** The vacuum pump connected to the blue bag and the plastic film with hoses. **(C)** A molded blue bag with a perforated hose on it.

that a vacuum can be uniformly built up, as shown in **Fig. 4.7.** The infrared external markers are then placed on the surface for initial patient setup.

For cervical or upper thoracic (T1–T3) spinal lesions, a thermal plastic head mask is also used to immobilize the head. The patient is supine with the arms on both sides, as this is the most comfortable and durable position for patients. For some patients with severe curvature of the vertebral column, a customized alpha cradle has been used to accommodate the special body curvature.

Image-Guided Immobilization and Repositioning

The accuracy and reproducibility of the BodyFix system on repositioning patients have been studied by several groups.[12,13]

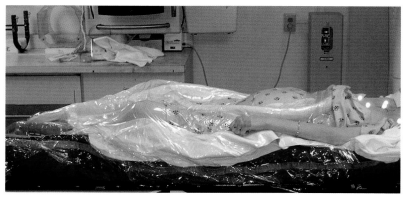

Figure 4.7 A patient is immobilized and infrared external markers are placed on the chest for thoracic spine radiosurgery using Novalis.

Nevinny-Sticke et al studied the repositioning accuracy of the BodyFix system with a simple two-dimensional/two-dimensional (2D/2D) manual image match method, which compared the orthogonal electronic portal images with their respective digital reconstructive radiographs during each fraction of treatment.[13] A total of 187 fractions in 10 patients with abdominal or pelvis lesions were analyzed. The mean three-dimensional (3D) positioning error was reported as 2.5 ± 1.1 mm, with a maximum shift of 10 mm observed. Fuss et al systematically studied the reproducibility of the BodyFix system on 36 lung or liver cancer patients who underwent fractionated stereotactic radiotherapy.[12] They first used multiple external markers and a root-mean-square (RMS) based scoring function to assess the spatial integrity of the vacuum cushion over the treatment course. The results demonstrated that the vacuum cushion deformed little over the course of treatment and under the pressure of the patient's weight. Next step was to verify positioning accuracy and reproducibility using a 3D/3D manual image match of internal bony landmarks between simulation and repositioning CTs. Fuss et al found that the mean deviation of anatomical landmark coordinates was −0.4 ± 3.9 mm, −0.1 ± 1.6 mm, and 0.3 ± 3.6 mm along the x- (lateral), y- (posteroanterior [PA]), and z-axes (longitudinal), respectively. There were 29.4% of setup CT images that had deviations > 5 mm along one or two (x- and z-) principal axes. The median and mean 3D magnitude vector of body translation in the BodyFix system was 4.0 mm and 4.8 ± 3.4 mm, respectively. In addition, mean patient body rotations about the x-, y-, and z-axes in the immobilization system were 0.9 ± 0.7, 0.8 ± 0.7, and 1.8 ± 1.6 degrees, respectively.

These results suggest that using external markers and the BodyFix system has some degree of position uncertainty. Therefore, image-guided target localization or other invasive immobilization and localization methods are required for spine radiosurgery. We have used the Novalis system for target localization in spine radiosurgery, which included two steps: (1) using external infrared markers and the BodyFix system to initially set up the patients, and (2) using the x-ray image-guided system with 2D/3D automatic image fusion to accurately localize the target. We could use the position differences between the external marker localization system and the x-ray image-guided system to evaluate the reliability of the BodyFix system. Our experience is consistent with the above results of translational deviation. We have studied body rotational differences between simulation and treatment in 52 spinal patients.[14] The average rotational deviation was 0.7 ± 1.8, 0.7 ± 1.5, and 0.7 ± 1.6 degrees along the AP, longitudinal, and lateral rotation axes. The following two factors may relate to variation. One is that the external markers on the patient surface were used in our study so that respiratory motion may affect the initial setup and hence the rotation. The other is that the lesions in our study ranged from cervical spine to the sacrum, compared with the lung and liver lesions in Fuss et al's study.

Besides the translational and rotational shifts, another parameter that is related to the reproducibility of the immobilization system is the position deformability. Just as a rotational deviation in the initial setup will affect the accuracy of 2D/2D image fusion, large position deformability can induce uncertainty for 2D/3D or 3D/3D image fusion. Therefore, in the image-guided radiotherapy, the position deformability is an especially important property for an immobilization device. This position deformability can be quantified by the RMS scoring function[12] to assess the integrity of the vacuum cushion, or by the variation of performing multiple automatic fusions for the simulation and setup images with different areas of interest for each fusion. We have compared the local position deformability using 2D/3D fusion between two patients who had lesions in different regions.[14] Patient A had an L3 lesion. Patient B had a T2 lesion. Both of them were immobilized with the BodyFix system as mentioned earlier. A head mask was also used for patient B. A pair of setup images was fused with the simulation CT image for 10 times using the BrainLab 2D/3D autofusion software. Each time a different area of interest in the images was selected for the fusion. **Table 4.1** shows the standard deviation of the fusion results for both patients in each translational and rotational direction. Patient B had remarkably larger variations than patient A, especially for translational shift in the z- (AP) axis. The 95% of confidence interval of the variation for patient B in the z-axis, which is about twice the standard deviation, was ± 1.6 mm. This suggests that the local position deformability for patient B, who had the spinal lesion close to the neck area, was significantly larger than that for patient A, who had a spinal lesion in the abdominal area.

It is our general experience that the local position deformability is larger in the neck area than in the low thoracic and abdominal area. Garg et al had reported significant cervical spine curvature changes for head and neck patients.[15] Indeed, the cervical spine curvature is highly dependent on the position of the head and shoulder. Careful attention should be paid to conformably mold the vacuum cushion for the posterior contour of the neck and shoulder and build sufficient rims around this area. A head and shoulder mask has been used to immobilize the area, but a randomized trial comparing the head mask with the head and shoulder mask showed no significant difference in terms of position reproducibility.[16] The position deformability was not compared between the two masks in this study. Therefore, further study may be

Table 4.1 Translational and Rotational Accuracy of 6-D Fusion at the Targets of L3 and T2 by Novalis Radiosurgery

Patient	Target Location	Translational Variation, SD (mm)			Rotational Variation, SD (degree)		
		x	y	z	α	β	γ
Patient A	L3	0.13	0.28	0.09	0.26	0.21	0.21
Patient B	T2	0.42	0.28	0.80	0.59	0.73	0.52

needed to determine if any of these positioning devices can improve the position deformability.

Patient Motion during Treatment

Patient motion can be divided into respiratory and nonrespiratory motion. Using fluoroscopy, Yin et al observed that respiratory motion had little effect on the vertebral column.[17] On the other hand, nonrespiratory motion, which is usually caused by uncontrolled physiologic behaviors, such as coughing, swallowing, or movement of air, or due to a patient's adjusting to a more comfortable position because he or she cannot tolerate staying in the same position for so long, could potentially move the spinal position. The spine radiosurgery treatment procedure, including the image-guided target localization and portal images verification, usually lasts 30 to 60 minutes. During this entire treatment procedure, the patient has to be kept in the same position to ensure accurate delivery of the radiation to the planned target.

We have recently studied patient position variations during the course of treatment for 25 consecutive patients undergoing spine radiosurgery.[18] After the patient position was finally set up with the image-guided localization system and verified with portal images, verification x-ray images were acquired at the beginning, in the middle, and at the end of dose delivery. The 2D/3D fusion software in the image-guided system was used to determine the position shifts. **Figure 4.8** shows the position variations for all 25 patients in three orthogonal directions. The overall variations were 0.10 ± 0.87,

0.21 ± 1.16, and 0.17 ± 1.02 mm in the AP, longitudinal, and lateral directions, respectively. This suggests that position variations during treatment were relatively small and that most of the patients tolerated the prolonged treatment without significant movement. However, there were two patients who had relatively large (~4 mm) lateral or longitudinal variation. By checking the position deformability of these two patients, we concluded that the large variations were mainly due to patient motion secondary to pain or uncomfortable body posture. Therefore, the therapists, the physicians, and the physicists should be vigilant about the potential patient motion. A suitable dose of pain medication can be given to the patient before treatment to reduce potential motions.

Taking verification kV x-ray images can also be used to routinely check the position change during the treatment. However, doing so cannot monitor the position continuously. In addition, taking verification images and performing the consequent 2D/3D fusion require extra time, which would be the trade-off for inducing more motions. The BrainLab ExacTrac system is able to monitor the patient surface motion during treatment through the infrared markers placed on the patient surface. However, the motion represented by the infrared markers is often the combination of respiratory motion and nonrespiratory motion. The amplitude of respiratory motion at the chest and abdominal surface can be up to 2 to 3 cm. Therefore, the nonrespiratory motion is often hidden under the respiratory motion and is thus difficult to detect. We are developing a nonrespiratory motion monitor technique that can separate the nonrespiratory motion

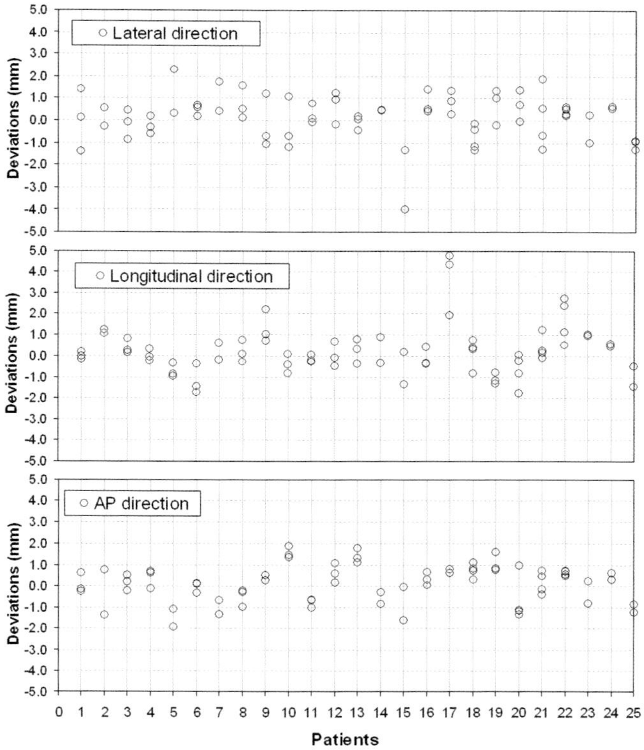

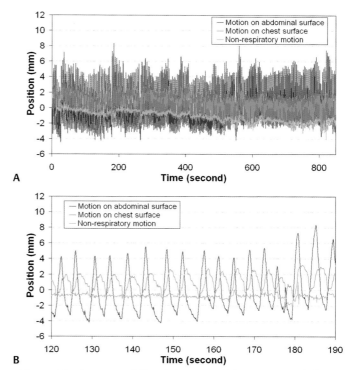

Figure 4.8 Position variations in the beginning, middle, and end of treatment for 25 patients in three orthogonal directions.

Figure 4.9 Long-term **(A)** and short-term **(B)** motion signals from chest and abdominal surfaces.

from the respiratory motion.[19] Two sets of motion signals at different areas with a large difference of respiratory amplitudes were used to derive the respiratory and nonrespiratory signals. As shown in **Fig. 4.9,** the respiratory ripples in the chest motion signal can be effectively removed, left with the nonrespiratory signal and irregular respiratory components. Such a system, if combined with the x-ray image-guided localization, can potentially be used to effectively monitor patient motion during spine radiosurgery.

References

1. Hamilton AJ, Lulu BA, Fosmire H, et al. Preliminary clinical experience with linear accelerator-based spinal stereotactic radiosurgery. Neurosurgery 1995;36(2):311–319.

2. Lohr F, Debus FJ, Frank C, et al. Noninvasive patient fixation for extracranial stereotactic radiotherapy. Int J Radiat Oncol Biol Phys 1999;45(2):521–527.

3. Wulf J, Hadinger U, Oppitz U, Olshausen B, Flentje M. Stereotactic radiotherapy of extracranial targets: CT-simulation and accuracy of treatment in the stereotactic body frame. Radiother Oncol 2000;57(2):225–236.

4. Yenice KM, Lovelock DM, Hunt MA, et al. CT image-guided intensity-modulated therapy for paraspinal tumors using stereotactic immobilization. Int J Radiat Oncol Biol Phys 2003;55(3):583–593.

5. Murphy MJ, Chang S, Gibbs I, Le Q-T, Martin D, Kim D. Image-guided radiosurgery in the treatment of spinal metastases. Neurosurg Focus 2001;11(6):e6.

6. Ryu SI, Kim D, Murphy MJ, et al. Image-guided frameless robotic stereotactic radiosurgery to spinal lesions. Neurosurgery 2001;49:838–847.

7. Ryu S, Yin FF, Rock J, et al. Image-guided and intensity-modulated radiosurgery for patients with spinal metastasis. Cancer 2003;97(8):2013–2018.

8. Shiu AS, Chang EL, Ye J-S, et al. Near simultaneous computed tomography image-guided stereotactic spinal radiotherapy: an emerging paradigm for achieving true stereotaxy. Int J Radiat Oncol Biol Phys 2003;57(3):605–613.

9. Adler JR, Murphy MJ, Chang SD, Hancock SL. Image-guided robotic radiosurgery. Neurosurgery 1999;44:1299–1307.

10. Murphy MJ, Chang SD, Gibbs IC, et al. Patterns of patient movement during frameless image-guided radiosurgery. Int J Radiat Oncol Biol Phys 2003;55(5):1400–1408.

11. Gerszten PC, Ozhasoglu C, Burton SA, et al. CyberKnife stereotactic radiosurgery for spinal lesions: clinical experience in 125 patients. Neurosurgery 2004;55(1):89–98.

12. Fuss M, Salter BJ, Rassiah P, Cheek D, Cavanaugh SX, Herman TS. Repositioning accuracy of a commercially available double-vacuum whole body immobilization system for stereotactic body radiation therapy. Technol Cancer Res Treat 2004;3(1):59–67.14750894

13. Nevinny-Stickel M, Sweeney RA, Balek J, Posch A, Auberger T, Lukas P. Reproducibility of patient positioning for fractionated extracranial stereotactic radiotherapy using a double-vacuum technique. Strahlenther Onkol 2004;180(2):117–122.

14. Jin J, Ryu S, Rock J, et al. Image-guided target localization for stereotactic radiosurgery: accuracy of 6D versus 3D image fusion. In Kondziolka D (ed). Radiosurgery, vol. 6. Basel, Karger, 2006;6:50–59.

15. Garg MK, Yaparpalvi R, Beitler JJ. Loss of cervical spinal curvature during radiotherapy for head-and-neck cancers: the neck moves, too. Int J Radiat Oncol Biol Phys 2004;58(1):185–188.

16. Sharp L, Lewin F, Johannson H, Payne D, Gerhardsson A, Rutqvist LE. Randomized trial on two types of thermoplastic masks for patient immobilization during radiation therapy for head-and-neck cancer. Int J Radiat Oncol Biol Phys 2005;61(1):250–256.

17. Yin FF, Ryu S, Ajlouni M, et al. Image-guided procedures for intensity-modulated spinal radiosurgery [technical note]. J Neurosurg 2004;101(Suppl 3):419–424.

18. Jin J, Ajlouni M, Ryu S, et al. Evaluation of residual patient position variation for spinal radiosurgery using the Novalis image guided system. Med Phys 2008;35(3):1087–1093.

19. Jin JY, Ajlouni M, Ryu S, et al. A technique of quantitatively monitoring both respiratory and non-respiratory motion in patients using external body markers. Med Phys 2007;34(7):2875–2881.

5

Imaging and Target Localization

Fang-Fang Yin, Zhiheng Wang, John P. Kirkpatrick, and Q. Jackie Wu

Imaging is a critical component for spine radiosurgery. It has a substantial impact on each step of the radiosurgical process. This chapter will describe the clinical roles of imaging in diagnosis, simulation, planning, localization, delivery, and assessment of spine radiosurgery.

◆ Imaging for Diagnosis

Vertebral body metastases occur in up to 40% of patients suffering from malignant cancer, and as many as one quarter of these will develop epidural spinal cord compression.[1] Although the most common tumors metastasizing to the spine are lung, breast, prostate, and renal cell carcinomas, almost any tumor can present with spinal metastases.[2,3] The thoracic spine is the most common site of epidural metastases, with 60 to 80% of disease occurring in this area. However, up to half of patients have disease in two or more regions. In the overwhelming majority of patients with vertebral body metastases and/or spinal cord compression, back pain is the first symptom.[2-4] At diagnosis, other common symptoms of spinal cord compression (in decreasing frequency) are weakness, autonomic dysfunction, and sensory deficits.[4] These symptoms are almost always accompanied by back pain.[1-4]

In general, magnetic resonance imaging (MRI) is the imaging modality of choice for diagnosing metastatic disease to the spine[1,5-8] because it provides superior definition of the extent of disease radially and axially, can help distinguish malignant from benign disease,[9,10] and is noninvasive. MRI has a specificity of 97 to 98%,[6,10] a sensitivity of 93%,[10] and a positive predictive value of 98%.[6] In a prospective study of 280 patients with suspected malignant spinal cord compression, Husband et al[6] found that 211 (75%) had epidural spinal cord or thecal sac compression. Of the patients with spinal cord compression, 25% had compression at two or more levels, and 69% of these involved more than one region of the spine. A paraspinal mass was found in 28% of patients, and only a third of these masses were detected on plain films. When radiotherapy fields were planned solely on the basis of plain films and neurological findings in 91 patients, the use of the subsequent MR images resulted in changes in 48 (53%) of these plans. A clinically significant change—primarily lengthening and/or widening of the field to include disease untreated on the initial "non-MRI" plan—was observed in 19 cases (21%).

Although a staging bone scan may provide an initial indication of the sites of spinal metastases, it is far less sensitive than MRI in detecting small or intermedullary lesions.[11] Computed tomography (CT) scans with bone and soft tissue windowing may suggest the presence of paraspinal, spinal, and epidural disease, but they are inferior to MRI in diagnosing the precise location of metastases. However, a CT scan remains essential to treatment planning and, in many cases, quality control. Although ^{18}F-FDG (^{18}F-2-deoxy-2-fluoro-D-glucose) positron emission tomography (PET)/CT may offer significantly better specificity than CT scanning alone in the diagnosis of malignant disease in the spine,[12] it lacks the spatial resolution of MRI and is not (yet) an established tool for treatment planning. PET also lacks sensitivity in detecting blastic lesions arising from prostate and breast cancer.[13,14]

Whereas diagnosis is often, unfortunately, delayed, prompt treatment of malignant spinal cord compression is essential to optimizing outcome.[15-21] In a prospective trial of patients with malignant spinal cord compression, Turner et al[20] found that palliative radiation therapy, delivered via a posteroanterior (PA) field to the involved spine of ambulatory patients, allowed over 80% to remain ambulatory postradiation therapy. However, only 2 of 16 nonambulatory patients became ambulatory postradiation therapy. Pain was significantly reduced in 22 of 30 patients (73%). In a similar prospective trial, Maranzano and Latini[17] found that "early diagnosis and treatment" (i.e., detection and radiation therapy of spinal cord compression prior to the onset of major neurologic deficits) was a significantly favorable predictor for the retention/recovery of the ability to walk. Complete or partial pain relief was observed in 54 (17%) of the patients undergoing radiation therapy. In a prospective trial of 139 male veterans with epidural compression who were treated with dexamethasone and radiotherapy, Zaidat and Ruff[21] found that starting radiation within 12 hours of the loss of ambulation was 6.86 times more likely to restore ambulation than if treatment began after 12 hours (p < .001). Somewhat paradoxically, Rades et al[19] noted that the functional outcome following radiotherapy for malignant spinal cord compression is significantly better in patients with a slow onset of motor deficits.

◆ Imaging for Planning

CT Imaging

CT, MR, and often PET imaging are used for treatment planning. CT is typically used as the gold standard for geometric target localization, along with soft tissue information provided by MRI. PET images are also used to provide supplemental functional information of the detected tumors. Subsequent to immobilization, simulation images are acquired to localize the target and critical organs/structures for radiation treatment planning.

Three-dimensional (3D) CT imaging is the preferred modality for radiation treatment simulation, as it provides accurate patient geometric information and electron density information for heterogeneity correction during the monitor unit calculation. The drawback of using CT for simulation is its relatively poor soft tissue contrast compared with MRI. Iodine-based contrast agents are typically used to improve the image contrast. After a treatment plan is generated, a set of digitally reconstructed radiographs (DRRs) are typically calculated in two orthogonal directions. The DRRs are used as references to check the treatment isocenter against the treatment portal images. The ideal slice thickness should be no more than 3 mm because a thicker slice tends to degrade the quality of the DRR images and decreases the localization accuracy.

MR Imaging

MR images can usually provide good soft tissue contrast, and thus are useful for delineating the tumor target. T1-weighted MR images are commonly used for spine radiosurgery.[22-25] Because MR images lack information about electron density and may suffer geometric distortion, they are usually regis-

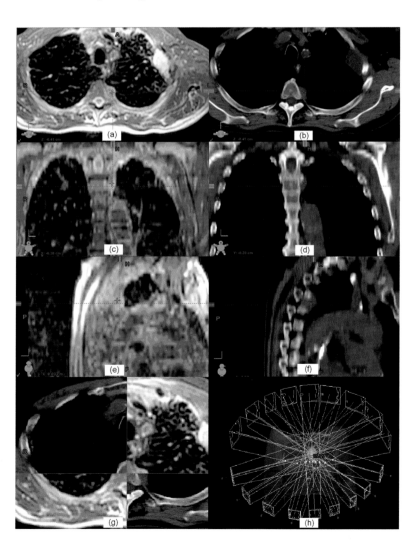

Figure 5.1 T1-weighted magnetic resonance imaging (MRI) **(a,c,e)** and the corresponding computed tomography (CT) images **(b,d,f)**. The fusion result can be checked with the MRI-CT hybrid images **(g)**. Beam orientation of an intensity-modulated radiation therapy plan for spine radiosurgery with three-dimensional rendering is shown in **h**.

tered to the simulation CT images for treatment planning. The soft tissue information in the MRI is fused to the CT to confirm target delineation. However, dose calculations are still performed based on the simulation CT images. **Figure 5.1** shows T1-weighted MR images on the left and the corresponding CT images on the right. Both MR and CT images are shown in three orthogonal orientations—axial, coronal, and sagittal views. After the MR and CT images are registered, the fusion result can be checked with the MR-CT hybrid images (**Fig. 5.1g**). Because tumors being treated with radiosurgery are usually small, high spatial resolution is required for MR images. The resolution is usually limited by slice thickness. A slice thickness of 1 mm should be used for small tumors.

Molecular Imaging

Sometimes, molecular imaging using PET images is used to help confirm the malignancy of an identified lesion. Regis-

tration of PET images with either CT or MR images is rather challenging due to different imaging information presented in these images. The use of PET/CT modality would enhance this correlation between CT and PET images because both types of images are acquired when the imaging object is at the same position. As described in the previous section, the sensitivity and specificity are not always 100%, and biopsy remains the only definitive diagnostic tool.

Planning Techniques

After 3D images are acquired and imported into a treatment planning system and the image registration is completed (if multimodality images are used), the target and critical organ volumes are then delineated based on CT, MRI, and/or other imaging modalities, such as PET. Either 3D conformal (both static and arc) or intensity-modulated radiation therapy (IMRT) beams can be used to deliver a highly conformal

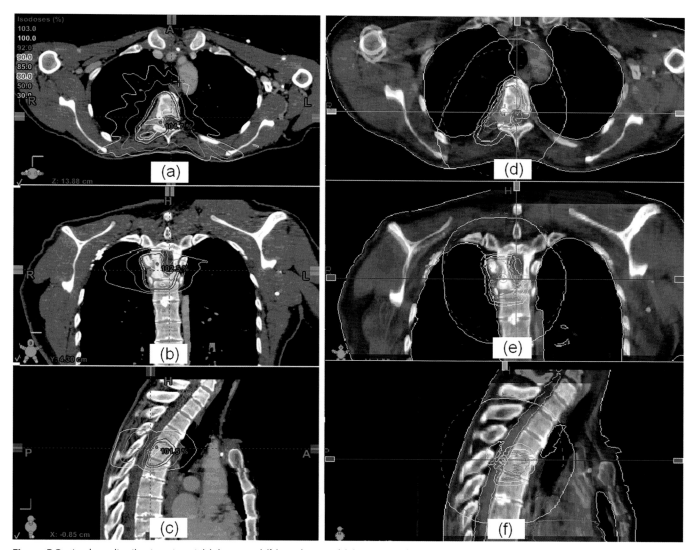

Figure 5.2 Isodose distributions in axial **(a)**, coronal **(b)**, and sagittal **(c)** views, and cone-beam computed tomography–guided target verification **(d–f)** for a spine radiosurgery case.

dose to the target.[26-33] For stationary conformal plans, a large number of beams should be used to conform the radiation to the target and achieve a rapid dose fall-off. Each beam can be conformed using a multileaf collimator (MLC) or other beam-shaping materials. For conformal arc beams, the radiation dose is delivered while the gantry rotates around the isocenter. When MLC is used on arc treatment, it can dynamically reshape the field to conform the beam to the target at each gantry angle. This technique is effective in conforming the geometry to the target, but it is not optimal for critical organ sparing. Compared with other techniques, IMRT can be used to deliver the radiation dose more precisely to the target while sparing critical organs. IMRT beams are modulated according to fluence maps, which are usually obtained through an inverse-planning process. During treatment delivery, the modulated beams are delivered according to an intensity map by moving the MLC either in a sliding-window mode or in a step-and-shoot mode. **Figure 5.1h** shows an example of an IMRT plan for spine radiosurgery using an Eclipse (Varian Medical Systems Inc., Palo Alto, California) treatment planning system with 120-leaf MLC. Nine IMRT beams are used to deliver the dose to the target volume. The dose to the spinal cord is minimized with IMRT. The corresponding isodose distributions are shown in **Fig. 5.2**.

◆ Imaging for Localization

Target localization is a critical process in radiosurgery for spinal tumors. It is essential to precisely deliver the planned radiation dose to the target. Any deviation in localization accuracy could lead to an unexpected deviation from the treatment intent. Radiographic imaging has proven to be one of the most effective methods for localization of spinal tumors. Recent developments in onboard imaging technology have substantially improved this verification technique. Conventional film imaging has been largely replaced by more efficient two-dimensional (2D) digital imaging, as well as more accurate 3D cone-beam computed tomography (CBCT).

2D Radiography

There are two approaches to acquire 2D radiographic images for target localization: megavoltage (MV) imaging using treatment beams and kilovoltage (kV) imaging using localization beams. Both are typically used for isocenter localization. Electronic portal imagers are commercially available that use MV beam in real time for target localization. This verification method has become the norm in many radiation therapy centers. However, some concerns with this technology remain to be addressed, including poor soft tissue contrast, high radiation dose from using MV beams, and the fact that MV portal images are not exactly congruent to simulation images because of the different physical principles of image formation. The desire to use a kV x-ray beam for patient positioning and target localization is becoming stronger as daily imaging is increasingly used for patient setup correction and target localization. Although several approaches

were developed decades ago, clinical implementation of kV imaging has become commercially available only within the last 5 years.

Whereas MV portal imaging uses the treatment beam, kV imaging requires an additional x-ray source for imaging. Various system configurations have been developed for in-room kV imaging for treatment target localization.[31] Some kV imaging systems are mounted on the treatment machines so that both x-ray tubes and detectors are movable relative to the patient. Others are mounted either on the ceiling or under the floor so that they are fixed relative to the patient. In terms of detector/source combinations, some systems consist of two x-ray tubes and two detectors, and others consist of a single x-ray tube and detector. At present, amorphous silicon (a-Si) flat-panel detectors are widely used for this purpose. The detectors used for MV photons have a metal build-up sheet, whereas kV detectors often use an antiscatter grid to improve image quality.

The term room-mounted systems pertains to those systems with the kV source-detector assemblies mounted onto the walls, ceiling, or floor of the treatment room. These systems are designed for stereoscopic projection and/or fluoroscopic imaging. Target localization will be based on bony landmarks or implanted radio-opaque markers as surrogates. Currently, two commercial vendors offer products where the room-mounted imaging subsystems are integrated with the treatment machines.[33,34] They are the CyberKnife system from Accuray Inc. (Sunnyvale, California) and the Novalis system from BrainLab AG (Feldkirchen, Germany). Both systems are primarily designed for stereotactic radiosurgery and stereotactic body radiotherapy. The CyberKnife system mounts two x-ray tubes on the ceiling and two standing detectors on the floor; the Novalis system mounts two x-ray tubes under the floor and two detectors on the ceiling. The a-Si flat-panel detectors with an active detector size of ~20 × 20 cm are used.

Gantry-mounted kV imaging is the key feature of the new line of medical accelerators that are specifically marketed for image-guided radiation therapy. The two available commercial products, Elekta Synergy from Elekta AB (Stockholm, Sweden) and the On-Board Imager from Varian Medical Systems Inc. (Palo Alto, California), are similar in configurations and operations.[35-37] Synergy-S (Elekta AB, Stockholm, Sweden) and Trilogy (Varian Medical Systems, Palo Alto, California) are the commercial designations of treatment machines that combine image guidance and radiosurgery capabilities. An x-ray tube and a-Si flat panel detector are mounted to the gantry orthogonally to the electronic portal imager. The Synergy x-ray system is mechanically attached to the gantry, whereas the x-ray imaging system in Trilogy is controlled by three robotic arms (one for the tube, one for the kV detector, and one for the MV detector). The active detector sizes are 40 × 40 cm (Synergy) and 40 × 30 cm (Trilogy). Their detector-element matrix sizes are 1024 × 1024 (Synergy) and 2048 × 1536 (Trilogy). The frame rate ranges from 7 to 15 frames per second.

With either a room-mounted or gantry-mounted system, 2D orthogonal kV images can be acquired for treatment localization. **Figure 5.3** shows a pair of orthogonal kV localization images acquired for a patient who underwent spine radiosurgery.

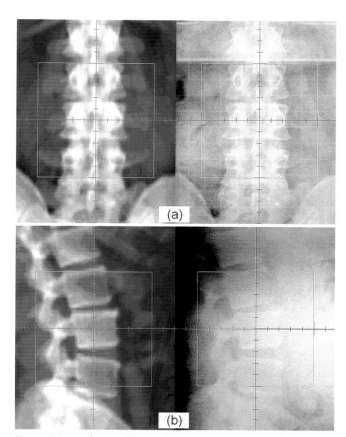

Figure 5.3 Orthogonal kV localization images acquired for a patient who underwent spine radiosurgery. **(a)** Anteroposterior view, with the digitally reconstructed radiograph (DRR) on the right and the kV radiograph on the left. **(b)** The DRR and kV radiographs for the right lateral view.

3D Computed Tomography

The visualization of anatomy in 2D radiographic images inherently suffers when multilayered anatomy is projected onto a single-image plane. Three-dimensional imaging techniques can be used to reconstruct individual slices, which substantially improve anatomical visibility and allows patient setup on the basis of daily soft tissue localization. CBCT is an extension of traditional fan-beam CT that encompasses the superoinferior imaging dimension. Whereas traditional fan-beam CT systems contain only a limited number of detector rows, CBCT is implemented with a rectangular flat-panel detector that usually contains several hundred to a few thousand rows. The x-ray source is also opened in the third dimension to irradiate the rectangular detector, and the beam is thus in the shape of a cone rather than a fan. As such, CBCT acquires a full 3D volumetric image during a single rotation of the source-detector tandem. On the other hand, fan-beam CT (i.e., helical CT) requires translation of the patient during scanning. Commercial CBCT systems generally allow for the reconstruction of a large volume (e.g., 25 × 25 × 17 cm) with submillimeter voxels, enabling all three dimensions to be viewed in high resolution. The resultant

CBCT localization volumes can be registered directly with planning-CT image data for highly accurate patient positioning.[31,38-40]

The conventional imaging method for radiation therapy treatment localization and verification is MV electronic portal imaging. As a step further, the projections of electronic portal images may also be reconstructed as MV CBCT.[37,41,42] When MV CBCT was first developed, the radiation dose required to acquire the whole set of projections could be hundreds of centigrays (cGy). With a state-of-the-art detector, the dose for MV CBCT can be reduced to 2 to 3 cGy.[41] Another MV CT technique that has been recently developed is tomotherapy.[24,43,44] The imaging process of MV CT is similar to the diagnostic kV CT, but with the x-ray source replaced by a rotating MV linear accelerator beam. Using tomotherapy, the radiation dose of MV CT is reduced to 1 to 2 cGy. Although the image contrast of MV CT or MV CBCT is relatively poorer than that of kV CT or kV CBCT, MV x-ray imaging has some advantages over kV x-ray imaging.[37,45] First, the treatment unit itself can generate MV x-rays for imaging. This not only simplifies the system, but it also enables the use of portal imaging for treatment verification during actual treatment delivery. Second, MV CT images are less noisy than kV CBCT for thick patients due to less radiation attenuation with the MV beam. Third, imaging artifacts associated with metal implants and other high-density materials are significantly reduced with MV CT images.

CBCT slices substantially improve anatomical visibility relative to 2D radiographic images, but CBCT image quality is somewhat inferior compared with traditional CT due largely to the increased scatter. When imaging a volume with traditional fan-beam CT geometry, each slice is irradiated independently, and any scatter traveling away from the slice of interest goes undetected. In a CBCT scan, the entire subject volume is irradiated simultaneously, and scatter creates cross-talk between each slice. Increased scatter during a CBCT acquisition has the doubly negative effect of increasing quantum noise while decreasing image contrast in the projection data. Thus, the contrast-to-noise ratio (CNR) in CBCT images is lower than the CNR in traditional CT images. Furthermore, scattered radiation creates large-scale "cupping" artifacts in axial CBCT slices, which artificially reduce the Hounsfield unit (HU) values of reconstructed voxels near the isocenter.

In addition, standard circular-orbit CBCT scans are prone to Defrise artifacts (or cone-beam artifacts), which result from incomplete sampling of the 3D problem due to the diverging source beam. These artifacts become more severe for larger cone angles. Motion artifacts can be more difficult to manage in gantry-based CBCT scans as well, due to the relatively long duration of a CBCT acquisition (> 1 min).

CBCT also shares common CT artifacts, such as ring artifacts caused by variability in the gain of different detector elements, cupping artifacts caused by beam hardening, and streak artifacts emanating from regions of high density caused by either beam hardening or photon starvation. If not properly accounted for, mechanical instability and geometric uncertainty can result in additional image artifacts, including a loss of resolution in CBCT reconstructions.

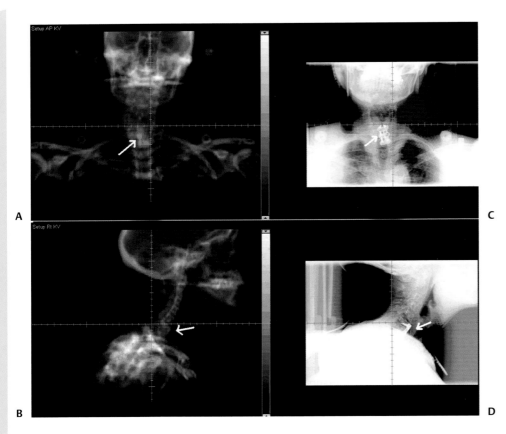

Figure 5.4 Marker localization with two-dimensional orthogonal onboard kV images. **(A)** Anteroposterior digitally reconstructed radiograph (DRR), **(B)** anteroposterior kV radiograph, **(C)** radiation therapy DRR, and **(D)** radiation therapy kV radiograph. Arrows indicate marker locations.

With 3D CBCT, it is possible to perform target localization using 3D soft tissue anatomy. The image-guided treatment procedure may be summarized as the following: (1) download 3D planning CT, along with contours to treatment station; (2) acquire CBCT images; (3) compare CBCT with planning CT using either bony or soft tissue information; (4) correct patient positioning if necessary; (5) acquire documentation images using either 2D or 3D images if correction is done; (6) initiate treatment; and (7) acquire post-treatment documentation images (optional). An example of CBCT-guided target verification for a spine radiosurgery case is illustrated in **Fig. 5.2D–F,** where the planning CT and CBCT are blended in three orthogonal views. The contours as drawn on the simulation CT images are also shown in the figure.

Implanted Markers

Implanted radio-opaque markers can be used as surrogators for target localization. These markers could be either metal seeds implanted just for radiation therapy localization or existing metal structures such as surgical screws or clips.[25,28,46,47] Both 2D orthogonal images and 3D CBCT images can be used for marker localization. **Figure 5.4** shows the marker localization with 2D orthogonal onboard kV images. The marker locations, indicated with a white arrow in each image, match well between DRR and orthogonal radiographs. A localization accuracy of ~1 to 2 mm can be achieved with orthogonal 2D kV radiographs. **Figure 5.5** shows the marker localization on 3D CBCT images in axial, coronal, and sagit-

tal views. The images are superimposed between CBCT and simulation CT. The marker location is indicated with a white arrow in each image. The marker location on the CBCT images matches well with the one on the simulation CT images. The contours, as transferred from the simulation CT images to the treatment console for 3D matching, are the target and spinal cord volumes. The contours are aligned well with the corresponding structures on the CBCT images, as shown in **Fig. 5.5.** A localization accuracy of < 1 mm can be achieved with onboard 3D CBCT images.

◆ Imaging for Assessment

The key elements in the appropriate follow-up of patients treated for spinal lesions are a thorough history and physical examination. The history should cover dose, pain medication type and usage, location and intensity of pain, steroid usage, bowel/bladder function, ambulatory status, ability to carry out activities of daily living, and activity level (yielding an assessment of performance status). The physical exam should entail a digital rectal exam and a thorough neurologic evaluation, including deep tendon reflexes, sensation to light touch, and a motor strength and gait assessment. Radiographic imaging is often used for treatment assessments. Spinal MRI may be useful to gauge the radiographic response to therapy, but it should be reserved for diagnosing recurrent disease associated with a distinct change in neurologic status. Plain films may also be useful for rapid evaluation of

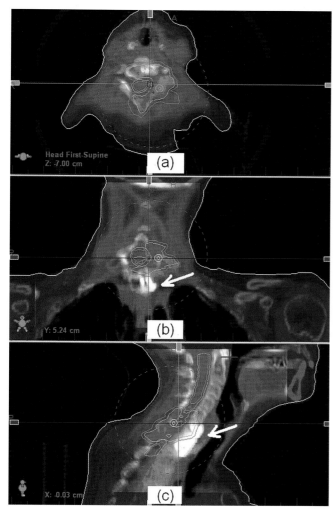

Figure 5.5 Marker localization on three-dimensional cone-beam axial **(a)**, coronal **(b)**, and sagittal **(c)** computed tomography images.

suspected vertebral body collapse. Tumor response to therapeutic radiation is often difficult to assess with anatomical imaging alone, and PET/CT images can provide valuable information to monitor the response to the treatment. **Figure 5.6** shows the PET/CT images of a patient acquired 3 months before the treatment, at the time of the treatment, and 2 months after the treatment.

◆ Image Analysis

Image Fusion

Image registration/fusion is the process of aligning images so that corresponding features can be easily correlated. There are two typical approaches to image fusion: manual and automatic. The manual image fusion method adjusts

the image transformation (translation and rotation), assuming a rigid body transformation between the image sets. Multiple fiducial markers and internal anatomical structures are often used to visually inspect the matching results. In routine clinical practice, radiation oncologists will typically perform manual image registration to do the following: (1) define tumor volumes for treatment planning (registration with standard anatomy), (2) assess the progression of disease or the effects of radiation therapy (registration with follow-up studies), (3) correlate structure with function (registration of multimodality images), and (4) access treatment positional variations (registration for correction of treatment setup variations). They perform this spatial alignment manually and subjectively, on the basis of their professional knowledge and experience. The images used cross a wide range of modalities, including CT, MRI, magnetic resonance spectroscopy (MRS), PET, CBCT, and radiographs.

During the past decade, considerable progress has been made in the development of algorithms for automatic image registration. Automatic image fusion uses a computer-matching process based on various mathematical analysis tools. These automatic methods can be roughly classified into four categories: (1) landmark-point–based registration, (2) edge-based registration, (3) moment-based registration, and (4) voxel-similarity measurement–based registration.[48-50]

The use of corresponding internal anatomical-point landmarks and "fiducial markers" in the two image sets is the most intuitive registration procedure. For a rigid structure, identification and localization of three landmarks are sufficient to establish the transformation between 3D image volumes, provided these points are not all in a straight line. In practice, however, it is common to use more than three landmarks.[48] Methods in the fourth category compare the intensity similarity voxel by voxel, using minimum intensity difference, cross-correlation, or intensity histograms. The voxel-intensity histogram–based methods are most popular and robust. They include joint entropy, correlation ratio, or mutual information because they are generally applicable to both intra- and intermodality registrations.

According to the types of transformation, image registration methods are also divided into rigid and nonrigid body methods.[51,52] Rigid body registration is widely used where the structures of interest are either bone or enclosed in bone. For the head region and vertebral bodies, rigid body registration has shown excellent accuracy. Rigid body registration has also been used for other regions of the body that are in the vicinity of bone (e.g., neck, pelvis, or leg), but the errors are likely to be larger. Often deformable registration for spine radiosurgery may not be required.

Image Management

Because a large number of images is used for imaging-guided treatment, data management becomes a critical issue. For planning images, the CT images are typically 0.514 MB/image, MRI 0.188 MB/image, and PET 0.034 MB/image. For localization images, the kV images are typically 1.54 MB/

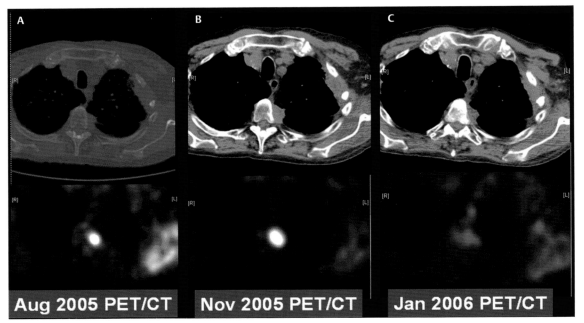

Figure 5.6 Positron emission tomography/computed tomography images that were acquired 3 months before treatment **(A)**, at the time of treatment **(B)**, and 2 months after treatment **(C)**.

image, MV portal images 0.386 MB/image, DRR images 0.514 MB/image, and CBCT images 0.514 MB/image. For a typical imaging-guided stereotactic body radiotherapy (SBRT) case, the image data are in the range of 600 MB to 1 gigabyte (GB). Sufficient disk space should be allocated. To effectively and accurately use all imaging data during spine radiosurgery, an image management system that integrates multimodality image datasets is highly desirable. This same system should be used for image and data storage, retrieval, manipulation, and display. It would improve not only the treatment efficiency but also the treatment accuracy by minimizing any mistakes in handling images.

Image Quality

Radiation therapy departments typically have very strict quality assurance (QA) protocols for treatment machine calibration and dose measurements. However, the expanded use of imaging modalities in radiation treatment also requires a thorough QA program to ensure image quality, imaging accuracy, and imaging dose. A QA program should be established that reflects the importance of the contribution of each component of the system to the accuracy of the patient's treatment. Some components should be checked daily, such as the alignment of the lasers and the HU accuracy in water. Others may be checked monthly, annually, or after significant upgrades to the system. Special phantoms have also been designed to assist with various aspects of QA. It is highly recommended that procedures for imaging-device calibration and routine QA protocols be developed prior to any clinical application.

References

1. Bryne T. Epidural disease. In: Black PM, Loeffler JS, eds. Cancer of the Nervous System. Philadelphia: Lippincott Williams & Wilkins; 2004.
2. Prasad D, Schiff D. Malignant spinal-cord compression. Lancet Oncol 2005;6(1):15–24.
3. Ratliff JK, Cooper PR. Metastatic spine tumors. South Med J 2004;97(3):246–253.
4. Gilbert RW, Kim JH, Posner JB. Epidural spinal cord compression from metastatic tumor: diagnosis and treatment. Ann Neurol 1978;3(1):40–51.
5. Cook AM, Lau TN, Tomlinson MJ, et al. Magnetic resonance imaging of the whole spine in suspected malignant spinal cord compression: impact on management. Clin Oncol (R Coll Radiol) 1998;10(1):39–43.
6. Husband DJ, Grant KA, Romaniuk CS. MRI in the diagnosis and treatment of suspected malignant spinal cord compression. Br J Radiol 2001;74(877):15–23.
7. Loughrey GJ, Collins CD, Todd SM, et al. Magnetic resonance imaging in the management of suspected spinal canal disease in patients with known malignancy. Clin Radiol 2000;55(11):849–855.
8. Woolard E. Vertebral body tumors. In: Black PM, Loeffler JS, eds.. Cancer of the Nervous System. Philadelphia: Lippincott Williams & Wilkins; 2004.
9. Chan JH, Peh WC, Tsui EY, et al. Acute vertebral body compression fractures: discrimination between benign and malignant causes using apparent diffusion coefficients. Br J Radiol 2002;75(891):207–214.
10. Li KC, Poon PY. Sensitivity and specificity of MRI in detecting malignant spinal cord compression and in distinguishing malignant from benign compression fractures of vertebrae. Magn Reson Imaging 1988;6(5):547–556.
11. Taoka T, Mayr NA, Lee HJ, et al. Factors influencing visualization of vertebral metastases on MR imaging versus bone scintigraphy. AJR Am J Roentgenol 2001;176(6):1525–1530.
12. Metser U, Lerman H, Blank A, et al. Malignant involvement of the spine: assessment by 18F-FDG PET/CT. J Nucl Med 2004;45(2):279–284.
13. Fogelman I, Cook G, Israel O, et al. Positron emission tomography and bone metastases. Semin Nucl Med 2005;35(2):135–142.

14. Hamaoka T, Madewell JE, Podoloff DA, et al. Bone imaging in metastatic breast cancer. J Clin Oncol 2004;22(14):2942–2953.

15. Levack P, Graham J, Collie D, et al. Don't wait for a sensory level—listen to the symptoms: a prospective audit of the delays in diagnosis of malignant cord compression. Clin Oncol (R Coll Radiol) 2002;14(6):472–480.

16. Loblaw DA, Laperriere NJ. Emergency treatment of malignant extra-dural spinal cord compression: an evidence-based guideline. J Clin Oncol 1998;16(4):1613–1624.

17. Maranzano E, Latini P. Effectiveness of radiation therapy without surgery in metastatic spinal cord compression: final results from a prospective trial. Int J Radiat Oncol Biol Phys 1995;32(4):959–967.

18. McLinton A, Hutchison C. Malignant spinal cord compression: a retrospective audit of clinical practice at a UK regional cancer centre. Br J Cancer 2006;94(4):486–491.

19. Rades D, Heidenreich F, Karstens JH. Final results of a prospective study of the prognostic value of the time to develop motor deficits before irradiation in metastatic spinal cord compression. Int J Radiat Oncol Biol Phys 2002;53(4):975–979.

20. Turner S, Marosszeky B, Timms I, et al. Malignant spinal cord compression: a prospective evaluation. Int J Radiat Oncol Biol Phys 1993;26(1):141–146.

21. Zaidat OO, Ruff RL. Treatment of spinal epidural metastasis improves patient survival and functional state. Neurology 2002;58(9):1360–1366.

22. Hamilton AJ, Lulu BA, Fosmire H, et al. Preliminary clinical experience with linear accelerator-based spinal stereotactic radiosurgery. Neurosurgery 1995;36(2):311–319.

23. Rock J, Kole M, Yin FF, et al. Radiosurgical treatment for Ewing's sarcoma of the lumbar spine: case report. Spine 2002;27(21):E471–E475.

24. Rock JP, Ryu S, Yin FF, et al. The evolving role of stereotactic radiosurgery and stereotactic radiation therapy for patients with spine tumors. J Neurooncol 2004;69(1–3):319–334.

25. Ryu SI, Chang SD, Kim DH, et al. Image-guided hypo-fractionated stereotactic radiosurgery to spinal lesions. Neurosurgery 2001;49(4):838–846.

26. Kavanagh BD, McGarry RC, Timmerman RD. Extracranial radiosurgery (stereotactic body radiation therapy) for oligometastases. Semin Radiat Oncol 2006;16(2):77–84.

27. Kavanagh BD, Timmerman RD. Stereotactic radiosurgery and stereotactic body radiation therapy: an overview of technical considerations and clinical applications. Hematol Oncol Clin North Am 2006;20(1):87–95.

28. Murphy MJ, Adler JR Jr, Bodduluri M, et al. Image-guided radiosurgery for the spine and pancreas. Comput Aided Surg 2000;5(4):278–288.

29. Shiu A, Parker B, Ye JS, et al. An integrated treatment delivery system for CSRS and CSRT and clinical applications. J Appl Clin Med Phys 2003;4(4):261–273.

30. Timmerman RD, Forster KM, Chinsoo Cho L. Extracranial stereotactic radiation delivery. Semin Radiat Oncol 2005;15(3):202–207.

31. Yin FF, Das S, Kirkpatrick J, et al. Physics and imaging for targeting of oligometastases. Semin Radiat Oncol 2006;16(2):85–101.

32. Yin FF, Ryu S, Ajlouni M, et al. Image-guided procedures for intensity-modulated spinal radiosurgery [technical note]. J Neurosurg 2004;101(Suppl 3):419–424.

33. Yin FF, Ryu S, Ajlouni M, et al. A technique of intensity-modulated radiosurgery (IMRS) for spinal tumors. Med Phys 2002;29(12):2815–2822.

34. Murphy MJ, Cox RS. The accuracy of dose localization for an image-guided frameless radiosurgery system. Med Phys 1996;23(12):2043–2049.

35. Jaffray DA, Chawla K, Yu C, Wong JW. Dual-beam imaging for online verification of radiotherapy field placement. Int J Radiat Oncol Biol Phys 1995;33(5):1273–1280.

36. Jaffray DA, Drake DG, Moreau M, et al. A radiographic and tomographic imaging system integrated into a medical linear accelerator for localization of bone and soft-tissue targets. Int J Radiat Oncol Biol Phys 1999;45(3):773–789.

37. Yin FF, Guan H, Lu W. A technique for on-board CT reconstruction using both kilovoltage and megavoltage beam projections for 3D treatment verification. Med Phys 2005;32(9):2819–2826.

38. Jaffray DA. Emergent technologies for 3-dimensional image-guided radiation delivery. Semin Radiat Oncol 2005;15(3):208–216.

39. Yin FF, Wang Z, Yoo S, et al. Integration of cone-beam CT in stereotactic body radiation therapy. Tech Cancer Res Treat 2008;7(2):133–140.

40. Letourneau D, Wong JW, Oldham M, et al. Cone-beam CT-guided radiation therapy: technical implementation. Radiother Oncol 2005;75(3):279–286.

41. Pouliot J, Bani-Hashemi A, Chen J, et al. Low-dose megavoltage cone-beam CT for radiation therapy. Int J Radiat Oncol Biol Phys 2005;61(2):552–560.

42. Groh BA, Siewerdsen JH, Drake DG, et al. A performance comparison of flat-panel imager-based MV and kV cone-beam CT. Med Phys 2002;29(6):967–975.

43. Forrest LJ, Mackie TR, Ruchala K, et al. The utility of megavoltage computed tomography images from a helical tomotherapy system for setup verification purposes. Int J Radiat Oncol Biol Phys 2004;60(5):1639–1644.

44. Langen KM, Zhang Y, Andrews RD, et al. Initial experience with megavoltage (MV) CT guidance for daily prostate alignments. Int J Radiat Oncol Biol Phys 2005;62(5):1517–1524.

45. Hansen EK, Larson DA, Aubin M, et al. Image-guided radiotherapy using megavoltage cone-beam computed tomography for treatment of paraspinous tumors in the presence of orthopedic hardware. Int J Radiat Oncol Biol Phys 2006;66(2):323–326.

46. Murphy MJ. Fiducial-based targeting accuracy for external-beam radiotherapy. Med Phys 2002;29(3):334–344.

47. Russakoff DB, Rohlfing TF, Adler JR Jr, et al. Intensity-based 2D–3D spine image registration incorporating a single fiducial marker. Acad Radiol 2005;12(1):37–50.

48. Hillard VH, Shih LL, Chin S, et al. Safety of multiple stereotactic radiosurgery treatments for multiple brain lesions. J Neurooncol 2003;63(3):271–278.

49. Maintz JB, Viergever MA. A survey of medical image registration. Med Image Anal 1998;2(1):1–36.

50. Crum WR, Hartkens T, Hill DL. Non-rigid image registration: theory and practice. Br J Radiol 2004;77(Spec No 2):S140–153.

51. Bellmann C, Fuss M, Holz FG, et al. Stereotactic radiation therapy for malignant choroidal tumors: preliminary, short-term results. Ophthalmology 2000;107(2):358–365.

52. Christensen GE, Carlson B, Chao KS, et al. Image-based dose planning of intracavitary brachytherapy: registration of serial-imaging studies using deformable anatomic templates. Int J Radiat Oncol Biol Phys 2001;51(1):227–243.

6

Treatment Delivery

D. Michael Lovelock and Cihat Ozhasoglu

Essential requirements for a delivery system to be used for spinal treatment include the following:

- The ability to image bony structures with high spatial accuracy
- The ability to deliver very conformal dose distributions that may be required to wrap around the spinal cord
- The ability to monitor the target position at frequent intervals during beam delivery to detect a possible shift in position
- The means to readily correct for such a shift

For the irradiation of deep-seated tumors of the spine, a variety of treatment machines that use linear accelerators (linacs) to generate high-energy photons are now in use. The most common radiosurgery systems are the Novalis system from BrainLab AG (Feldkirchen, Germany) and the CyberKnife system from Accuray Inc. (Sunnyvale, California). Novalis uses a micro-multileaf collimator for beam shaping with one isocenter, whereas Cyberknife employs a robotic computer-controlled gantry with multiple isocenters. Other sophisticated arrangements of a linac-mounted gantry with various image-guidance methods are being developed. Another system called Hi Art, from TomoTherapy Inc. (Madison, Wisconsin), features a 6 MV linac mounted on a computed tomography (CT)–like gantry. The imaging systems associated with the various treatment machines vary considerably. Some are capable of three-dimensional (3D) volumetric imaging; others are capable of rapidly verifying target position during treatment. Implanted fiducial markers may also be required for some patients, depending on the imaging technique used.

Because of the close proximity of the spinal cord, even small patient movements that may occur after the final pretreatment imaging could result in the delivered dose to the spinal cord being higher than that planned. It is therefore important to be able to verify in 3D the target position at regular times during dose delivery. On a conventional linac, this can be done by stopping treatment and acquiring either a pair of localization images taken at different gantry angles or a cone-beam scan. Delivery using the TomoTherapy machine would be done in several passes. These can be interleaved with passes using the imaging beam. Therapy machines equipped with in-room imaging systems are capable of acquiring a pair of radiographs in a few seconds. When coupled with a means of rapidly registering the radiographs with the corresponding reference images and automatically implementing the corresponding correction, in effect the system can compensate for any small movements the patient may make during treatment.

The clinical effort required to localize the target during treatment, then correct the patient position, depends on the treatment delivery platform. Careful patient immobilization will reduce the chances of movement during dose delivery, especially necessary because frequent target position verification is slow and time consuming. Clinical procedures differ widely. **Table 6.1** compares features important to high-dose spinal radiotherapy for four different delivery systems.

The remainder of this chapter describes some of the clinical experiences gained from two centers, each of which has been using radiosurgery to treat patients with paraspinal disease for 6 years or more. Although the two centers use very different treatment platforms, a CyberKnife and a conventional linac equipped with kV imaging, both perform hypofractionated and high-dose (24 Gy) single-fraction treatments. Each has developed techniques and clinical procedures necessary to safely deliver these complex treatments.

◆ Clinical Experience from the University of Pittsburgh Medical Center

The CyberKnife is an image-guided whole-body stereotactic radiosurgery system that consists of a 6 MV compact linac mounted to a robotic arm that is coupled through a control loop to a digital diagnostic x-ray imaging system. The robotic arm can point the radiation beam anywhere in space

Table 6.1 Comparison of Features of Delivery Systems Important in High-Dose Spinal Radiotherapy

Feature	Linac with MV or kV CBCT	CyberKnife	Novalis with in-room kV	TomoTherapy
Field-shaping method	Dynamic or stop-and-shoot IMRT	Multiple isocenters delivered using typically 100–150 anterior noncoplanar beams	Dynamic or stop-and-shoot IMRT	Helical fan beam IMRT continuously delivered from all beam directions
Important dimensions associated with treatment beams	Leaf width at isocenter: Varian: 5 mm Elekta: 10 mm Siemens: 10 mm	Cylindrical collimators used; diameters used for spinal treatments typically 20–25 mm	Leaf width at isocenter: 3 mm Maximum field size: 10 × 10 cm	Minimum width of fan beam: 10 mm
Imaging equipment	MV portal imaging kV imaging systems: source and imager mounted on gantry kV beam direction at 90 degrees to MV beam	Dual in-room kV imagers	Dual in-room kV imagers	Helical 3D scan using ~4 MV fan beam
Images	Fluoroscopy, radiographs, portal images, cone-beam volumetric imaging	Orthogonal radiographs from fixed directions	Orthogonal radiographs from fixed directions	Volumetric MV images
Method used to correct target misalignment after registration of localization images (2D or 3D)	Translational corrections sent to couch remotely; rotational corrections possible if robotic couch top available	Patient position not changed; translational and rotational corrections used to modify directions of subsequent beams	Translational corrections sent to couch remotely; rotational corrections available if robotic couch top installed	Cranial-caudal and anteroposterior corrections applied remotely; left-right corrections applied manually in room
Time required to localize and correct target position during treatment	Minutes	< 5 seconds	Seconds	Minutes

Abbreviations: CBCT, cone-beam computed tomography; IMRT, intensity-modulated radiation therapy; linac, linear accelerator; 3D, three-dimensional; 2D, two-dimensional.

with six degrees of positioning freedom, without being constrained to a conventional isocenter.[1-4] The CyberKnife was developed to overcome the geometrical limitations of gantry-based systems and to eliminate the need for application of invasive frames. **Figure 6.1** depicts the basic components of the CyberKnife:

- Compact 6 MV X-band linac mounted to a robotic arm
- Two orthogonal flat-panel amorphous silicon digital x-ray detectors with a resolution of 0.3 mm/pixel. One diagnostic x-ray source is mounted to the ceiling for each panel detector.
- Robotic treatment couch with six degrees of freedom (translations along all three axes, roll, yaw, and pitch)

Spine Tracking

To ensure safe delivery of high doses of radiation to spinal tumors, the position of the tumor needs to be tracked continually throughout the radiosurgery procedure. The CyberKnife system's software is capable of tracking spinal tumors based on fiducial markers implanted in or near the tumor or by registering the position of one or two vertebrae close to the tumor. These two different techniques are described briefly below.

Six-Degree Fiducial Tracking

Prior to treatment, each patient is implanted with four to six fiducial markers, which act as radiographic landmarks for

the image guidance system. The fiducials are 0.8 × 5 mm cylindrical gold seeds or 2 × 6 mm stainless steel screws. They are typically implanted percutaneously in or near vertebrae under fluoroscopic guidance; the pedicles are the most common location. By placing fiducials in bony structures, one can significantly reduce the chance of fiducial migration. Three fiducials are necessary to define a full spatial transformation in all six degrees of freedom of target translation and rotation. Fiducials are implanted rostrally and caudally to the lesion so that the tumor is approximately centered within them. They are placed such that they are 2 cm or more apart and arranged in a noncoplanar configuration. For spine radiosurgery, rotational tracking accuracy can be important; therefore, we aim to use at least four fiducials because four fiducials yield much better tracking accuracy than three, whereas more than five fiducials give little further improvement[5] (**Fig. 6.2**).

Following the implantation of fiducial makers, the patient returns for the planning CT. The patient is placed in a supine position in a conformal alpha cradle or Vac-Lok (MEDTEC, Orange City, Iowa) bag during CT scanning as well as during treatment. CT images are acquired with a slice thickness of 1.25 mm to include the lesion of interest as well as the fiducials. Because the fiducial markers are 5 mm or longer, they are visible in one to five consecutive slices, depending on their orientation. During treatment planning, the fiducials are located and their positions identified in three dimensions on the CT dataset.

On the day of treatment, the patient is positioned supine in the same immobilization device that was used for the CT

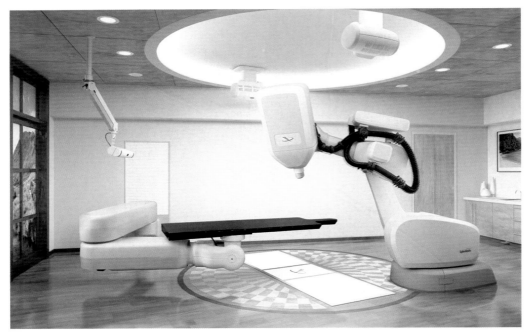

Figure 6.1 The main components of the CyberKnife robotic radiosurgery system: compact 6 MV X-band linear acceleratorlinac mounted to a robotic arm; two flat-panel in-floor x-ray detectors positioned opposite to the diagnostic x-ray sources mounted to the ceiling; and a robotic treatment couch with six degrees of freedom. (Courtesy of Accuray Inc., Sunnyvale, California.)

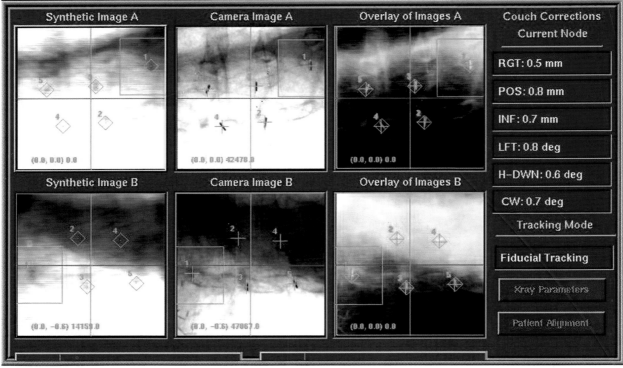

Figure 6.2 A snapshot from the CyberKnife console computer taken during treatment of a patient with a spinal lesion. The synthetic images are digitally reconstructed radiographs (DRRs) generated from the patient's computed tomography scan. The "diamonds" in the DRRs indicate the position of the gold markers. The camera images are the near-real-time x-ray images taken during the treatment. The green crosses in these images depict the positions of the gold fiducial markers as determined by real-time automatic image-processing algorithms. "Couch corrections" indicate how much one needs to move the couch to set up the patient exactly as he or she was scanned. Note that these corrections are six dimensional (three translations and three rotations).

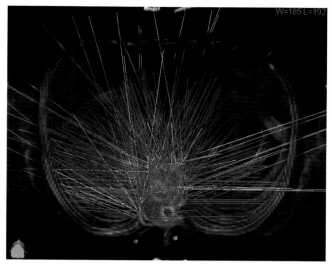

Figure 6.3 Beam directions for a plan of a patient with a lesion at T9. Beams with nonzero dose are shown in cyan. The tumor and spinal cord are outlined in red and green, respectively. This plan had 147 beams.

scan study. Two diagnostic orthogonal x-ray images ("live" images) are taken synchronously using the x-ray sources mounted to the ceiling and the flat-panel detectors positioned opposite the sources. CyberKnife tracking software processes the live images and extracts coordinates of the fiducial makers, then compares them to the position of the fiducials in digitally reconstructed radiographs (DRRs). Discrepancies between the two sets of values are reported as "couch corrections" to the operator. The operator can use these values to move the couch remotely from the operating console room. The patient is positioned with six degrees of freedom, three translations (inferosuperior, anteroposterior, and left/right) and three rotations (roll, yaw, and pitch). Once the fiducial markers are identified and verified by the operator at the beginning of the treatment, the determination of the patient position is a completely automated process. It takes only 2 to 4 seconds to produce a pair of orthogonal images and determine the patient position. It typically takes 10 to 20 minutes to set up a patient, although one may sometimes have difficult setups that take longer. For example, visualization of the fiducial markers in live images may prove to be a difficult task when large patients are imaged due to the limited penetrating power of the diagnostic x-ray sources.

Once the initial setup is complete, radiation treatment may commence. A typical CyberKnife treatment has 100 to 150 beams[6,7] (**Fig. 6.3**). Each beam enters from a different trajectory and typically has 200 monitor units (MU) or less. Because the linac has a dose rate of 600 MU/min, it takes 20 seconds or less to deliver the dose associated with each beam. The patient position can be verified by imaging the patient before the dose for each beam that is delivered. In this fashion, CyberKnife can continually correct for any deviation in patient position from the planning CT throughout the treatment. **Figure 6.4** shows the changes in patient position during a spine radiosurgery treatment for a patient with a lesion at L4. Note that the patient position has deviated from the planning CT position by only 0.71 mm based on the last diagnostic x-ray image taken. However, because the robot moves the radiation beam to compensate for this deviation, in theory, the targeting error is reduced to its residual systematic component. For static targets such as spinal lesions, the CyberKnife system has been shown to have overall submillimeter radiation delivery accuracy.[8-10] The CyberKnife robot can move the radiation beam to compensate for patient movements of up to 1 cm along each axis. The robot can also rotate the beam to compensate for target rotations of up to 1 degree about each axis. If the patient movement exceeds these limits, the system automatically turns off the radiation beam, and the treatment can only be resumed after the patient is moved back into the ideal position. The typical treatment time for a single-fraction radiosurgical procedure is 30 to 60 minutes.

Six-Degree Skeletal Structure Tracking

Although fiducial-based spine tracking has proven to be clinically feasible and safe for the radiosurgical treatment of spinal lesions,[11-18] implantation of the fiducial markers is invasive and lengthens the treatment time. In addition, the placement of fiducials in the cervical spine can be risky. The CyberKnife system allows fiducial-free spine tracking via Xsight software. Xsight has been developed to eliminate the need for fiducial markers, as it is capable of tracking bony landmarks such as the vertebrae directly without requiring surrogate markers.[19,20]

Figure 6.5 shows a snapshot of the console screen for an L4 spinal lesion that was treated using Xsight spine tracking software. In this figure, "synthetic images" are DRRs that are derived from the planning CT. "Camera images" are orthogonal "live" x-ray images taken during treatment. The green mesh region of interest (ROI) is the center of the planning CT,

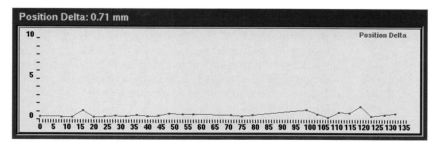

Figure 6.4 "Position delta" is the deviation of the patient's position during treatment from the planning computed tomography position. The vertical axis shows the deviation in millimeters, and the horizontal axis indicates the beam number. Position delta was 0.71 mm when this patient was imaged for the last time. The patient moved only a few millimeters throughout the treatment, which is typical of most spine treatments.

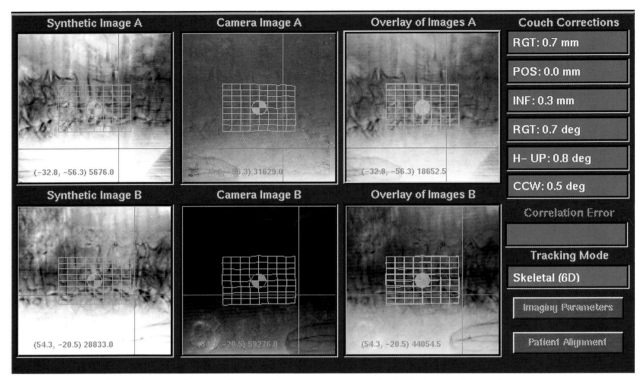

Figure 6.5 A snapshot of the console screen for an L4 lesion that was treated using Xsight tracking software.

indicated by the yellow circle. The mesh is a 9 × 9 grid representing 81 nodes or points of interest. The blue mesh in the live images is slightly deformed, indicating that the target position is not exactly the same as it was in the planning CT. Each node in the grid of the live images is registered to the corresponding node in the DRRs to accurately determine the patient's treatment position and couch corrections.

By registering the live images to DRRs, the target pose (tumor position and orientation) is determined. Xsight spine tracking software uses intensity-based two- (2D) and three-dimensional (3D) image registration to determine the target pose. The technical details of the Xsight software have been presented elsewhere.[19–21] It takes 2 to 4 seconds to determine the position of the patient and report the couch corrections to the operator using Xsight software. Thus, spine tracking via Xsight is as efficient as fiducial-based spine tracking. Xsight, like fiducial-based tracking, has also been shown to have submillimeter tracking accuracy.[10,19] Besides the tracking technique, the clinical workflow for Xsight treatments is the same as the fiducial-based spine treatments.

Clinical Experience

As of November 2006, some 900 spinal lesions had been treated at the University of Pittsburgh Medical Center (Pittsburgh, Pennsylvania) using the CyberKnife. Most of these cases were treated in a single fraction with 16 to 20 Gy to the 80% isodose line using fiducial-based tracking. Since it

was installed in October 2005, the Xsight software has been in routine clinical use at the center. Our published clinical outcome results have been impressive.[13–18] CyberKnife spine radiosurgery has proven to be a safe new treatment modality for spinal tumors, primarily because of its near-real-time x-ray imaging system and highly accurate robotic beam-pointing capability.

◆ Clinical Experience from Memorial Sloan-Kettering Cancer Center

CT-Guided Treatments Using the Stereotactic Body Frame

Stereotactic body radiotherapy for patients with paraspinal disease started at the Memorial Sloan-Kettering Cancer Center (New York) in February 2000. The initial treatment facility consisted of a high-energy linac (21EX, Varian Medical Systems Inc., Palo Alto, California) equipped with an MV portal imager. A CT scanner, installed in the same bunker, was positioned such that the couch of the CT scanner and the couch of the treatment machine could be positioned end to end. Both couches were fitted with a simple rail system to facilitate the easy transfer of an immobilized patient from one to the other.

A stereotactic body frame (SBF) and immobilization system was developed to allow CT-based image-guided treatments.[22] A stereotactic coordinate system, constructed from aluminum rods, similar to that developed by Lax et al,[23] allowed the body frame coordinates of specific features of the bony anatomy in the vicinity of the target to be determined in the pretreatment CT scan. These were compared with the corresponding coordinates from the planning CT scan to determine the setup errors. To immobilize the patient, the SBF used a set of small pressure plates that pressed against the lateral pelvis and rib cage, the anterior pelvis at the hips, and, optionally, the sternum. All the pressure plate positions were reproducible from fraction to fraction.

Five-fraction (5 × 4 Gy) and single-fraction (1 × 24 Gy) treatments were delivered using CT guidance. An early finding was that a strictly stereotactic approach to setup did not always ensure that the target was correctly positioned just prior to treatment. After the CT-guided setup, corrections were sometimes made using image guidance based on orthogonal MV localization images. This effect, presumably due to the patient's shifting within the frame during transfer, has also been described by Wulf et al.[24]

Image Guidance and the Memorial Body Cradle

The need to treat patients with primary bone disease to a dose of 66 to 70 Gy delivered in conventional 1.8 Gy fractions using image guidance for every fraction led to the development of a second immobilization system, the Memorial Body Cradle (MBC). It was designed for the rapid setup and immobilization of patients using image guidance. As such, it has external scales for initial setup using the MBC coordinates but has no CT or magnetic resonance (MR) fiducial system. Patients are immobilized in the MBC in the virtual simulation suite. After the CT scan, the physician contours the target, and an isocenter is chosen. The cradle coordinates of the isocenter are recorded using the room lasers of the virtual simulator prior to the patient's being tattooed. The tattoos are used to assist in the subsequent setups of the patient in the cradle, in particular to check for correct positioning in the cradle and for rotation about the cranial-caudal axis. The cradle coordinates are used for the initial setup of the patient prior to imaging. Design goals for the MBC were the following:

- Allow positioning of the patient to within 2 mm of the planned position
- Simplify the patient setup, making it possible for therapists to perform it in about 10 minutes
- Allow for customization for each patient, but also high patient throughput
- Be compatible with and provide for patient setup and immobilization in MR and positron emission tomography (PET)–CT scanners
- Maximize patient comfort while immobilized

Early in the project, the importance of patient comfort was realized. For this reason, patients in the MBC are immobilized with their arms at their sides. The design of the MBC features four sturdy paddles that press against the patient's sides at the hips and chest below the axilla. The paddle positions are customized for each patient and can be adjusted to accommodate patients ranging in size from small 12-year-olds to 350-pound adults. No anterior pressure plates are used. Much attention is given to patient comfort. A custom cushion made using expanding foam kits (alpha cradle) extending from the neck to either the thighs or the ankles, custom head cushions, and, when necessary, custom elbow support cushions are all used to fit the cradle to each individual (**Fig. 6.6**).

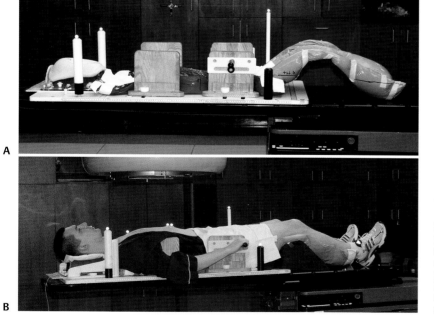

Figure 6.6 (A,B) The Memorial Body Cradle (MBC). Four paddles press against the sides of the patient at the hips and at the chest below the axilla. The expanding foam cushion forms itself around the paddles and to the patient's posterior contour. The knees are raised, and a custom cushion is used to support the head. For treatment sites in the cervical spine, a face mask can be used.

The initial use of the MBC with standard fractionation provided an opportunity to safely evaluate its performance. Pre- and post-treatment imaging was used to determine target shifts with respect to the cradle during treatment. Although initially intended for use with standard fractionation, the MBC is now used for all paraspinal treatments, including the high-dose (24 Gy) single-fraction deliveries that can take 2 hours or more. Post-treatment imaging, still done for all single-fraction treatments, is used as an ongoing quality assurance test of the entire clinical procedure.

Monitoring Patients during Treatment

The approach taken has been to use modest immobilization and to provide patients with whatever is necessary to help them stay comfortable and still throughout treatments. As such, the cradle cannot guarantee perfect immobilization. Thus, instead of trying to further constrain a patient to improve immobilization, we monitor the patient's position within the cradle using an infrared stereoscopic camera during the treatment session (**Fig. 6.7**). Small infrared reflectors are taped to the patient's skin during setup. These generally are placed close to the underlying bone, such as over the clavicles, sternum, costal cartilages, or hips, as near as possible to the cranial caudal position of the target vertebra. Generally, three or four reflectors are used and are placed to

include positions left and right of the center line to monitor possible rotational shifts. Four additional reflectors attached to the cradle form a pattern recognized by the camera control software. The software, developed in-house, first computes the mean position of each patient marker through several breathing cycles around the time the first pretreatment images are acquired. Each patient reflector is tracked until the end of the treatment. The therapists are provided with a real-time readout of the difference between the current reflector position and its initial mean position using a moving trace. The reflectors are tracked in the coordinate system of the cradle; therefore, they are not affected by shifts or rotations of the linac couch. Although the markers generally exhibit respiratory motion, the baselines are easy to discern. If the baselines show a drift or a sudden change in position, the therapists stop treatment and reimage the patient. If necessary, the target position is corrected by shifting the couch. The system is used only for the monitoring of intrafractional motion, not for setup. A report generated for each tracking session is included in the patient's chart.

Geometric Accuracy of the Imaging Process

Prior to the establishment of the Memorial Sloan-Kettering image-guided radiotherapy program, an assessment was made of the accuracy of the overall imaging process and

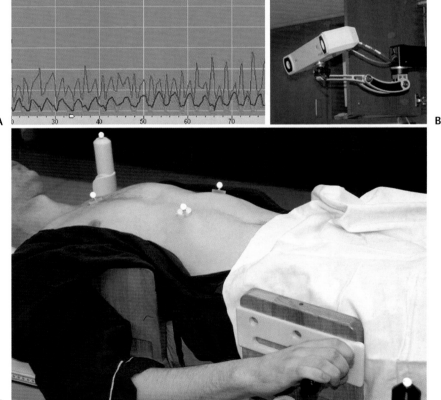

Figure 6.7 Monitoring a patient during treatment using the Memorial Body Cradle. **(A)** The real-time trace of each reflector's motion. Here the blue and green traces, from the reflectors on the left and right lower ribs, were used to monitor the patient's position. The red trace was from a reflector on the patient's stomach. **(B)** The wall-mounted camera. **(C)** The small infrared reflectors taped to the patient.

what, if any, improvements could be made. This was a factor in determining the goal of being able to position a bony target to within 2 mm of its planned position.

Uncertainties associated with the imaging process can be divided into their systematic and random components. Systematic errors can arise from the small mechanical misalignments associated with the imaging system; these may be a function of gantry and collimator angles, for example. If a phantom with a sharply defined target is imaged and perfectly aligned with its reference image, the delivered dose distribution may still be displaced from that planned because of residual systematic errors. During the first 3 years of the paraspinal treatment program, most patients were treated on a conventional high-energy linac equipped with an MV portal imager. Registration was done manually using software supplied by the vendor (PortalVision, Varian Medical Systems). In preparation for registration, outlines of anatomical features to be used for registration are traced onto an overlay of a reference image generated from the planning CT scan. The field outline is placed on a second overlay layer. At the time of target localization, the anatomy overlay is positioned over the MV image such that the drawn features are aligned with the corresponding features in the image. The location of the isocenter in the image is set by aligning the field overlay with a grid with a 2 cm spacing that is projected onto the image by a graticule tray inserted into the head of the linac. The setup error is related to the difference in position of the two overlays.

The largest contributor to the systematic error was found to be the position of the graticule with respect to the radiation beam. Routine monthly quality assurance (QA) reviews keep the graticule to within 1 mm of the field edge defined by the jaws. The jaws themselves are kept to within 1 mm of the correction position, as defined by a light field on graph paper. However, it is possible that much of the 2 mm error tolerance could arise from this single contributor.

A change in the QA procedures reduced the uncertainty in graticule placement to < 1 mm. First, because all spinal stereotactic body radiotherapy (SBRT) fields are delivered using intensity-modulated radiation therapy (IMRT), the graticule was referenced to the multileaf collimator (MLC) (120-leaf Millennium MLC, Varian Medical Systems) instead of the jaws. Losasso[25] described film-based procedures that are used to set the MLC positions to within approximately 0.2 mm of the correct position with respect to the axis of collimator rotation. The accuracy of the MLC-defined field edge as a function of the gantry angle is also known to be constant to within a few tenths of a millimeter. In practice, we have found it possible to maintain very tight tolerances on both the MLC positions with respect to the axis of collimator rotation and the gap width, an important parameter for dynamic delivery. The procedure used to align the graticule tray with the MLC-defined field was changed from a visual inspection of exposed film to a profile analysis of a high-resolution image acquired using the MV imager (**Fig. 6.8**). This reduced uncertainty of graticule to field location to approximately 0.5 mm.

After the installation of an onboard kV imaging system (Varian Medical Systems), paraspinal treatments were done using kV image guidance, using either orthogonal radio-

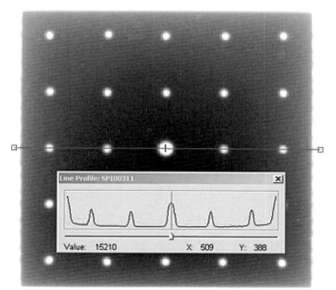

Figure 6.8 An MV portal image of a 10 × 10 cm field defined using a Millennium MLC (Varian Medical Systems) with a graticule tray inserted. The profile tool allows the central fiducial mark to be located with respect to the field edges to within ± 0.25 mm.

graphs or cone-beam scanning. Analysis of an Institutional Review Board–approved protocol demonstrated that setups of patients being treated for paraspinal disease using cone-beam image guidance was consistent with the setups performed using orthogonal MV imaging.[26] A comprehensive QA procedure has been published for a gantry-mounted kV imaging system.[27] One potential source of systematic error in this system is the displacement of the origin of the kV imaging system from the radiation isocenter. This has been tracked over the 3 years since installation.[28] The displacement has been found to be small (~1 mm) and constant. Initially, these small offsets were incorporated into the in-house registration software. After an upgrade of the vendor software and recalibration of the hardware, the offsets were found to be about 0.5 mm in each direction, essentially small enough to be neglected.

Random errors typically arise in the registration process itself. Poor quality reference or localization images where the features of the vertebra to be registered are indistinct, may lead to difficult registrations that may be operator dependent and vary day to day. As such, such contributions to the overall error are difficult to quantify. One measure taken at the start of the program to improve the quality of the reference images, both 2D and 3D, was to reduce the slice spacing and thickness of the CT scans from 3 to 2 mm.

The second measure, used for all 2D imaging, both MV and kV, was to require that there be fiducial markers attached to the spine. Many patients have had surgery during which titanium hardware is attached to the spine to brace it. The titanium, which generally spans the target, serves as a useful fiducial structure. Patients without titanium hardware undergo the implantation of approximately six gold seeds into the posterior elements of the vertebrae. Generally, two

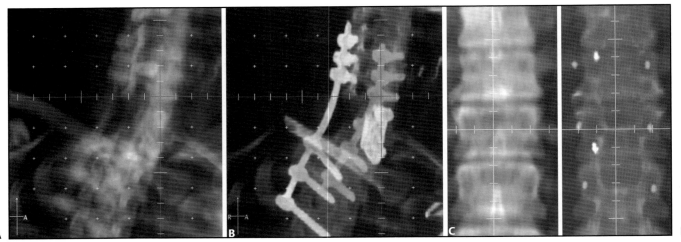

A   B   C   D

Figure 6.9 A comparison of reference images made using a digitally composited radiograph (DCR) in which the opacity of voxels with computed tomography numbers corresponding to metal has been increased. **(A)** A conventional digitally reconstructed radiography (DRR) of a patient with titanium hardware. **(B)** The corresponding DCR. **(C)** DRR of a patient with six gold fiducials (not visible). **(D)** The corresponding DCR, with the fiducials circled.

seeds per vertebra are implanted into the target vertebra and the adjacent superior and inferior vertebrae. The procedure is done under local anesthesia in the interventional radiology department. We have made use of a feature in the virtual simulation software (AcQSim, Philips Medical Systems, Bothell, Washington) called a digitally composited radiograph (DCR). In a DCR, the opacities of the voxels with CT numbers corresponding to the gold or titanium are increased. As can be seen in **Fig. 6.9,** the reference images constructed in this way are superior to the more conventional DRRs and allow for accurate and robust registration.

Fractionation, Dose, and Imaging Technique

Several fractionation schemes are now used at Memorial Sloan-Kettering for paraspinal treatments. Primary bone diseases, such as osteosarcoma, chordoma, and chondrosarcoma, are treated with conventional fractionation to 66 or 70 Gy. Patient immobilization and image guidance are used for all 35 fractions. Salvage treatments, used when patients have had prior radiotherapy and have experienced failure of local control, were treated to 20 Gy delivered in five fractions. This dose has been escalated to 30 Gy delivered in five fractions. Patients with metastatic disease with no prior radiotherapy to the target are treated with a single fraction of 24 Gy. Two-dimensional imaging with fiducial markers are used for all standard and hypofractionated cases. Cone-beam guidance is used for all single-fraction cases. All treatments are planned using IMRT with an in-house treatment planning system. The intensity-modulated beams are delivered using a dynamic sliding window technique.

◆ Conclusion

The linac with gantry-mounted 2D and 3D imaging capability, when coupled with an immobilization system and real-time infrared monitoring of patient position during treatment, has proved to be a very effective delivery platform. Patients can be positioned and maintained to within about 2 mm for the duration of treatment, allowing the delivery of tightly conformal dose distributions to the target while maximally sparing the spinal cord.

References

1. Adler JR, Murphy MJ, Chang S, Hancock S. Image-guided robotic radiosurgery. Neurosurgery 1999;44:1299–1306.
2. Murphy MJ, Adler JR, Bodduluri M, et al. Image-guided radiosurgery for the spine and pancreas. Comput Aided Surg 2000;5:278–288.
3. Coste-Maniére É, Olender D, Kilby W, Schulz RA. Robotic whole body stereotactic radiosurgery: clinical advantages of the CyberKnife integrated system. J Med Robot Comput Assist Surg 2005;1(2):28–39.
4. Romanelli P, Schweikard A, Schlaefer A, Adler J. Computer aided robotic radiosurgery. Comput Aided Surg 2006;11(4):161–174.
5. Murphy MJ. Fiducial-based targeting accuracy for external-beam radiotherapy. Med Phys 2002;29(3):334–344.
6. Schweikard A, Bodduluri M, Adler JR. Planning for camera-guided robotic radiosurgery. IEEE Trans Robot Automat 1998;14:951–962.
7. Tombropoulos RZ, Adler JR, Latombe J-C. CARABEAMER: a treatment planner for a robotic radiosurgical system with general kinematics. Med Image Anal 1999;3:237–264.
8. Murphy MJ. The accuracy of dose localization for an image-guided frameless radiosurgery system. Med Phys 1996;23:2043–2049.
9. Chang SD, Main W, Martin DP, Gibbs IC, Heilbrun MP. An analysis of the accuracy of the CyberKnife: a robotic frameless stereotactic radiosurgical system. Neurosurgery 2003;52(1):140–147.
10. Ho AK, Fu D, Cotrutz C, et al. A study of the accuracy of CyberKnife spinal radiosurgery using skeletal structure tracking. Neurosurgery 2007;60:147–156.
11. Ryu SI, Chang SD, Kim DH, et al. Image-guided hypo-fractionated stereotactic radiosurgery to spinal lesions. Neurosurgery 2001;49(4):838–846.
12. Murphy MJ, Chang S, Gibbs I, et al. Image-guided radiosurgery in the treatment of spinal metastases. Neurosurg Focus 2001;11:E6.
13. Gerszten PC, Ozhasoglu C, Burton SA, Kalnicki S, Welch WC. Feasibility of frameless single-fraction stereotactic radiosurgery for spinal lesions. Neurosurg Focus 2002;13:E2.

14. Gerszten PC, Ozhasoglu C, Burton SA, et al. CyberKnife frameless stereotactic radiosurgery for spinal lesions: clinical experience in 125 cases. Neurosurgery 2004;55(1):89–99.

15. Gerszten PC, Ozhasoglu C, Burton SA, et al. CyberKnife frameless single-fraction stereotactic radiosurgery for tumors of the sacrum. Neurosurg Focus 2003;15:E7.

16. Gerszten PC, Burton SA, Ozhasoglu C, et al. Stereotactic radiosurgery for spinal metastases from renal carcinoma. J Neurosurg Spine 2005;3:288–295.

17. Gerszten PC, Germanwala A, Burton SA, Welch WC, Ozhasoglu C, Vogel WJ. Combination kyphoplasty and spinal radiosurgery: a new paradigm for pathological fractures. J Neurosurg Spine 2005;3:296–301.

18. Gerszten PC, Burton SA, Ozhasoglu C, Welch WC. Radiosurgery for spinal metastases: clinical experience in 500 cases from a single institution. Spine 2007;32:193–199.

19. Muacevic A, Staehler M, Drexler C, Wowra B, Reiser M, Tonn J-C. Technical description, phantom accuracy, and clinical feasibility for fiducial-free frameless real-time image-guided spinal radiosurgery. J Neurosurg Spine 2006;5:303–312.

20. Fu D, Kuduvalli G, Maurer CR, Allison JW, Adler JR. 3D target localization using 2D local displacements of skeletal structures in orthogonal X-ray images for image-guided spinal radiosurgery. J Comp Assist Radiol Surg 2006;1:198–200

21. Fu D, Kuduvalli G. Enhancing skeletal features in digitally reconstructed radiographs. In: Reinhardt JM, Pluim JPW, eds. SPIE Medical Imaging 2006: Image Processing. 2006:61442M-1-61442M-6

22. Yenice KM, Lovelock DM, Hunt MA, et al. CT image guided intensity-modulated therapy for paraspinal tumors using stereotactic immobilization. Int J Radiat Oncol Biol Phys 2003;55(3):583–593

23. Lax I, Blomgren H, Naslund I, Svanstrom R. Stereotactic radiotherapy of malignancies in the abdomen: methodological aspects. Acta Oncol 1994;33(6):677–683.

24. Wulf J, Hadinger U, Oppitz U, Olshausen B, Flentje M. Stereotactic radiotherapy of extracranial targets: CT-simulation and accuracy of treatment in the stereotactic body frame. Radiother Oncol 2000;57(2):225–236

25. LoSasso TL. Acceptance testing and commissioning of IMRT. In: A Practical Guide to Intensity-Modulated Radiation Therapy. Madison, WI: Medical Physics Publishing; 2003:123–146.

26. Kriminski S, Lovelock DM, Amols H, Ali I, Yamada Y. Comparison of cone beam computed tomography with MV imaging for paraspinal radiosurgery patient alignment and position verification. Int J Radiat Oncol Biol Phys 2006; 66(3, Suppl 1)S146

27. Yoo S, Kim GY, Hammoud R, et al. A quality assurance program for the on-board imager. Med Phys 2006;33(11):4431–4447

28. Lovelock DM, LoSasso T, Ali I, et al. Quantifying the geometric accuracy of the on-board imager over a one year period. Med Phys 2006; 33(6):2000

7

Quality Assurance in Spine Radiosurgery

Timothy D. Solberg and Paul M. Medin

In the 50-plus years since it was first introduced, stereotactic radiosurgery, high-dose irradiation of cranial neoplasms delivered in a single fraction, has become a standard of care in the treatment of brain tumors, vascular malformations, functional disorders, and pain. Modern radiosurgery can be performed noninvasively yet with an extremely high degree of accuracy and on an outpatient basis. Within the past 10 years, the success of radiosurgery as a clinical treatment has given rise to optimism that similar gains may be achievable in extracranial sites. In particular, several parallels exist in the nature and management of neoplasms involving the spine. Histologies commonly treated with stereotactic radiosurgery, including schwannomas, meningiomas, arteriovenous malformations, and metastatic disease, also occur frequently in the spine. Management of both cranial and spinal disease is a standard part of the neurosurgical training curriculum.

Radiosurgery for spinal disease poses several challenges that are unique. Since its inception, the clinical practice of clinical radiosurgery has relied on rigid skull fixation for localization of intracranial structures. Targets outside the skull, however, are not readily amenable to fixation using rigid frames. Thus, issues of patient positioning, immobilization, reproducibility, and potentially even intrafraction motion present significant challenges in accurate localization and subsequent dose delivery. These practical challenges are exacerbated by the close proximity of the spinal cord, a particularly radiation-sensitive structure in which radiation-induced myelopathy has profound consequences. As late-responding tissues, spinal myelopathies may not manifest themselves for months after treatment. Additionally, although there are 50 years' worth of clinical data covering the cranial radiosurgery experience, the total number of spinal cases treated worldwide is less than 5000. All of these factors highlight the importance of targeting and dosimetric accuracy and place a high burden on the quality assurance (QA) process.

◆ Description of Spine Radiosurgery Systems

A methodology for clinical radiosurgery for targets involving and adjacent to the spine was first described by Hamilton and Lulu.[1] The system consisted of a shallow rigid box, with lateral dimensions compatible with computed tomography (CT) imaging. Patients were placed within the box in a prone position, and under anesthesia, small clamps were attached to one or two spinous processes adjacent to the intended target. These clamps were rigidly attached to two semicircular metal arches secured to the box. The stereotactic space was defined relative to a small radio-opaque sphere using the coordinate system of the CT scanner. Treatment room lasers were subsequently used to align the sphere with the isocenter of the linear accelerator (linac). Imaging, planning, and treatment were performed in a single setting with rigid fixation for the duration of the procedure. The authors used radio-opaque spheres hidden within phantoms and animal cadavers to assess localization uncertainties, reported to be 2.0 mm in a worst case scenario. The "hidden target" test, commonly referred to as a Winston-Lutz test after the authors who first described the procedure in cranial radiosurgery applications, remains the gold standard for assessing target localization.[2] This prototype spinal system was subsequently used in the treatment of nine patients, all of whom had recurrent spinal disease.[3,4] Doses delivered were understandably conservative, ranging from 8 to 10 Gy, with distributions constructed in such a way that no portion of the spinal cords received > 3 Gy. An attempt to commercially market the "Arizona" spinal radiosurgery system proved unsuccessful.

Several specialized systems for performing spinal radiosurgery have been described since the initial Arizona experience. Ryken et al modified an infrared (IR)-based navigation system to facilitate ultrasound-guided targeting of paraspinal tumors.[5] System applicability was limited to soft tissue tumors located on the dorsal aspect of the spinal column; disease involving the bony vertebrae, the most common site for metastatic spread, could not be localized due to inherent limitations of ultrasound imaging. The authors subsequently described the treatment of a single patient presenting with a recurrent metastatic squamous cell carcinoma at the level of T11; a dose of 15 Gy was delivered to the 80% isodose line. To date, this is the only publication on this particular technique.

Medin et al proposed a minimally invasive localization technology that allowed for high-dose, single-fraction irradiation of soft tissue or bony spinal tumors.[6] Briefly, under local anesthesia, three small radio-opaque markers were permanently affixed within the vertebral and spinous processes. Patients received a subsequent CT scan in which the target was identified and contoured. Simultaneously, biplanar radiographs were obtained in which the implanted markers were identified. Both imaging procedures utilized an external localization box from which a coordinate system was established. Within this coordinate system, the locations of the implanted fiducials were determined from the biplanar radiographs, and the location of the target isocenter was determined from the CT scan. Prior to treatment, biplanar radiographs were repeated with the patient in the treatment position. The implanted fiducials were identified, and the isocenter position was calculated based on the geometric relationship between the target and implanted markers obtained at the time of CT imaging. In this manner, accurate target localization could be performed despite the fact that (1) the patient had moved from the time of the initial CT and (2) the target could not be directly visualized in the treatment room.

The authors went on to experimentally evaluate the overall system accuracy. Phantoms were constructed to evaluate the integrity of absolute spatial dimensions and to study the effect of marker and target spacing. The largest targeting error observed was 1.17 mm, with most combinations tested resulting in targeting errors well below 1 mm. The methodology was subsequently evaluated in a swine model. Results indicated that (1) the implant procedure was simple to perform, requiring < 30 minutes time to complete; (2) implanted markers were readily distinguishable from normal anatomy on radiographs; (3) once implanted, markers stayed fixed and did not move relative to the intended target or to one another; (4) with the swine in a supine position, markers did not move with normal or forced respiration; and (5) there was little loss in targeting accuracy when markers associated with one vertebra were used to target adjacent vertebrae. This system represented a true milestone in accurate, minimally invasive stereotaxis of a wide range of neoplasms associated with the spine.

Two additional single-institution systems for spine radiosurgery have been described in the literature. Yenice et al constructed a stereotactic body frame to facilitate immobilization and localization.[7] The frame incorporates CT localization fiducial plates that define a coordinate system to localize patient anatomy with respect to the frame. Unique to the

design, the patient is initially set up in a vertical standing position, after which the frame and patient are tilted backward into a horizontal treatment position. It is believed that this manner of setup provides for better daily reproducibility of internal anatomy. The system is also designed to facilitate daily CT imaging, which is performed just prior to each treatment. The authors were able to demonstrate a localization accuracy of within 1 mm in any direction, which they concluded was sufficient to ensure that the maximum dose to the spinal cord was within 10 to 15% of the planned value. Daily CT imaging was eventually replaced with localization based on electronic portal imaging, with little loss of targeting accuracy.[8]

A similar system for spine radiosurgery was described by Shiu et al.[6,9] Patients were immobilized in a full-body stereotactic frame and received localization/verification CT scans immediately prior to treatment. This was facilitated by a CT on rails installed in the treatment room. With daily CT imaging, the authors evaluated the overall deviation from the intended isocenter was within 1 mm for each treatment. Furthermore, they determined the effect of respiration on spinal targeting accuracy and concluded that, for supine patients, there was no significant movement.

Since these initial attempts, two commercial systems have been developed and widely adopted for spine radiosurgery. The first, the CyberKnife system (Accuray Inc., Sunnyvale, California), is a robotic radiosurgery system originally designed to treat cranial tumors without a stereotactic head frame.[10–12] The CyberKnife consists of a 6 MV X-band linear accelerator attached to a robotic arm that can move about the patient with six degrees of freedom, coupled with two diagnostic x-ray units projecting on two opposing amorphous silicon detectors. The biplanar imaging system provides the capabilities for frameless stereotactic radiosurgery.[13] Because the imaging system is permanently mounted in the treatment room, targeting can be performed without the need for additional "localization boxes." The integrated image guidance system employed by the CyberKnife provides the capabilities for stereotactic irradiation of extracranial sites.[14]

Murphy et al described modifications to the CyberKnife to facilitate stereotactic irradiation of spinal tumors.[15] For the cervical spine, image registration based on bony anatomy is performed between in-room images and digitally reconstructed radiographs (DRRs) obtained from the planning CT. In the thoracic and lumbar spine, however, much of the bony anatomy is superimposed upon itself in the oblique projections, making image-based registration difficult. For these anatomical sites, the authors implant fiducial markers in the bony spine adjacent to the target of interest. The fiducial markers are readily localized on x-ray images from which the target position can subsequently be determined. In contrast to the methodology described by Medin et al,[6] markers were inserted in the vertebral bodies (as opposed to the spinous and vertebral processes), and the reference marker locations were derived from CT images (as opposed to radiographs).

Yin et al have described a methodology for stereotactic spinal irradiation using the second commercial system, the Novalis system (BrainLab AG, Feldkirchen, Germany).[16] The

Novalis system incorporates an IR component for patient monitoring and a stereoscopic x-ray component for localization of extracranial targets. The IR component includes two ceiling-mounted cameras that detect the three-dimensional (3D) positions of IR reflective markers placed on the surface of the patient. The IR signal is continuously updated every 50 msec. Although studies by Wang et al have demonstrated that the position of each IR-reflecting sphere can be determined to be < 0.3 mm, with overall CT-defined targeting accuracy in rigid objects on the order of 3 mm at the 95% confidence level, issues of marker reproducibility and patient motion preclude the use of the IR system for accurate stereotaxis.[17] The kV x-ray component consists of two floor-mounted x-ray tubes and two opposing amorphous-silicon (a-Si) flat-panel detectors mounted to the ceiling. Each x-ray tube/detector pair is configured to image through the linac isocenter with a coronal field of view of about 18 cm in both the superoinferior and left-right directions at the isocenter.

The Novalis x-ray localization system can be operated in two modes: matching of implanted radio-opaque markers in a manner similar to that of the CyberKnife, and automated registration of x-ray and DRRs using an iterative edge-matching algorithm. A comprehensive evaluation of targeting accuracy has been reported by Verellen et al.[18]

The principle of 3D localization using a pair of two-dimensional (2D) projections is called stereophotogrammetry, and has found application is many fields, including human growth and motion analysis,[19-22] joint repair and prosthesis fabrication,[23] computer-aided analysis of facial expressions,[24] and the study of ocular disorders.[25] Menke et al and Schlegel et al employed video stereophotogrammetry as a means of evaluating the repositioning accuracy of a specially designed head holder for fractionated radiotherapy.[26,27] The principles of stereophotogrammetry were first applied to x-ray localization by Selvik.[19]

◆ Quality Assurance of Target Localization

Quality assurance for spine radiosurgery procedures can be divided into two primary tasks: QA of the localization and delivery systems and patient-specific QA. Of these, ensuring accuracy in target localization is a foremost priority. In contrast to cranial radiosurgery, external surrogates (i.e., the head frame) do not provide an adequate basis for accurate targeting. Thus, the clinical spine radiosurgery process is based explicitly on image guidance. Assessing image guidance capabilities in vivo is difficult at best; therefore, anthropomorphic phantoms must be used.

In cranial stereotactic radiosurgery, the Winston-Lutz test, also known as a hidden target test, is a universally accepted methodology for assessing targeting accuracy.[2,28] Briefly, a small radio-opaque sphere is positioned at the presumed linac isocenter. A series of beams/eye images are obtained by rotating the gantry and couch through various angles. By observing where the projection of the ball falls relative to the central axis of the beam, any offset from the presumed isocenter can be determined.

While at the University of California, Los Angeles, we adopted a similar approach for assessing target localization in spine radiosurgery. We have constructed an anthropomorphic torso phantom composed primarily of solid water, with a vertebral column that covers the cervical through lumbar spine, as well as low-density lung regions. At various levels, small radio-opaque spheres have been embedded to serve as hidden targets (**Fig. 7.1**). In commissioning the spine radiosurgery process for clinical use, all procedural steps are performed with the phantom in a manner identical to that for patients. First, the phantom receives a CT scan from which one or more isocenters (radio-opaque spheres) are defined. A treatment plan is constructed, and the CT data and corresponding isocenter location are transferred to the image guidance workstation. The phantom is placed on the treatment table, and a pair of x-rays are obtained. The x-rays are fused with DRRs obtained from the planning CT, from which a translation necessary to position the sphere at the treatment isocenter is calculated (**Fig. 7.2**). Once positioned, a series of beams/eye images are acquired and evaluated using software that automatically identifies the radiation field and image of the ball and determines the offsets of their corresponding centers (**Fig. 7.3**).

Verellen et al performed a similar hidden target assessment on the Novalis unit located at their institution.[18] For localization based on x-ray/DRR fusion, they observed an average targeting accuracy of 0.41 mm with a standard deviation of 0.92 mm in 40 repeated hidden target tests. When implanted markers were used for localization, average targeting accuracy improved to 0.28 mm with a standard deviation of 0.36 mm. The authors also suggested a rigorous series of tests to characterize localization capabilities in a variety of situations:

- Localization accuracy in the absence of any shifts (localization reproducibility)
- Localization accuracy with a known translation in individual dimensions
- Localization accuracy with known translations in three dimensions
- Localization accuracy with known rotation about one of the principle axes
- Localization accuracy in the presence of known translations and a rotation about one of the principle axes
- Localization accuracy in the presence of known translations and known rotations

In contrast, Murphy et al compared dose profiles measured using a 2D thermoluminescent dosimeter (TLD) array with those computed by the planning system.[15] In this manner, several sources of uncertainty, including imaging, planning, fiducial registration, and delivery, were evaluated simultaneously. Results demonstrated a root-mean-square (RMS) targeting error of ~0.7 mm along each axis. In a subsequent study, Yu et al repeated the study in anthropomorphic phantoms of the head and torso.[29] Five implanted markers were used for localization and registration purposes, and radiochromic film was used to measure the delivered dose distributions, which were compared with planned distributions as in the earlier study. In 16 phantom treatments performed at three participating

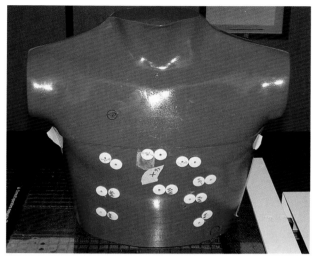

A

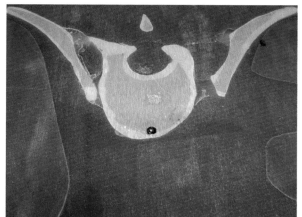

B

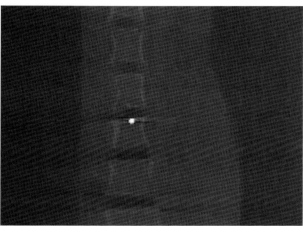

C

Figure 7.1 **(A)** An anthropomorphic phantom used for evaluating targeting accuracy in spinal radiosurgery. **(B)** Small radio-opaque spheres are embedded in the phantom and used as objects for "hidden target" tests. **(C)** A coronal reconstruction of the planning computed tomography scan.

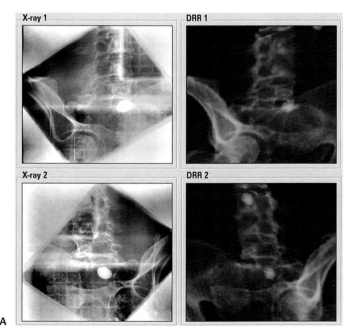

A

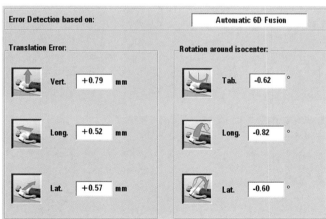

B

Figure 7.2 **(A)** In the treatment room, a pair of positioning x-rays is obtained and fused with the digitally reconstructed radiographs. **(B)** Based on a six-dimensional fusion algorithm, the translations and rotations necessary to position the phantom at isocenter are calculated.

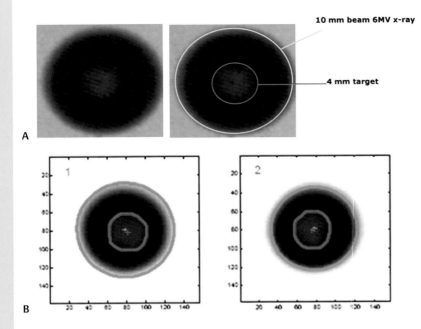

Figure 7.3 **(A)** An example of the hidden target assessment, showing an image of a radio-opaque sphere 4 mm in diameter within a circular radiation field 10 mm in diameter. The sphere and radiation field are automatically identified using a software application, and the offsets between the corresponding centers are calculated. **(B)** An analysis of an anteroposterior and lateral image pair from one hidden target experiment.

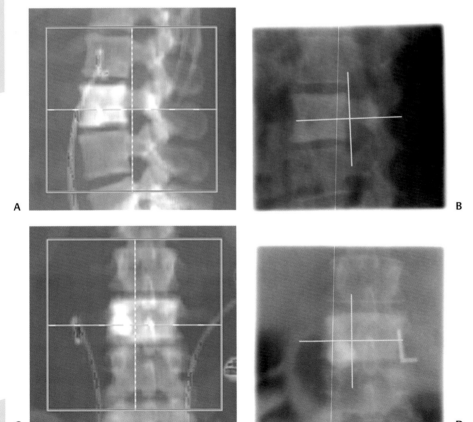

Figure 7.4 **(A–D)** Anteroposterior and lateral films are acquired and compared with corresponding digitally reconstructed radiographs prior to any spinal radiosurgery treatment.

institutions, a mean targeting error of 0.68 mm (σ = 0.29 mm) was observed. Unfortunately, a targeting assessment based on anatomical landmarks was not performed.

Independent and redundant verification is crucial to ensuring accurate target localization. At our institution, we perform two specific tasks prior to every patient treatment. First, table heights and other shifts from known landmarks are determined from the treatment planning system and used as a qualitative verification of target position. In our experience, these values are typically within 1 cm or less, which is more than adequate for verifying that the appropriate vertebrae are targeted, or ensuring against right-left errors. Additionally, anteroposterior and lateral port films are acquired and compared against DRRs (**Fig. 7.4**). This provides additional localization assurance, though not at the submillimeter level that can be achieved through x-ray stereophotogrammetry.

Secure patient immobilization is critical in spine radiosurgery, particularly as treatment times can often take over an hour. Many practitioners prefer to use the BodyFix stereotactic system (Medical Intelligence Medizintechnik GmbH, Schwabmünchen, Germany). The BodyFix system consists of a full-length vacuum bag that creates a precise mold of the patient's body. This can be complemented by a translucent plastic sheet placed on top of the patient and subsequently evacuated to restrict voluntary and involuntary movement. An example of this device is shown in **Fig. 7.5**. At our institution, it is also common to embed a standard head mask in the vacuum bag, particularly when treating targets in the cervical and thoracic spine. All spine radiosurgery patients are treated with arms at their sides. This provides better anatomical reproducibility as well as patient comfort.

Even with excellent immobilization, it is important to periodically verify a patient's positioning during a spine radiosurgery procedure. With the Novalis system, continuous monitoring of the patient's position can be performed using the IR system. Because the IR markers are placed on a patient's surface, however, they respond to respiratory motion, which limits the system's localization ability to only a few

millimeters. For their CyberKnife treatments, Ryu et al perform repeat imaging, 20 to 30 times per fraction, as a direct means of verifying target positioning.[30] At our institution, we regularly reconfirm target position between beams or during other natural interruptions (e.g., when the couch is rotated) using the Novalis x-ray system.

◆ Dosimetric Considerations

Although the methodology described by Murphy et al evaluates localization and dosimetric characteristics together, QA of dose delivery is generally addressed separately from localization accuracy, as this allows each to be evaluated in greater detail.[15] The task of dosimetric verification involves comparing prescribed doses. Both absolute dose and relative dose distributions must be verified, regardless of the delivery methodology used. At our institution, conformal fields or dynamic conformal arcs are preferred for more regularly shaped tumors that do not wrap around the spinal cord. These treatment options are more expedient and require fewer monitor units to deliver than intensity-modulated radiation therapy (IMRT). However, IMRT is needed in many spine radiosurgery cases to adequately spare the spinal cord.

In any case, dosimetric verification requires mapping a patient's treatment parameters onto a phantom in which quantitative measurements can be performed. At our institution, a combination of film and ionization chamber measurements are performed prior to every patient treatment to verify the absolute dose delivered to the target as well as the overall dose distribution. The importance of patient-specific pretreatment QA has been emphasized by other authors.[15] The specific methodology used at our institution was presented in detail by Agazaryan et al.[31] Absolute dose and composite dose distributions are measured in one of two phantoms: the Benchmark IMRT Phantom (MED-TEC, Orange City, Iowa) is used for targets that are surrounded by largely homogeneous tissue, such as targets in the lumbar spine. The Thorax

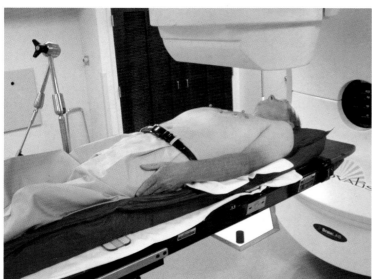

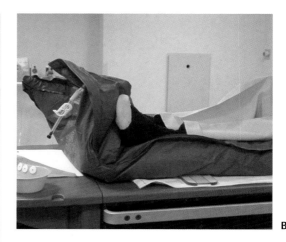

Figure 7.5 A spine radiosurgery patient in the BodyFix system. Note that the arms are at the patient's sides **(A)**, and the end is molded to conform to the feet **(B)**.

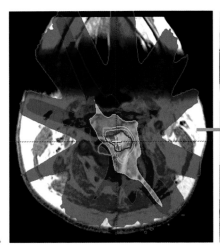 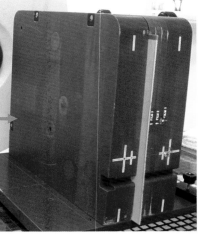 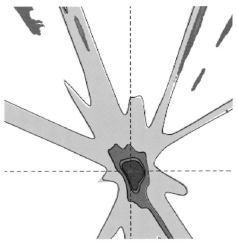

A
B

Figure 7.6 **(A)** Dose distributions for targets located in the cervical and lumbar spine are mapped onto a homogeneous solid water phantom for dosimetric analysis. Software is used to superimpose the film measurements and calculated dose and quantitatively compare the two distributions. **(B)** Results are shown, with the calculated 90, 80, 50, and 20% isodose lines (solid black lines) superimposed on the corresponding dose levels from film measurements (color wash). Green areas indicate regions where the 3% dose and 3 mm distance criterion was exceeded.

IMRT Phantom (CIRS Inc., Norfolk, Virginia) is used for targets that require irradiation through a lung. Both phantoms are constructed with multiple axial planes for film measurements and with multiple inserts for ionization chambers. After a treatment plan has been completed, the Novalis planning software is used to map all parameters from the patient plan to a CT scan of the appropriate phantom. In-phantom dose distributions are exported for subsequent comparison with film measurements. Composite dose distributions are measured in the axial plane at the isocenter using EDR2 film (Eastman Kodak Corp., Rochester, New York.). The dynamic range of EDR2 film (≤ 5 Gy) is exceeded in most single-fraction applications; therefore, monitor units delivered must be scaled downward by an appropriate factor. In IMRT applications, such scaling can change the final distribution, though such changes are insignificant.

Following delivery, films are digitized and compared with the calculated dose distributions with the aid of software dedicated to this task.[31] The measured and calculated dose distributions are superimposed and positioned graphically using shift, rotate, and mirror tools, or by specifying isocenter coordinates and fiducial marks on the film. Dose difference, distance to agreement, and the gamma index (the minimum scaled multidimensional distance between a measurement and a calculation point determined in combined dose and distance space) are calculated.[32] At our institution, we have defined our acceptability criteria as 3% dose difference and 3 mm distance, and gamma is normalized accordingly. The results of dosimetry for single-fraction radio-

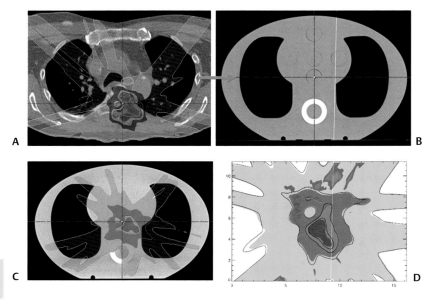

A
B
C
D

Figure 7.7 Seven intensity-modulated radiation therapy (IMRT) fields were used to develop the treatment plan **(A)**, in which the target was covered by the 95% isodose line while keeping the spinal cord below 50%. The patient's plan was subsequently mapped onto the Thorax IMRT Phantom from CIRS Inc. **(B)**, producing the dose distribution shown in **C. (D)** Resulting film measurements are shown in color wash superimposed on results from treatment planning calculations (*solid lines*). The 90, 80, 50, and 20% isodose regions are displayed. Areas where the acceptability criterion of 3% dose and 3 mm distance-to-agreement was exceeded, as measured by the multidimensional gamma parameter, are shown in the green overlay.

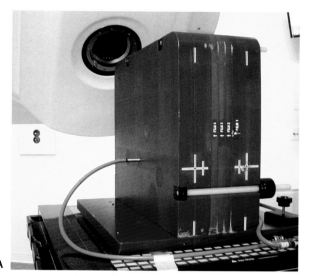 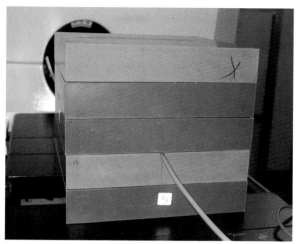

A   B

Figure 7.8   The absolute dose should be verified using a calibrated ionization chamber and can be evaluated in a variety of phantoms. **(A)** Benchmark™ IMRT QA Phantom (CIVCO Medical Solutions, Orange, Iowa.) **(B)** Solid Water (Gammex, Inc., Middleton, Wisconsin).

surgery to a C-spine target are shown in **Fig. 7.6.** Shown are the 90, 80, 50, and 20% isodose levels, with the calculation in solid black lines and the corresponding isodose lines from film measurements in color wash. Dark green areas indicate regions where the 3% dose and 3 mm distance criterion was exceeded. Small areas of disagreement are common, as the criteria adopted for comparison are quite stringent.

Figure 7.7 shows a seven-field IMRT plan designed to treat a vertebral body metastasis within the thoracic spine. Because some of the beams pass through the lung, the CIRS phantom was used for dosimetric purposes. Absolute dosimetry for every patient's composite plan is performed using a 0.015 cm³ ionization chamber inserted in an appropriate phantom (**Fig. 7.8**). The acceptability criterion adopted in our clinic is ± 3%. In our experience, absolute dose agreement at this level, even when tissue heterogeneities are encountered, is readily achievable.

Whenever possible, localization and dosimetric verification parameters should be performed through a record-and-verify system, using patient-specific parameters. In this manner, potential errors can be detected before they are propagated to the patient.

◆ Conclusion

Spine radiosurgery is an effective therapy that is quickly becoming popular and more widely available, with a growing body of encouraging clinical data. The fact that there have been few reported neuropathies to date is a tribute to the care and dedication of the early spine radiosurgery adopters. Nevertheless, the inherent radiation sensitivity of the spinal cord, the potential for debilitating side effects, and the paucity of dose response data to single-fraction delivery place demands on the accuracy of target and dose localization that are unprecedented within the radiotherapy experience. Fortunately, there are ample guidelines in the literature to assist

spine radiosurgery practitioners in establishing procedures and acceptability criteria needed to ensure the highest quality of care.

References

1. Hamilton AJ, Lulu BA. A prototype device for linear accelerator-based extracranial radiosurgery. Acta Neurochir Suppl (Wien) 1995;63:40–43.
2. Lutz W, Winston KR, Maleki N. A system for stereotactic radiosurgery with a linear accelerator. Int J Radiat Oncol Biol Phys 1988;14:373–381.
3. Hamilton AJ, Lulu BA, Fosmire H, Stea B, Cassady JR. Preliminary clinical experience with linear accelerator-based spinal stereotactic radiosurgery. Neurosurgery 1995;36:311–319.
4. Hamilton AJ, Lulu BA, Fosmire H, Gossett L. LINAC-based spinal stereotactic radiosurgery. Stereotact Funct Neurosurg 1996;66:1–9.
5. Ryken TC, Meeks SL, Traynelis V, et al. Ultrasonographic guidance for spinal extracranial radiosurgery: technique and application for metastatic spinal lesions. Neurosurg Focus 2001;11:E8.
6. Medin PM, Solberg TD, DeSalles AAF, et al. Investigations of a minimally invasive method for treatment of spinal malignancies with linac stereotactic radiation therapy: accuracy and animal studies. Int J Radiat Oncol Biol Phys 2002;52:1111–1122.
7. Yenice KM, Lovelock DM, Hunt MA, et al. CT image-guided intensity modulated therapy for paraspinal tumors using stereotactic immobilization. Int J Radiat Oncol Biol Phys 2003;55:583–593.
8. Lovelock DM, Hua C, Wang P, et al. Accurate setup of paraspinal patients using a noninvasive patient immobilization cradle and portal imaging. Med Phys 2005;32:2606–2614.
9. Shiu AS, Chang EL, Ye J, et al. Near simultaneous computed tomography stereotactic spinal radiotherapy: an emerging paradigm for achieving true stereotaxy. Int J Radiat Oncol Biol Phys 2003;57:605–613.
10. Adler JR, Cox RS. Preliminary clinical experience with the CyberKnife: image guided stereotactic radiosurgery. In: Alexander E, Kondziolka D, Loeffler JS eds, Radiosurgery. Basel: Karger; 1996:316–326.
11. Adler JR, Chang SD, Murphy MJ, et al. The CyberKnife: a frameless robotic system for radiosurgery. Stereotact Funct Neurosurg 1997;69:124–128.
12. Adler JR, Murphy MJ, Chang SD, et al. Image-guided robotic radiosurgery. Neurosurgery 1999;44:1299–1306.
13. Murphy MJ. An automatic six-degree-of-freedom image registration algorithm for image-guided frameless stereotaxis radiosurgery. Med Phys 1997;24:857–866.

14. Schweikard A, Glosser G, Bodduluri M, et al. Robotic motion compensation for respiratory movement during radiosurgery. Comput Aided Surg 2000;5:263–277.

15. Murphy MJ, Adler JRJr, Bodduluri M, et al. Image-guided radiosurgery for the spine and pancreas. Comput Aided Surg 2000;5:278–288.

16. Yin FF, Ryu S, Ajlouni A, et al. A technique of intensity-modulated radiosurgery for spinal tumors. Med Phys 2002;29:2815–2822.

17. Wang LT, Solberg TD, Medin PM, et al. Infrared patient positioning for stereotactic radiosurgery of extracranial tumors. Comput Biol Med 2001;31:101–111.

18. Verellen D, Soete G, Linthout N, et al. Quality assurance of a system for improved target localization and patient set-up that combines real-time infrared tracking and stereoscopic X-ray imaging. Radiother Oncol 2003;67:129–141.

19. Selvik G. Roentgen stereophotogrammetric analysis. Acta Radiol 1990;31:113–126.

20. Axelsson P, Johnsson R, Stromqvist B. Mechanics of the external fixation test of the lumbar spine: a roentgen stereophotogrammetric analysis. Spine 1996;21:330–333.

21. Carman AB, Milburn PD. Conjugate imagery in the automated reproduction of three dimensional coordinates from two dimensional coordinate data. J Biomech 1997;30:733–736.

22. Peterson B, Palmerud G. Measurement of upper extremity orientation by video stereometry system. Med Biol Eng Comput 1996;34:149–154.

23. Kearfott KJ, Juang RJ, Marzke MW. Implementation of digital stereo imaging for analysis of metaphyses and joints in skeletal collections. Med Biol Eng Comput 1993;31:149–156.

24. Waters K, Terzopoulos D. The computer synthesis of expressive faces. Philos Trans R Soc Lond B Biol Sci 1992;335:87–93.

25. Johnson CA, Keltner JL, Krohn MA, et al. Photogrammetry of the optic disc in glaucoma and ocular hypertension with simultaneous stereo photography. Invest Ophthalmol Vis Sci 1979;18:1252–1263.

26. Menke M, Hirschfeld F, Mack T, et al. Stereotactically guided fractionated radiotherapy: technical aspects. Int J Radiat Oncol Biol Phys 1994;29:1147–1155.

27. Schlegel W, Pastyr O, Bortfeld T, et al. Stereotactically guided fractionated radiotherapy: technical aspects. Radiother Oncol 1993;29:197–204.

28. Winston KR, Lutz W. Linear accelerator as a neurosurgical tool for stereotactic radiosurgery. Neurosurgery 1988;22:454–464.

29. Yu C, Main W, Taylor D, et al. An anthropomorphic phantom study of the accuracy of CyberKnife spinal radiosurgery. Neurosurgery 2004;55:1138–1146.

30. Ryu SI, Chang SD, Kim DH, et al. Image-guided hypo-fractionated stereotactic radiosurgery to spinal lesions. Neurosurgery 2001;49:838–845.

31. Agazaryan N, Solberg TD, DeMarco JJ. Patient specific quality assurance for the delivery of intensity modulated radiotherapy. J Appl Clin Med Phys 2003;4:40–50.

32. Low DA, Harms WB, Mutic S, Purdy JA. A technique for the quantitative evaluation of dose distributions. Med Phys 1998;25:656–661.

Clinical Application of Spine Radiosurgery

8

Target Delineation and Dose Prescription

Samuel Ryu and Peter C. Gerszten

Radiosurgery is defined as the delivery of a large, highly conformal dose of radiation to a localized area using a stereotactic approach. One of the defining characteristics of radiosurgery is the rapid fall-off of the radiation dose distribution outside the target volume, allowing for the delivery of a large dose to the target while avoiding the adjacent normal tissue. It is for this reason that radiosurgery requires precise targeting of the target volume. In this context, the accurate delineation of the target tumor is the first and perhaps most critical step in the clinical application of radiosurgery.

The process of target tissue delineation should be based on the physical and biological characteristics of radiosurgery, requiring a detailed knowledge and understanding of the particular tumor growth patterns and imaging. In addition, there is both voluntary and physiologic motion of extracranial target sites. Most physiologic motion is secondary to inspiration and expiration. Although there also may be minor organ movements that are related to arterial pulsation or transient elevated intracranial pressure, the spinal cord and vertebrae move relatively little with respiration when a patient is in a supine position. Because physiologic movement of the spine is negligible, including this variable of uncertainty in the determination of the margin for the planning target volume is generally not performed. Nevertheless, the accuracy of patient immobilization and treatment must be carefully considered in the design and planning of each target volume.

The proper use of imaging technology is important in delineating the target volume. Image fusion of computed tomography (CT) and magnetic resonance imaging (MRI) is frequently employed in spine radiosurgery. Commercial fusion algorithms are available, using the image stretching method to compensate for different spine curvatures. A preferred method is an image fusion of the involved spine without image modification, although the curvature of the entire spinal column may not match precisely. The MRI must be fused with the planning CT, with the region of interest at the center of both studies. In some cases of bone-only disease involvement, the planning CT images may provide better target delineation than MR images. Avoiding the extra step of obtaining an MRI for fusion planning certainly decreases the overall cost of the treatment and eliminates another test for the patient. Most patients have already undergone diagnostic MRI prior to radiosurgery treatment that provides sufficient anatomical information for contouring purposes. Functional imaging studies such as 18-fluorodeoxyglucose (FDG)–positron emission tomography (PET) to assist in target delineation for spine tumors are currently being explored.

◆ Target Delineation

Radiosurgery Treatment Decision Algorithm

Conventional treatment for spine metastases has included the use of palliative radiotherapy, which usually involves one or two rostral and caudal vertebral bodies in addition to the involved vertebrae, employing various fractionation schedules, most commonly 30 Gy in 10 fractions.[1] When there is an epidural tumor extension that causes rapid neurological deterioration, open surgical decompression has been favored.[2,3] Recently, more aggressive first-line direct decompressive surgery followed by radiotherapy led to a superior outcome over conventional fractionated radiotherapy alone in patients with symptomatic spinal cord compression from metastatic cancer.[4] The results of this study emphasize the important role of achieving local tumor control in spine metastases patients with epidural compression of neural structures. In a similar fashion, the goal of spine radiosurgery is to improve local tumor control by delivering a high biological dose of radiation to the delineated target.

Because many patients with spine metastases have functional problems related to the spine involvement, in addition to complex medical and oncologic issues, the treatment should be well tailored to the individual patient's medical and psychosocial needs, with an emphasis on the patient's functional outcome. Indeed, there are many long-term survivors with spine metastases. A recent meta-analysis of spinal metastases reported an overall 1-year survival rate of 40 to 50%.[5] An analysis of radiosurgery for solitary spine metastases also showed a similar survival rate, with varying median survival time according to different tumor histology. The median survival time of patients with breast and prostate primaries and multiple myeloma far exceeds 12 months.[6] This fact supports the use of aggressive local treatment to maintain long-term tumor control, as has been demonstrated to be the case for radiosurgery for brain metastases.[7]

The primary goal of spine radiosurgery is to maximize local tumor control of the involved spine while palliating symptoms. Therefore, the intent of radiosurgery is to treat the entire visible gross tumor in the spine. The treatment algorithm pathway of radiosurgery for spine metastases at the Henry Ford Hospital (Detroit, Michigan) is illustrated in **Fig. 8.1.** Radiosurgery is most frequently used to treat solitary spine metastasis (**Fig. 8.1a**). Any soft tissue extension of the tumor causing epidural compression or a paraspinal mass is included in the target volume. Likewise, two contiguous spine levels can be treated with radiosurgery (**Fig. 8.1b**). In addition, radiosurgery may be used to treat separate lesions that are not adjacent to one another (**Fig. 8.1c**). When there is diffuse spine involvement with one or two levels of more clinical significance either by symptoms or by epidural compression (**Fig. 8.1d**), radiosurgery can be

used as a boost to those specific vertebral bodies concurrent with conventional external beam radiotherapy. Target delineation in these cases should be the same as for other solitary metastases. In cases of more diffuse metastatic spine involvement, conventional external beam radiotherapy or radionuclide therapy is indicated instead of radiosurgery (**Fig. 8.1e**). With increased experience, we have found that patients with diffuse spine metastases can also be treated successfully with single-fraction radiosurgery, thus avoiding protracted fractionated radiotherapy, if the symptomatic area is identifiable both radiographically and clinically. In patients who experience a rapid neurological deterioration resulting from direct compression of the spinal cord or cauda equina by either epidural tumor or retropulsed bone, open surgical decompression is indicated. Radiosurgery has been employed successfully in these postoperative cases with a similar type of target delineation as for solitary metastases.[8] In a similar manner to postoperative cases, radiosurgery may be used by combining the overall management of the lesion with pretreatment minimally invasive procedures such as vertebroplasty and kyphoplasty.[9]

Vertebral Metastasis with or without Epidural or Paraspinal Extension

Several target volumes must be considered in the spine radiosurgery treatment plan. The gross tumor volume (GTV) represents all tumor that is visible on imaging studies. The clinical target volume (CTV) is the volume likely to contain microscopic disease. Because of the rapid dose fall-off inherent to radiosurgery, if the CTV is not included in the target delineation, the patient may have a less than satisfactory clinical and radiographic response. In spine radiosurgery, the planning target volume (PTV) often equals the CTV with no margin accounting for setup error and target motion. There are many factors that influence the process of making decisions on the radiosurgery target volume, including tumor factors, normal tissue constraints, and host factors. These factors are summarized in **Table 8.1.**

In delineating the radiosurgery target volume, there are generally two different types of practices currently employed. The first practice is to include the entire vertebral body and soft tissue component within the target volume, more consistent with the classic teaching of non-imaged-guided conventional external beam irradiation. The other practice is to include only the GTV that is visible on either CT or MRI and not the entire bone. There is currently no consensus on the use of one contouring practice over the other. There are limited data as to whether one method is superior in terms of local tumor control, symptomatic response, or recurrence.

At both the Henry Ford Hospital and the University of Pittsburgh Medical Center (Pittsburgh, Pennsylvania) spine radiosurgery programs, it is the current practice to delineate the target volume to include the entire involved vertebral body and both pedicles of the affected vertebrae. When there is paraspinal or epidural extension of the tumor, the involved vertebra or vertebrae and the gross tumor are included in the target volume as well. The reason to employ this method

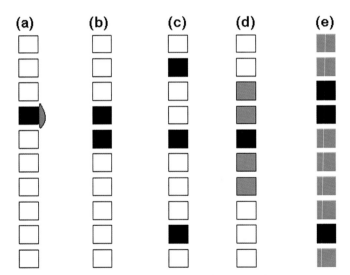

(a)　**(b)**　**(c)**　**(d)**　**(e)**

Figure 8.1 The decision protocol of radiosurgery for spine metastases. **(a)** A solitary spine metastasis is treated with radiosurgery. Any soft tissue extension of the tumor causing epidural compression or a paraspinal mass is included in the target volume. **(b)** Two contiguous spine levels may be treated with radiosurgery. **(c)** Noncontiguous lesions are treated with radiosurgery. **(d)** Diffuse spine involvement with one or two levels of more clinical significance either by symptoms or by epidural compression, radiosurgery can be used as a boost to conventional radiotherapy. **(e)** In widespread diffuse spine involvement, radiosurgery can be used for epidural compression or clinical significance in conjunction with conventional radiotherapy.

Table 8.1 Factors in the Determination of Target Volume

Tumor factors
    Tumor histology
    Extent and number of spine levels involved
    Shape of the tumor
    Systemic disease status

Normal tissue constraints
    Spinal cord
    Kidney
    Bowel
    Esophagus
    Lung

Host factors
    Prior irradiation to the target
    Concurrent systemic therapy
    Comorbidity
    Performance status
    Estimated survival time

is based on the understanding that the metastatic process likely will involve the medullary bone within the involved vertebral body. Tumor cells within the bone marrow have been found in > 30% of patients with even early breast cancer.[10] This would imply that the presence of micrometastasis may be even greater in the bone marrow when the spine is invaded by the gross tumor. The microstructure of the bone marrow renders it particularly vulnerable to tumor cell accumulation and bone invasion. Multiple capillaries near the endosteal bone margin become contiguous with a rich venous sinusoidal system with a capacity 6 to 8 times that of the osseous arterial system. It is thought that metastases to bone are mostly hematogenous, yet the skeletal blood flow represents only 4 to 10% of cardiac output. The high incidence of spread within bone tissue is attributed to this microstructure of bone.[11] By including the clinically involved spine within the target volume for radiosurgery, the failure outside the target volume (i.e., at the immediately adjacent spinal level) was < 5% in one clinical series.[12]

This method of target delineation is illustrated in **Fig. 8.2.** There can be several different scenarios of spine involvement. Involvement of the actual body of the vertebra is the most common type of spine metastasis (**Fig. 8.2A**). In this case, the entire involved vertebral body and both pedicles

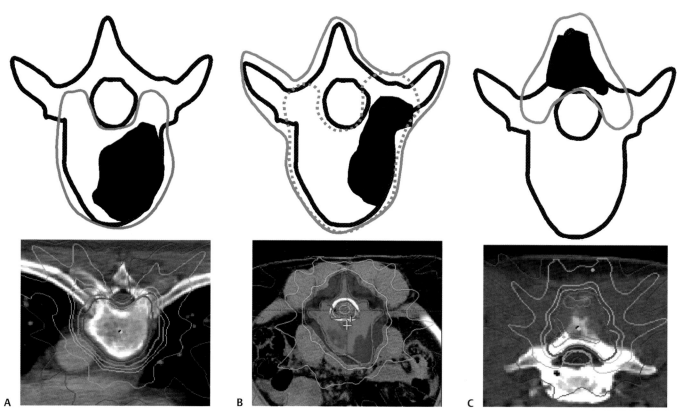

A   B   C

Figure 8.2 The target volume definition of radiosurgery for spine metastases. **(A)** Involvement of the body of the vertebra is the most common type of spine metastasis. The entire vertebral body and both pedicles are included in the radiosurgery plan. **(B)** Vertebral body involvement can be treated either to the entire vertebra (vertebral body and dorsal elements) or in the same fashion as in **A** and **C** but with a generous margin (*dotted line*). **(C)** For involvement of dorsal elements, the target volume is the dorsal elements only (spinous process and lamina), including both pedicles, while sparing the vertebral body.

are included in the radiosurgery plan, as shown. **Figure 8.2C** demonstrates an example of the treatment of the dorsal elements (spinous process and lamina), including both pedicles, while sparing the vertebral body. Vertebral body involvement, such as that shown in **Fig. 8.2B,** can be treated either to the entire bony element (vertebral body and dorsal elements) or in the same fashion as in **Fig. 8.2A** and **C,** but with a generous margin.

In rare cases, radiosurgery targeting of the GTV only is used when the spinal cord is significantly dose limiting or when the treatment is strictly for palliation of symptoms.

Target Delineation in the Postoperative Setting

Experience with postoperative radiosurgery for spine metastases has been published.[8] In this series, surgical treatment varied depending on the extent of bony involvement and the need for spinal stabilization after decompression and tumor resection. The radiosurgery target volume (CTV) was delineated as the tumor bed and the surgical cavity in the same fashion as that shown in **Fig. 8.2.** It is frequently difficult to delineate the target volume due to the altered anatomical landmarks after surgery and the surgical instrumentation that causes image distortion. It is also not known what adverse consequences such large doses have on bony fusion. In this study of a postoperative radiosurgery treatment, 65% of patients experienced improvement in pain, and 66% experienced improvement in functional status. A CT myelogram is necessary only in those rare cases in which the spinal instrumentation obscures the anatomy (**Fig. 8.3**).

Primary Tumors of the Spine

Experience with radiosurgery for the treatment of primary malignant tumors of the spine or the spinal cord is limited.

Surgery is often the primary treatment. These tumors are uncommon, and treatment decision making may vary depending on the clinical circumstances, largely by judicious selection and a multimodality combination of surgery, fractionated radiotherapy, and chemotherapy. Most of the primary malignant tumors of the spine, such as sarcomas and chordomas, have a high rate of local recurrence, and most are relatively radioresistant.

Because surgery is usually the chief treatment for primary spine tumors, radiosurgery may be used postoperatively as a boost to the grossly involved area with or without fractionated external beam radiotherapy to the surgical bed. For these tumors, radiosurgery seems to be a reasonable adjuvant therapeutic modality that might improve the local tumor control by increasing the total delivered radiation dose compared with standard fractionated external beam radiotherapy. If the surgical cavity is sufficiently small, it may also be treated with radiosurgery. An example of this type of treatment is shown in **Fig. 8.4.** The patient had an osteogenic sarcoma at T4 with an extension into the epidural area. The patient initially underwent open surgery and subtotal tumor resection. Postoperative radiosurgery was delivered with intensity modulation to the surgical cavity (16 Gy) and to the gross residual tumor (20 Gy).

In cases of radiosurgery for benign tumors, target delineation is more straightforward. Only the GTV is targeted for treatment. A margin is not necessary for radiation dose planning.

Delineation of Normal Structures

The most important normal tissue at risk for radiation toxicity in spine radiosurgery is the spinal cord. Planning CT images with 1 to 3 mm slice thickness are used for delineation of the spinal cord with or without MRI fusion. In particular,

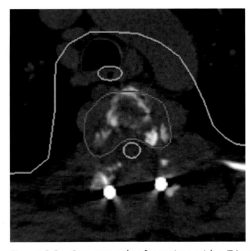

Figure 8.3 Case example of a patient with a T4 multiple myeloma lesion. The patient had presented with a spinal cord compression and underwent an open decompression and posterior arthrodesis. The tumor, spinal cord, esophagus, and lungs have been contoured. The titanium rods are clearly visible and do not interfere with the anatomy of the spinal cord or vertebral body tumor.

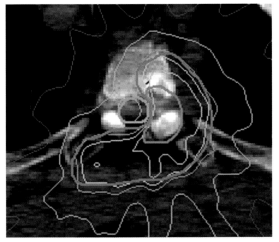

Figure 8.4 Osteogenic sarcoma case. This patient had osteogenic sarcoma involving the paraspinal region with epidural extension at T4. The patient had partial resection of the tumor. The clinical target volume (surgical cavity and gross residual tumor, *purple line*) was treated with a single fraction of 16 Gy, and the GTV (gross tumor volume, *pink line*) was boosted to a dose of 20 Gy.

for cases in which the tumor extends into the spinal canal and directly abuts or compresses the spinal cord, MRI fusion may be required to confidently determine the precise location of the spinal cord. The spinal cord may be delineated by fusion of simulation CT images with T1-weighted gadolinium enhanced or T2-weighted MR images. At the Henry Ford Hospital, the spinal cord volume is consistently defined as the volume extending from 6 mm above to 6 mm below the radiosurgery target. With this definition of spinal cord volume, an average dose of 10 Gy was given to the 10% volume of the spinal cord at the involved spine segment, and this was well tolerated.[6] Definitions for the cauda equina or the region of the filum terminale and radiation dose constraints are the same as those for the spinal cord. At the University of Pittsburgh Medical Center, a different technique is employed for single-fraction treatment. Every attempt is made to keep the maximum dose to the spinal cord < 8 Gy, and the total spinal cord volume receiving > 8 Gy is carefully considered on a case-by-case basis. At the level of the cauda equina, the entire spinal canal is contoured as the critical structure of neural tissue (**Fig. 8.5**), and the maximum dose of 10 Gy is allowed.

Other normal tissues are defined depending on the level of the involved vertebral body being treated. Normal tissue, such as the pharynx, esophagus, bowel, or kidney, should be carefully delineated for the radiation planning as "critical structures" that are considered in the inverse treatment planning algorithms. Vascular structures, such as the aorta, carotid arteries, vertebral arteries, and vena cava, are not usually delineated as critical structures, unless there is concern of tumor invasion. There is no general consensus about the single-dose tolerance of normal tissues.

◆ Radiosurgery Dose

Similar to the process of target delineation, the selection of radiosurgery dose is based on many factors, including tumor factors, normal tissue tolerance, and the clinical goals of treatment. Some common factors that need to be considered are summarized in **Table 8.2**. The most common clinical indications for spine radiosurgery include pain, progressive

Table 8.2 Factors for Radiosurgery Dose Selection

Tumor factors
  Histology
  Dimension (size) of the target
  Shape of the target
Normal tissue tolerance
  Prior irradiation
  Concurrent systemic therapy
Clinical goals
  Pain improvement
  Local tumor control
  Prevention of tumor recurrence
  Prevention of tumor progression
  Improvement in neurological dysfunction

neurological deficit, and radiographic tumor progression, as well as a primary or definitive treatment. The doses necessary to achieve these different clinical goals for the same tumor histology may vary.

Dose Prescription for Pain

The optimum dose of radiosurgery necessary to achieve acceptable pain control or tumor response is not known at this time. Experience with radiosurgery for renal cell carcinoma spine metastases demonstrated that the pain response was more consistent and durable at median tumor doses > 14 Gy delivered in a single fraction.[13] The pain control or improvement was also higher (96%) with single doses ≥ 16 Gy in patients with breast cancer spine metastases.[14] In an interim analysis of a phase II trial at the Henry Ford Hospital, various factors affecting the patient outcomes after spine radiosurgery were analyzed, including age (< 66 vs ≥ 66 years old), Karnofsky performance status (< 70 vs ≥ 70), tumor histology, presence of neurological deficits, presence of systemic metastases other than the spine, number of spinal lesions (one vs multiple), dose of radiosurgery (< 14 vs ≥ 14 Gy), and concurrent systemic chemotherapy. None of these factors reached statistical significance in this cohort of patients. However, there was a strong trend toward increased pain

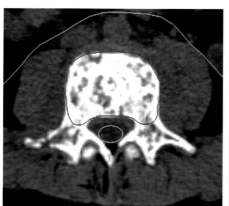
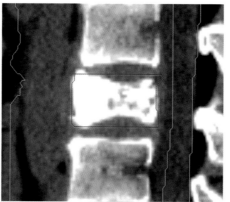

Figure 8.5 Case example of an L3 osteogenic sarcoma demonstrating in the axial (**A**) and sagittal (**B**) projections of the planning computed tomography scan how the entire thecal sac is contoured as the cauda equina critical structure.

A

B

control with a higher radiation dose of ≥ 14 Gy delivered in a single fraction. Pain control was > 80% for patients in the ≥ 14 Gy group compared with the lower dose group.[15]

A radiation dose response relationship for pain control may exist following radiosurgery for spine metastases. A meta-analysis of 10 randomized trials containing single-fraction radiotherapy for painful bone metastasis showed single-fraction radiation (median 8 Gy, range 8–10 Gy) achieved a complete pain response of 33.4% and an overall response rate of 62.1%.[16] Radiosurgery experiences have been reported with a single fraction of higher radiosurgery doses for spinal metastasis.[13–15,17,18] The results of pain control by various radiation doses[19–24] and radiosurgery at the Henry Ford Hospital phase II trial and the University of Pittsburgh are summarized in **Table 8.3**. The majority of the spine metastases consistently responded to the higher doses of radiosurgery regardless of the histology. Although there is no clear consistency and the results cannot be directly compared with each other, these results suggest a trend toward a higher overall pain control when using higher radiation doses.

The duration of pain control after radiosurgery is another important parameter, but the data are more limited. An accurate assessment of the durability of pain control is extremely difficult because these patients often develop further systemic tumor spread as well as new spine metastases with longer follow-up. It is therefore difficult to assess whether the pain is recurrent at the same treated vertebral body or from another metachronous metastasis in the adjacent vertebrae. The survival time of these patients may be relatively short, so that follow-up information is often not sufficient to interpret the response. As shown in **Table 8.3,** pain control after radiosurgery seems more durable with higher radiation doses. An updated report from the prospective Dutch Bone Metastasis Study comparing a single fraction of 8 Gy

reported a pain response rate of 87% and the duration of pain control as 17 weeks in patients surviving > 52 weeks.[24] With a single dose at 8 Gy, the initial response rate was 56% in the Radiation Therapy Oncology Group (RTOG) trial for painful bone metastases.[22] However, the retreatment rate was 18% in a 36 months' follow-up.[25] In the interim analysis of the Henry Ford Hospital phase II trial, the actuarial median duration of pain control was 13.3 months and the 1-year actuarial pain control was 84% in patients who were treated using radiosurgery doses ≥ 14 Gy.[15] There were no patients who had to have retreatment. The dose–pain control relationship needs to be explored further for both the rate and the total duration of pain control. Although the data are limited, the experiences in the literature suggest that spine radiosurgery appears to result in a higher rate of pain control and a durable pain control from spinal metastases compared with conventional external beam irradiation techniques.

Dose Prescription for Tumor Control

Tumors of the spine may be divided into two anatomical locations for purposes of radiosurgery target delineation and dose planning: paraspinal and epidural.[1,2] Although paraspinal tumors can be treated in a straightforward fashion with higher doses of radiosurgery, epidural tumors are more difficult to deal with due to their intimate location adjacent to the spinal cord or cauda equina. A dose guideline for spine radiosurgery can be derived from the experience with brain radiosurgery. However, there are a few unique differences between brain and spine radiosurgery. The RTOG guideline has been used for radiosurgery for brain metastases.[26] This guideline was developed largely based upon the spherical shape of the tumor within the brain and in part on the use of radiosurgery cone systems. Compared with tumors of the

Table 8.3 Dose Response of Pain to Single-Fraction Radiosurgery

Reference	Single Dose	Overall Pain Response (%)	Complete Response (%)	Time to Pain Relief	Duration of Pain Control
Hoskin et al[19]	8 Gy	69	39		4 months
Dutch study[20,24]	8 Gy	85		4 weeks	4 months
Royal Marsden[21]	8 Gy	78	57		
RTOG 9714[22]	8 Gy	65	15		
Gaze et al[23]	10 Gy	83	39		2.9 months
Henry Ford phase II[15]	≥ 12 Gy	60	39		
Henry Ford phase II[15]	≥ 14 Gy	82	50	2 weeks	13.3 months
Henry Ford phase II[15]	≥ 16 Gy	> 80	59		
Henry Ford phase II[15]	≥ 18 Gy	> 90			
University of Pittsburgh[14]	19 Gy* (15–22.5 Gy)	96			
University of Pittsburgh[18]	20 Gy* (15–25 Gy)	89			
University of Pittsburgh[13]	20 Gy* (17.5–25 Gy)	89			
University of Pittsburgh[17]	22 Gy	92			

* Mean dose with range in parentheses.
Abbreviation: RTOG, Radiation Therapy Oncology Group.

brain, the shape of tumors within the spine are rather irregular, and the target volumes tend to be much larger. The mean volume for spine radiosurgery target volumes is about 10 times greater than the intracranial radiosurgery targets (e.g., 32–200 cm^3 vs 3–20 cm^3). Spinal cords are usually located in the concave position of the target and often surrounded by the tumors, as shown in **Fig. 8.2.** Therefore, radiation intensity modulation is almost invariably needed. In addition, the management of radiation complication (notably radiation necrosis) is even more limited in the spinal cord than in the brain, where surgical resection of necrosis can still be used. Because of these reasons, a fractionated radiation regimen is also used. The fractionation pattern also varies in different institutions, but most of them generally follow the conventional fractional doses.[27] We used single-fraction radiosurgery for control of soft tissue tumors in the spine.

Although patient numbers are currently insufficient to show a statistically significant difference, there is a trend toward improved local tumor control when higher radiation doses are used in spine radiosurgery. It remains unclear whether tumors of different histologies exhibit different dose responses. Tumors that are relatively radiosensitive, such as non-small cell lung cancer and breast cancer, appear to have excellent local tumor control rates with a prescribed minimum dose of 16 Gy to the tumor margin. In the case of breast metastasis, the maximum dose (D_{max}) of 20 Gy provided a 100% radiographic local control rate and was well tolerated, without a single case of radiation-induced myelitis.[14] The more radioresistant tumors such as renal cell carcinoma may be more prone to failure following lower doses. In a series of 60 renal cell carcinoma spine radiosurgery cases, 6 patients failed spine radiosurgery and went on to open surgical decompression. The D_{max} was 17.5 Gy, below the mean D_{max} of 20.0 Gy for the entire cohort.[13] In a series of 36 melanoma spine metastases, all failures occurred in cases when the maximum prescribed dose was equal to or less than the mean maximum tumor dose of 22 Gy.[17]

Although there is no systematic report of spine radiosurgery specifically for epidural compression, sufficient experience has been accumulated to use radiosurgery for mild to moderate epidural compression of the spinal cord or cauda equina, both with and without neurological deficit. Obviously, in each case the overall clinical condition and degree of neurological dysfunction must be taken into consideration. In an interim analysis of a phase II study of radiosurgery in the setting of epidural compression, complete follow-up imaging studies were available in 62 cases for evaluation of radiographic tumor response. The objective tumor response rate was 93%. Radiosurgery "failure" was seen in only 11% of cases. Although there was no statistically significant difference due to the small sample size, minimum radiosurgery prescribed doses of 16 to 20 Gy achieved better tumor control than when lower doses were used. However, in some cases of epidural compression, it is more difficult to achieve a higher dose of radiation due to the close proximity of the tumor to the radiosensitive spinal cord. A more detailed analysis of radiosurgery in the setting of spinal cord compression is described in Chapter 12.

Dose Prescription for Recurrent Tumors

Spine radiosurgery is frequently employed as a "salvage therapeutic technique" when a tumor of the spine or spinal cord has progressed despite conventional external beam irradiation or an attempt of open surgical resection. For this reason, most reported clinical series of spine radiosurgery have included cases in which the lesion and surrounding structures have already received irradiation. The selection of radiosurgery dose for recurrent metastases is mainly based on the concern of the risk of spinal cord toxicity because of its exposure to prior irradiation. There is also concern of prior irradiation to other structures as well, including the esophagus, lungs, kidneys, and bowel. The radiosurgery dose is selected considering the interval from the previous radiotherapy, the target volume and shape in relationship to the position of the spinal cord, the patient's general condition, and the patient's symptoms.[28,29] Of all these factors, the most important is the time interval and total dose from prior radiation treatment.

At the Henry Ford Hospital, when the interval is > 1 year, the same dose is prescribed as for treatment-naive spine tumors as described above. If the affected vertebral level received radiation within 6 months of radiosurgery, the dose was reduced by 2 Gy, using the dose guideline of 10 Gy to the 10% partial volume of the spinal cord.[6] With this dose guideline, complete pain relief was achieved in 39%, partial pain relief in 26%, and stability in 19% of the patients. There was progression of pain in 6% despite the salvage radiosurgery. For the responding patients, pain relief was usually achieved within 10 to 14 days. In patients with neurological deficits prior to radiosurgery, complete or partial functional recovery was seen in six of eight patients (unpublished data).

At the University of Pittsburgh Medical Center, a slightly different approach is employed in the dose prescription of previously irradiated lesions. In our clinical experience, 70% of malignant cases treated with radiosurgery received prior conventional radiotherapy. Therefore, these cases represent a clear majority of the clinical experience. Rather than decreasing the maximum prescribed dose that is necessary for successful alleviation of clinical symptoms and good local tumor control, we more carefully design the treatment plan to decrease the dose to the critical structures. In some cases, this requires a longer treatment using a smaller collimator. For tumors with epidural extension that directly compresses the spinal cord, the CTV may be brought "inward" to allow for an acceptable dose to the spinal cord. Employing this technique, we have not had a single case of radiation myelitis in the series of previously irradiated tumors with acceptable clinical outcomes.

Dose Prescription for Primary Tumors of the Spine and Spinal Cord

The radiosurgery doses prescribed for primary malignant and benign tumors of the spine and spinal cord should be similar to their counterparts when such histologies occur within the cranium. Doses used to treat intracranial chordomas and acoustic neuromas are widely agreed upon. In contrast, given that these lesions represent a very small percentage of the total spine radiosurgery clinical experience and the necessary follow-up is much longer than for metastatic disease, there is much less agreement as to proper dose prescriptions. The use of fractionation in such cases is also not generally agreed upon. The fractionation pattern varies at different institutions. Despite these differences, initial clinical results are promising. At the University of Pittsburgh, 61 benign intradural tumors have been treated with single-fraction radiosurgery. Tumor histology included neurofibroma (30 cases), schwannoma (20 cases), and meningioma (11 cases). Sixteen patients had neurofibromatosis type 1, and 9 patients had neurofibromatosis type 2. The mean D_{max} was 22 Gy. This same dose is prescribed for all three histologies. This dose allowed for long-term radiographic control in 93% of cases, with a median follow-up of 28 months.[30] In the Stanford experience, the mean D_{max} in the series of 55 cases (comprising neurofibromas, schwannomas, and meningiomas) was 25 Gy, but the researchers divided their treatments into two to five fractions. This dose provided an equally excellent long-term control rate in all patients.[31] Radiosurgery for intramedullary tumors with hemangioblastomas and ependymomas with one to three fractionated doses of 18 to 25 Gy also showed encouraging radiographic results.[32] The experience of single-fraction radiosurgery for 34 primary spine tumors, including 7 intramedullary tumors, at the Henry Ford Hospital showed that the symptoms and neurological status were improved in 56% and stabilized in 28%. One-year radiographic local tumor control rate (defined as the lack of progression) was 94% after radiosurgery of 12 to 18 Gy for different histologies. Of these, complete response was seen in 26%, partial response in 26%, and stable findings in 42% (unpublished data).

◆ Conclusion

Target delineation and dose prescription are two important initial steps in spine radiosurgery treatment. There are several significant differences in target delineation for intracranial and spine tumors. The CTV and the GTV are currently being defined somewhat differently at different spine radiosurgery centers. However, including in the CTV part of the normal-appearing vertebral body outside the GTV is probably prudent. Such target delineation has translated into excellent clinical outcomes. An ideal dose prescription for spine radiosurgery has likewise not been defined. It has yet to be determined if tumor response is relatively independent of histology, as has been demonstrated to be the case for intracranial radiosurgery. A radiosurgery dose response rate by tumor histology may have more to do with the patterns of microscopic local tumor invasion than with radiobiological sensitivity. With reported overall clinical tumor response rates of > 90% from different centers using different delivery technologies, it will be difficult to define the ideal dose without a large cooperative trial. The recommendations of dose prescriptions presented in this chapter appear to provide good clinical response with minimal risk of long-term radiation-induced complications.

References

1. Tong D, Gillick L, Hendrickson FR. The palliation of symptomatic osseous metastasis: final results of the study by the Radiation Therapy Oncology Group. Cancer 1982;50:893–899.
2. Loblaw DA, Laperriere NJ. Emergency treatment of malignant extradural spinal cord compression: an evidence-based guideline. J Clin Oncol 1998;16:1613–1624.
3. Siegal T, Siegal T. Surgical decompression of anterior and posterior malignant epidural tumors compressing the spinal cord: a prospective study. Neurosurgery 1985;17:424–432.
4. Patchell RA, Tibbs PA, Regine WF, et al. Direct decompressive surgical resection in the treatment of spinal cord compression caused by metastatic cancer: a randomised trial. Lancet 2005;21:1–6.
5. Chow E, Harris K, Fung K. Successful validation of survival prediction model in patients with metastases in the spinal column. Int J Radiat Oncol Biol Phys 2006;65:1522–1527.
6. Ryu S, Jin JJ, Jin RY, et al. Partial volume tolerance of spinal cord and complication of single dose radiosurgery. Cancer 2007;109:628–636.
7. Kondziolka D, Martin J, Flickinger J, et al. Long term survivors after gamma knife radiosurgery for brain metastases. Cancer 2005;104:2784–2791.
8. Rock J, Ryu S, Shukairy MS, et al. Postoperative stereotactic radiosurgery for malignant spinal tumors. Neurosurgery 2006;58:891–898.
9. Gerszten PC, Germanwala A, Burton SA, et al. Combination kyphoplasty and spinal radiosurgery: a new treatment paradigm for pathologic fractures. J Neurosurg Spine 2005;3:296–301.
10. Singletary SE, Larry L, Tucker SL, Spitzer G. Detection of micrometastatic tumor cells in bone marrow of breast carcinoma patients. J Surg Oncol 1991;47:32–36.
11. Weiss L. Dynamic aspects of cancer cell populations in metastasis. Am J Pathol 1979;97:601–608.
12. Ryu S, Rock J, Rosenblum M, Kim JH. Pattern of failure after single dose radiosurgery for single spinal metastasis. J Neurosurg 2004;101:402–405.
13. Gerszten PC, Burton SA, Ozhasoglu C, et al. Stereotactic radiosurgery for spine metastases from renal cell carcinoma. J Neurosurg Spine 2005;3(4):288–295.
14. Gerszten PC, Burton SA, Welch WC, et al. Single fraction radiosurgery for the treatment of breast metastases. Cancer 2005;14(10):2244–2254.
15. Ryu S, Jin R, Jin JY, et al. Pain control by image-guided radiosurgery for solitary spinal metastasis. J Pain Symptom Manage 2008;35:292–298.
16. Wu JS, Wong JR, Johnson M, Bezjak A, Whelan T. Cancer Care Ontario Practice Guidelines Initiative Supportive Care Group. Meta-analysis of dose-fractionation radiotherapy trials for the palliation of painful bone metastases. Int J Radiat Oncol Biol Phys 2003;55:594–605.
17. Gerszten PC, Burton SA, Quinn AE, Agarwala SS, Kirkwood JM. Single fraction radiosurgery for the treatment of spinal melanoma metastases. Stereotact Funct Neurosurg 2006;83:213–221.
18. Gerszten PC, Burton SA, Belani CP, et al. Radiosurgery for the treatment of spinal lung metastases. Cancer 2006;107:2653–2661.
19. Hoskin P, Price P, Easton D, et al. A prospective randomised trial of 4 Gy or 8 Gy single doses in the treatment of metastatic bone pain. Radiother Oncol 1992;23:74–78.
20. Steenland ES, Leer J, van Houwelingen H, et al. The effect of a single fraction to multiple fractions on painful bone metastases: a global analysis of the Dutch Bone Metastasis Study. Radiother Oncol 1999;52:101–109.
21. Bone Pain Trial Working Party. 8 Gy single fraction radiotherapy for the treatment of metastatic skeletal pain: randomized comparison with a multifraction schedule over 12 months of patient follow-up. Radiother Oncol 1999;52:111–121.
22. Hartsell WF, Scott CB, Bruner DW, et al. Randomized trial of short- versus long-course radiotherapy for palliation of painful bone metastases. J Natl Cancer Inst 2005;97:798–804.
23. Gaze MN, Kelly CG, Kerr GR, et al. Pain relief and quality of life following radiotherapy for bone metastases: a randomised trial of two fractionation schedules. Radiother Oncol 1997;45:109–116.
24. Linden YM, Steenland E, van Houwelingen HC, et al. Patients with a favourable prognosis are equally palliated with single and multiple fraction radiotherapy: results on survival in the Dutch Bone Metastasis Study. Radiother Oncol 2006;78:245–253.
25. Konski A, DeSilvio M, Hartsell W, et al. Continuing evidence for poorer treatment outcomes for single male patients: retreatment data from RTOG 97-14. Int J Radiat Oncol Biol Phys 2006;66:229–233.

26. Shaw E, Scott C, Souhami L, et al. Radiosurgery for the treatment of previously irradiated recurrent primary brain tumors and brain metastases: initial report of radiation therapy oncology group protocol 90–05. Int J Radiat Oncol Biol Phys 1996;34:647–654.

27. Bilsky MH, Yamada Y, Yenice KM, et al. Intensity-modulated stereotactic radiosrugery of paraspinal tumors: preliminary report. Neurosurgery 2004;54:823–830.

28. Ryu S, Gorty S, Kazee AM, et al. "Full dose" re-irradiation of human cervical spinal cord. Am J Clin Oncol 2000;23:29–31.

29. Ang KK. Radiation injury to the central nervous system: clinical features and prevention. Front Radiat Ther Oncol 1999;32:145–154.

30. Gerszten PC, Ozhasoglu C, Burton SA, et al. CyberKnife frameless single-fraction stereotactic radiosurgery for benign tumors of the spine. Neurosurg Focus 2003;14(5):E16. AQ3

31. Dodd RL, Ryu MR, Kamnerdsupaphon P, et al. CyberKnife radiosurgery for benign intradural extramedullary spinal tumors. Neurosurgery 2006;58:674–685.

32. Ryu SI, Kim DH, Chang SD. Stereotactic radiosurgery for hemangiomas and ependymomas of the spinal cord. Neurosurg Focus 2003;15(5):E10.

9

Radiosurgery of Spinal Metastases

Peter C. Gerszten and Steven A. Burton

Standard treatment options for spinal metastases include radiotherapy alone, radionuclide therapy, radiotherapy plus systemic chemotherapy, hormonal therapy, or surgical decompression and/or stabilization followed by radiotherapy.[1] The role of radiation therapy in the treatment of metastatic tumors of the spine is well established and is often the initial treatment modality.[1-7] The goals of local radiation therapy in the treatment of spinal tumors have been palliation of pain, prevention of local disease progression and subsequent pathologic fractures, and stoppage of progression or reversal of neurological compromise.[8] Patients with metastatic spine tumors are often debilitated and at a high risk for surgical morbidity.[9] For patients with limited life expectancies from their underlying disease, high surgical complication rates with subsequent decrease in quality of life are most unacceptable.

The primary factor that limits radiation dose for local vertebral tumor control with conventional radiotherapy is the relatively low tolerance of the spinal cord to radiation. Conventional external beam radiotherapy lacks the precision to deliver large single-fraction doses of radiation to the spine near radiosensitive structures such as the spinal cord. It is the low tolerance of the spinal cord to radiation that often limits the treatment dose to a level that is far below the optimal therapeutic dose.[2,10,11] Radiotherapy may provide a less than optimal clinical response because the total dose is limited by the tolerance of the spinal cord. Precise confinement of the radiation dose to the treatment volume, as is the case for intracranial radiosurgery, should increase the likelihood of successful tumor control and clinical response at the same time that the risk of spinal cord injury is minimized.[11-19]

The idea of single-fraction radiotherapy for symptomatic bone metastases is not new. During the past 2 decades, several clinical trials have compared the relative efficacy of various dose-fractionation schedules in producing pain relief for symptomatic bone metastases.[20-25] Studies have previously determined the clinical efficacy of single-fraction therapy for painful bone metastases.[26] Both a Radiation Therapy Oncology Group (RTOG) phase III trial and a meta-analysis found no significant difference in complete and overall pain relief between single-fraction and multifraction palliative radiation therapy for bone metastases.[20,26] Most of these trials used 8 Gy in a single fraction. However, none of these trials were specifically evaluating spinal metastases.

Stereotactic radiosurgery has been shown to be very effective in controlling intracranial metastases, independent of histology.[27-33] Radiosurgery has been demonstrated to be an effective treatment for brain metastases, either with or without whole-brain radiation therapy, with an 85 to 95% control rate. The emerging technique of spine radiosurgery represents a logical extension of the current state-of-the-art radiation therapy. Stereotactic radiosurgery for tumors of the spine has more recently been demonstrated to be accurate, safe, and efficacious.[11,14,15,17-19,34-39] Since Hamilton et al[36] first described the possibility of linear accelerator–based spinal stereotactic radiosurgery in 1995 for spinal metastases, multiple centers have attempted to pursue large fraction conformal radiation delivery to spinal lesions using a variety of technologies.[11,14-19,34-42] Researchers have shown the feasibility and clinical efficacy of spinal hypofractionated stereotactic body radiotherapy for metastases.[11,13-19,43] Others have demonstrated the effectiveness of protons for spinal and paraspinal tumors.[44] There has been a rapid increase in the use of radiosurgery as a treatment alternative for malignant tumors involving the spine. Recent technological developments, including imaging technology for three-dimensional localization and pretreatment planning, the advent of intensity-modulated radiation therapy (IMRT), and a higher degree of accuracy in achieving target dose conformation while sparing normal surrounding tissue, have allowed clinicians to expand radiosurgery applications to treat malignant vertebral body lesions within close proximity of the spinal cord and cauda equina.

Overview of Spine Radiosurgery Treatment for Metastases

The spine radiosurgery procedure can be divided into four distinct components: immobilization and/or fiducial implantation,[1] computed tomography (CT) imaging for treatment planning and generation of digitally reconstructed radiographs (DRRs),[2] treatment planning,[3] and dose delivery.[4] Spine radiosurgery may be performed entirely in an outpatient setting. The patient is placed in a supine position in a conformal alpha cradle during CT imaging as well as during treatment. CT images are acquired using 1.25 mm slices to include the lesion of interest as well as all fiducials or necessary bony landmarks. Planning CT images may be acquired using the addition of intravenous (IV) contrast enhancement. However, contrast is often not necessary for lesions that are completely within the bony elements. In fact, bony windowing is often more helpful for lesion localization and treatment planning than soft tissue windowing for many spinal lesions. For patients with allergies to IV contrast or renal function that precludes contrast, nonenhanced CT imaging is performed with little difficulty in determining precise lesion anatomy.

Each spinal radiosurgical treatment plan is devised jointly by a team comprising a neurosurgeon, a radiation oncologist, and a medical physicist. In each case, the radiosurgical treatment plan is designed based on tumor geometry, proximity to the spinal cord or cauda equina and other critical structures, and location within the spinal column. The lesion is outlined based on CT imaging or from a magnetic resonance (MR) fusion capability. In our series of the first 625 patients with spinal metastases, the mean tumor volume was 46 cc (range 0.20–264.0 cc). This is more than 10 times the average volume of intracranial lesions treated using radiosurgery at our institution, the University of Pittsburgh Medical Center.

Dose Prescriptions

The tumor dose is determined based on the histology of the tumor, spinal cord or cauda equina tolerance, and previous radiation quantity to normal tissue, especially the spinal cord. There is no large experience to date with spine radiosurgery or hypofractionated radiotherapy that has previously developed optimal doses for these treatment techniques. Other centers, employing intensity-modulated, near-simultaneous, CT image–guided stereotactic radiotherapy techniques, have used doses of 6 to 30 Gy in one to five fractions.[15,16,19,45–47] We initially chose to use a single-fraction radiosurgery technique as opposed to fractionate therapy because of our experience with intracranial radiosurgery principles using the Leksell Gamma Knife (Elekta AB, Stockholm, Sweden). Given the good clinical response as well as the lack of adverse consequences to normal tissue, including the spinal cord, we have continued to employ a single-fraction treatment paradigm for our spine radiosurgery program.

In our series, maximum tumor dose was maintained at 12.5 to 22.5 Gy delivered in a single fraction (mean 20 Gy).[48] The appropriate dose or fractionation schedule for spine radiosurgery for metastatic tumors has not been determined. At our institution, the tumor dose is prescribed to the 80% isodose line. A maximum tumor dose of 20 Gy, or 16 Gy to the tumor margin, appears to provide a good tumor control with no radiation-induced spinal cord or cauda equina injury. Spine radiosurgery was found to be safe at doses comparable to those used for intracranial radiosurgery without the occurrence of radiation-induced neural injury. In our experience with spinal metastases, there has been no clinically or radiographically identifiable acute or subacute spinal cord damage attributed to the radiation dose with a follow-up period long enough to have seen such events were they to occur.[3,49–54]

Dose and fractionation schedules differ by institution. The Memorial Sloan-Kettering group used a maximum dose of 20 Gy delivered in five fractions.[15,47] The Georgetown group used a mean dose of 21 Gy in three fractions.[55] The MD Anderson group used 30 Gy in five fractions.[12,16] The Henry Ford Hospital group used a 6 to 8 Gy boost after conventional irradiation (25 Gy in 10 fractions).[19] Finally, De Salles et al reported a mean dose of 12 Gy.[17]

There is little experience regarding the tolerance of the human spinal cord to single-fraction doses, and the tolerance of the spinal cord to a single dose of radiation has not been well defined.[19,56] Spinal cord tolerance related to IMRT techniques has also not yet been addressed. Therefore, one must still rely on clinical data derived from external beam irradiation series in which the entire thickness of the spinal cord was irradiated. Radiation-induced spinal cord injury, or myelitis, is one of the most dreaded complications related to spine radiosurgery. The true tolerance of the human spinal cord to radiation is not known. The TD 5/5 (the dose at which there is a 5% probability of myelitis necrosis at 5 years from treatment) for 5, 10, and 20 cm lengths of the spinal cord in standard fractionation has been estimated by Emami et al as 5.0, 5.0, and 4.7 Gy, respectively.[57] These dose levels are estimates based on extrapolations of datasets that date back to 1948. These estimations have been widely adopted in clinical practice. To minimize the risk of spinal cord necrosis, the radiation tolerance with standard fractionation traditionally has been stated to be 45 to 50 Gy. A dose of 45 to 50 Gy in standard fractionation (1.8–2.0 Gy per fraction) is well within the radiation tolerance of the spinal cord (TD 5/5); 8 Gy in a single fraction delivered to a long segment of the spinal cord has been given without reported myelopathy.[58]

In a review of 172 patients treated with fractionated radiotherapy to the cervical and thoracic spine at the University of California, San Francisco (total dose of 40–70 Gy fractionated over a 2- to 3-week period), Wara et al reported nine cases of radiation-induced myelopathy.[54] Three out of nine patients had mild cervical cord neurological deficits without any significant long-term symptoms. The length of the spinal cord that was exposed to radiation ranged from 4 to 22 cm. Hatlevoll et al reported a series of 387 patients with bronchial carcinoma treated with a split-course regimen using large single fractions.[51] Seventeen patients developed radiation myelitis with an average total dose of 38 Gy. Kim and Fayos reported 7 patients with transverse myelopathy from a group of 109 patients treated with definitive radiotherapy for head and neck cancers to a total dose of 57 to 62 Gy with an average field size of 10 × 10 cm.[3] Abbatucci et al reported 8 (of 203) cases of radiation-induced myelopathy with a total radiation dose of 54 to 60 Gy to the cervical and thoracic spine.[49] McCunniff and Liang reported only 1 case of radiation myelopathy out of 652 patients who had received > 60 Gy using standard fractionation.[52] Phillips and Buschke reported 3 cases of transverse myelitis in 350 patients treated with tumors to the chest to a total radiation dose of 33.0 to 43.5 Gy.[53]

For each spine radiosurgery case, the spinal cord or cauda equina is outlined as a critical structure. At the level of the cauda equina, the spinal canal is outlined. Therefore, at the level of the cauda equina, the critical volume is the entire spinal canal and not actual neural tissue. A limit of 8 Gy is set as the maximum spinal cord dose for treatment planning calculations. For the cauda equina, this limit is raised to 10 Gy. A limit of 2 Gy is set as the maximum dose to each of the kidneys. A limit of 8 Gy is set as the maximum dose to the bowel. This becomes important in the treatment of lower thoracic and lumbar vertebral lesions, even more so if the patient has undergone a nephrectomy or received nephrotoxic chemotherapy.

◆ Spine Radiosurgery Indications and Clinical Outcomes

The spine radiosurgery program at the University of Pittsburgh Medical Center began in 2001 with the implementation of extracranial image-guided radiosurgery technology. Our institution's experience currently represents the largest spine radiosurgery series in the world.[59–62] This new modality was initially introduced into the treatment paradigm for spinal tumors to a subset of the center's oncology patient population who did not meet the criteria for other forms of therapy, including conventional radiotherapy and the latest in open surgical techniques. The indications for spine radiosurgery at the center have evolved over time and will continue to evolve as clinical experience increases. This is similar to the evolution of indications for intracranial radiosurgery that occurred in the past.

Table 9.1 summarizes the candidate lesions for spine radiosurgery. **Table 9.2** lists the current indications for radiosurgery for spinal metastases. **Table 9.3** summarizes the characteristics of our first 625 patients treated with a single-fraction radiosurgery technique. Ages ranged from 18 to 85 years (mean 56 years). The most common metastatic tumors (in descending order of frequency) were renal cell, breast, lung, colon, and melanoma. These five histopathologies represent over 60% of our total metastatic cases. **Table 9.4** presents the long-term pain improvement and long-term radiographic control rates for the four most common histopathologies.[48] **Figures 9.1** to **9.3** demonstrate several examples of spine radiosurgery used in clinical practice.

Table 9.1 Candidate Lesions for Spine Radiosurgery

Well-circumscribed lesions
Minimal spinal cord compromise
Radioresistant lesions that would benefit from a radiosurgical boost
Residual tumor after surgery
Previously irradiated lesions precluding further external beam irradiation
Recurrent surgical lesions
Lesions requiring difficult surgical approaches
Relatively short life expectancy as an exclusion criterion for open surgical intervention
Significant medical comorbidities precluding open surgical intervention
Lesions not requiring open spinal stabilization techniques

Table 9.2 Indications for Radiosurgery for Spinal Metastases

Pain
Primary treatment modality
Prevention of tumor progression
Radiation boost
Progressive neurologic deficit
Residual tumor after surgery
Postsurgical treatment of residual disease
Postsurgical tumor progression

Table 9.3 Characteristics of the University of Pittsburgh Medical Center Experience for Spine Metastases (N = 625)

Characteristic number of cases
  Previous external beam irradiation: 422
Primary indications for radiosurgery treatment
  Pain: 395
  Primary treatment modality: 96
  Tumor progression: 66
  Progressive neurologic deficit: 42
  Postsurgical treatment: 19
  Radiation boost: 7
Level treated
  Cervical: 84
  Thoracic: 262
  Lumbar: 145
  Sacral: 134
Tumor and dose characteristics
  Mean tumor volume: 46 cm³ (range 0.20–264.0 cm3)
  Median tumor volume: 29 cm³
  Mean maximum dose: 20 Gy (range 12.5–25 Gy)
  Mean volume of spinal canal dose > 8 Gy: 0.6 cm³

Table 9.4 Summary of the University of Pittsburgh Medical Center Experience for Pain and Radiographic Outcome for the Four Most Common Histopathologies (N = 337)

Histopathology	Long-term Pain Improvement (%)	Long-term Radiographic Control (%)
All patients	86	88
Renal cell	94	87
Breast	96	100
Lung	93	100
Melanoma	96	75

Pain

The most frequent indication for the treatment of spinal tumors is pain, and pain was the primary indication for spine radiosurgery in 70% of our cases. Radiation is well known to be effective as a treatment for pain associated with spinal malignancies. Conventional external beam irradiation may provide less than optimal pain relief because the total dose is limited by the tolerance of adjacent tissues (e.g., the spinal cord). Spine radiosurgery was found to be highly effective at decreasing pain in this difficult patient population, with an overall long-term improvement of pain in 374 of the 435 cases (86%), depending on the primary histopathology (**Table 9.4**). Long-term pain improvement was demonstrated in 96% of women with breast cancer, 96% of patients with melanoma, 94% of patients with renal cell carcinoma, and 93% of lung cancer cases.[59-61] Pain usually decreases within weeks after treatment, and occasionally within days. Spine radiosurgery is also effective at alleviating radicular pain caused by tumor compression of adjacent nerve roots. In some cases, post-treatment imaging revealed pathologic fractures, likely the cause of pain and the reason for radiosurgical failure. Such fractures require either open or closed internal fixation to alleviate the pain due to spinal instability.

The most thorough published work to date on pain control and quality of life improvement after spine radiosurgery has been from Georgetown University Hospital.[55] Using visual analog scales (VASs) for pain assessment and the 12-item Short Form Health Survey (SF-12), radiosurgery was demonstrated to statistically improve pain control and maintain quality of life with follow-up to 24 months. Early adverse events in the researchers' experience were infrequent and minor. The Memorial Sloan-Kettering group demonstrated a 90% excellent palliation of symptoms, with a median

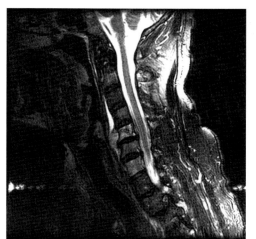

A

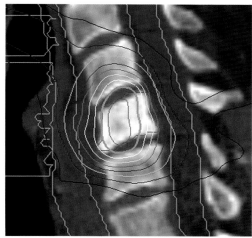

B

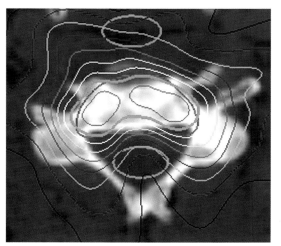

C

Figure 9.1 A 50-year-old man who presented with pain due to a right apical lung tumor. His initial treatment included chemotherapy and local irradiation. His cervical spine was treated previously with 30 Gy in 10 fractions, with temporary improvement of neck pain without radiculopathy for 3 months. Because of the recurrence of symptoms, he was referred for spine radiosurgery. **(A)** Gadolinium-enhanced sagittal magnetic resonance imaging revealed a destructive lesion of the C5 vertebra without significant spinal canal compromise. Sagittal **(B)** and axial **(C)** projections of the isodose lines of the treatment plan. The 80% isodose line represents the prescribed dose of 16 Gy, the tumor volume was 7.7 cm³, and the spinal cord received a maximum point dose of 8 Gy. The patient reported complete pain relief within 1 month.

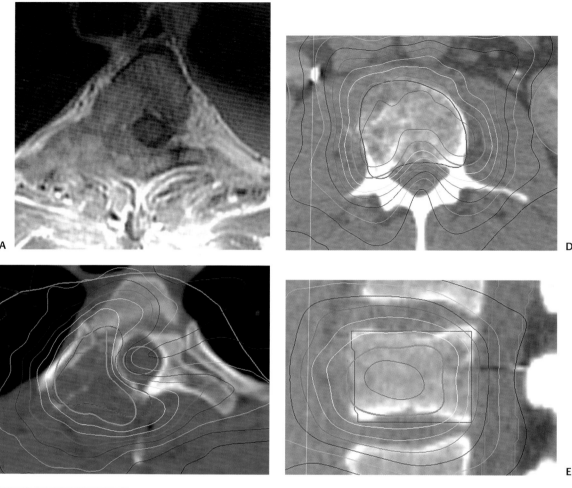

A

B

D

E

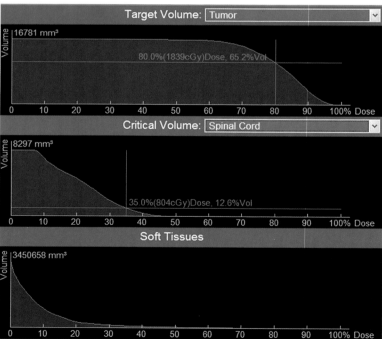

Target Volume: Tumor

16781 mm³

80.0%(1839cGy)Dose, 65.2%Vol

0   10   20   30   40   50   60   70   80   90   100% Dose

Critical Volume: Spinal Cord

8297 mm³

35.0%(804cGy)Dose, 12.6%Vol

0   10   20   30   40   50   60   70   80   90   100% Dose

Soft Tissues

3450658 mm³

0   10   20   30   40   50   60   70   80   90   100% Dose

C

Figure 9.2 **(A)** A 42-year-old man had painful melanoma metastases of the T3 and L2 vertebral bodies. He had not received prior irradiation to either lesion. The treatment plans were designed to treat the tumor with a prescribed dose of 18 Gy that was calculated to the 80% isodose line; the maximum tumor dose was 22.5 Gy. **(B)** For the T3 lesion, the tumor volume was 16.8 cm³, and the spinal cord received a maximum dose of 10 Gy (bold red line = contoured tumor; light orange line = 80% isodose line; yellow line = 60% isodose line; dark purple line = 40% isodose line at the edge of the spinal cord thecal sac). **(C)** The dose-volume histogram. There is conformality of the isodose line around the spinal cord. **(D,E)** For the L2 lesion, the tumor volume was 46.5 cm³, and the cauda equina received a maximum dose of 10 Gy. The patient experienced complete pain relief from both lesions within 2 weeks of treatment.

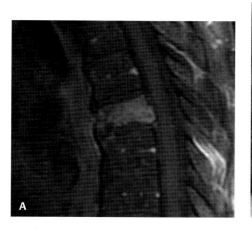 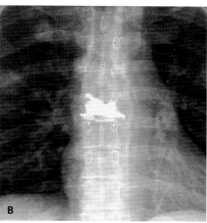 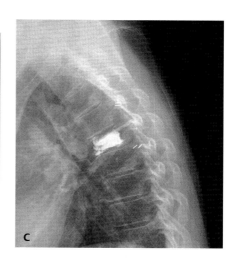

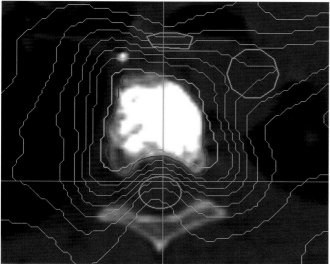

Figure 9.3 **(A)** Gadolinium-enhanced axial magnetic resonance image obtained in a 57-year-old woman with metastatic renal cell carcinoma, revealing an isolated symptomatic T6 pathologic compression fracture. A percutaneous kyphoplasty procedure was performed to allow for immediate stabilization of the painful fracture. **(B,C)** Anteroposterior and lateral plane radiographs revealing the methylmethacrylate placed during kyphoplasty. The four gold fiducial markers that allow for image guidance can be seen in the pedicles of T5 and T7. **(D,E)** Axial and sagittal projections of the isodose lines of the treatment plan. The 80% isodose line represents the prescribed dose of 18 Gy, the tumor volume is 17.9 cm³, and 0.02 cm³ of the spinal cord received > 8 Gy.

follow-up of 12 months.[47] Other series reported similar pain improvement results.[11,14,16–19,63]

Radiographic Tumor Progression

Spine radiosurgery is frequently used to treat radiographic tumor progression after the failure of conventional irradiation treatment. Most of these lesions have received irradiation with significant spinal cord doses, precluding further conventional irradiation delivery. Spine radiosurgery is frequently employed to treat lesions that have previously been treated with other forms of irradiation. The ideal lesion should be well circumscribed so that the lesion can be easily outlined (contoured) for treatment planning. In our series,[25]

overall long-term radiographic tumor control was 88% for all cases (**Table 9.4**). Radiographic tumor control differed based on primary pathology: breast (100%), lung (100%), renal cell (87%), and melanoma (75%). Yamada et al reported a 90% long-term radiographic control rate.[47] Similar radiographic control rates have been reported by others.[11,15–17,46,55]

Currently, spine radiosurgery is often employed as a "salvage" technique for those cases in which further conventional irradiation or surgery is not appropriate. As greater experience is gained, the technique will likely evolve into an initial upfront treatment for spinal metastases in certain cases (e.g., oligometastases). This is similar to the evolution that occurred over the past decade in the treatment of intracranial metastases using radiosurgery.

Primary Treatment Modality or Boost

In our series, 96 patients underwent spine radiosurgery as their primary treatment modality (meaning no prior irradiation to the lesion). Many of these lesions were in the same patient already being treated for a symptomatic lesion. The second asymptomatic lesion was treated with radiosurgery to avoid further irradiation to the neural elements as well as to avoid further bone marrow suppression. The benefits for this treatment option include a single treatment with minimal radiation dose to adjacent normal tissue. In addition, a much larger radiobiologic dose can often be delivered compared with external beam irradiation. When used as a primary treatment modality, long-term tumor control was demonstrated on follow-up imaging in 90% of cases (in all breast, lung, and renal cell carcinoma metastases and 75% of melanoma metastases).[59,60] Degen et al reported a 100% tumor control rate in lesions that had not previously undergone irradiation.[55] Radioresistant tumors (e.g., renal cell carcinoma, melanoma, sarcoma) may be treated with spine radiosurgery after conventional irradiation with or without IMRT for a boost treatment with equal long-term radiographic control. Ryu et al found this to be a highly effective treatment paradigm.[19,47]

Progressive Neurological Deficit

Spine radiosurgery may be used to treat patients with progressive neurological deficits when open surgical intervention is felt to be contraindicated. In most of these cases, conventional irradiation has already been delivered to the symptomatic spinal lesion. In our series, 36 of 42 patients (86%) with a progressive neurological deficit prior to treatment experienced at least some clinical improvement. In most of these cases, open surgical decompression was precluded because of medical comorbidities. Yamada et al reported 90 and 92% palliation of symptoms in patients treated for weakness and paresthesias, respectively.[47] Degen et al reported neurological deficits improved in 16 patients, were unchanged in 24 patients, and worsened in 11 patients in their series.[55]

After Open Surgery

If a tumor is only partially resected during an open surgery, radiosurgery may be used to treat the residual tumor at a later date. The spinal tumors can be removed away from neural structures, allowing for immediate decompression, the spine can be instrumented if necessary, and the residual tumor can be safely treated at a later date with radiosurgery, thus further decreasing surgical morbidity. Anterior corpectomy procedures in certain cases can be successfully avoided by posterior decompression and instrumentation alone followed by radiosurgery to the remaining anterior lesion. With the ability to effectively perform spine radiosurgery, the current surgical approach to these lesions might change. Given the steep fall-off gradient of the target dose, such treatments can be given early in the postoperative period as opposed to the usually significant delay before standard external beam irradiation is permitted. Open surgery for spinal metastases

will likely evolve in such a way as to avoid neurological deficits and minimize surgical morbidity.

Rock et al specifically evaluated the combination of open surgical procedure with adjuvant radiosurgery.[64] They found this to be a successful treatment paradigm that was associated with a significant chance of stabilizing or improving neurological function. The technique was well tolerated and associated with little to no morbidity.[64] Our experience with radiosurgery combined with open surgery has found it to be safe and highly successful in the treatment of the residual tumor bed.

◆ Contraindications to and Complications Associated with Spine Radiosurgery

There are several relative contraindications to spine radiosurgery. These include evidence of overt spinal instability,[1] neurological deficit resulting from bony compression of neural structures,[2] and previous radiation treatment to spinal cord tolerance dose.[3] With time and further clinical experience, these contraindications will be better understood and defined.

With a follow-up of > 60 months, there have been no clinically detectable neurological signs that could be attributable to the acute or subacute radiation-induced spinal cord injury in our series of metastatic spinal lesions. Post-treatment MR images failed to reveal any changes suggestive of radiation-induced spinal cord toxicity. Complications associated with radiosurgery are generally self-limited and mild. Potential complications include transient esophagitis, dysphagia, paresthesias, diarrhea, and a temporary flare-up of tumor-related pain. One concern that has been raised regarding radiosurgery for spinal metastases is that adjacent levels are not included in the radiation field. One possibility is that the tumor can progress within the adjacent levels. In our series, there were no cases of tumor progression at the immediate adjacent levels, justifying the treatment of the involved spine only. Other authors have also found this not to be the case.[38]

◆ Advantages of Radiosurgery for Spinal Metastases

Further experience with spine radiosurgery and careful patient follow-up will better define the clinical efficacy of this new treatment modality. There are several theoretical advantages to using a stereotactic radiosurgery technique as a primary treatment modality for spinal tumors. Early treatment of these lesions prior to the patient's becoming symptomatic and the stability of the spine threatened has obvious advantages.[17] Conformal radiosurgery avoids the need to irradiate large segments of the spinal cord. Early stereotactic radiosurgery treatment of spinal lesions may obviate the need for extensive spinal surgeries for decompression and fixation in these already debilitated patients. It may also avoid the need to irradiate large segments of the spinal column, known to have a deleterious effect on bone marrow reserve in these patients. Avoiding open surgery as well as preserving bone marrow function facilitates continuous chemotherapy in this patient population. Furthermore, improved local control such as has been the case with intracranial radiosurgery could translate into more effective palliation and potentially longer survival.

An advantage to the patient of using single-fraction radiosurgery is that the treatment can be completed in a single day rather than over the course of several weeks, which is not inconsequential for patients with a limited life expectancy. The technique may be useful to capitalize on possible advantages of radiosensitizers. In addition, cancer patients may have difficulty with access to a radiation treatment facility for prolonged, daily fractionated therapy. A large single fraction of irradiation may be more radiobiologically advantageous to certain tumors such as sarcomas, melanomas, and renal cell metastases compared with prolonged fractionated radiotherapy. Clinical response such as pain or improvement of a neurological deficit may also be more rapid with a radiosurgery technique. Finally, the procedure is minimally invasive compared with open surgical techniques and can be performed in an outpatient setting.

◆ Conclusion

Spine radiosurgery is now feasible, safe, and clinically effective for the treatment of metastatic spinal tumors. It represents a logical extension of the current state-of-the-art radiation therapy. Furthermore, it has the potential to significantly improve local control of cancer of the spine, which could translate into better palliation. Another advantage to the patient is that irradiation can be completed in a single day rather than over several weeks, something that is not inconsequential for patients with a limited life expectancy. In addition, cancer patients may have difficulty with access to a radiation treatment facility for prolonged, daily fractionated therapy. The major potential benefits of radiosurgical ablation of spinal lesions are relatively short treatment time in an outpatient setting combined with potentially better local control of the tumor with minimal risk of side effects. Spine radiosurgery offers a new and important alternative therapeutic modality for the treatment of spinal metastases in medically inoperable patients, previously irradiated sites, and for lesions not amenable to open surgical techniques or as an adjunct to surgery.

References

1. Gerszten PC, Welch WC. Current surgical management of metastatic spinal disease. Oncology 2001;14:1013–1024.
2. Faul CM, Flickinger JC. The use of radiation in the management of spinal metastases. J Neurooncol 1995;23:149–161.
3. Kim YH, Fayos JV. Radiation tolerance of the cervical spinal cord. Radiology 1981;139:473–478.
4. Markoe AM, Schwade JG. The role of radiation therapy in the management of spine and spinal cord tumors. In: Rea GL, ed. Spine Tumors. Rolling Meadows, IL: American Association of Neurological Surgeons; 1994:23–35.
5. Shapiro W, Posner JB. Medical vs surgical treatment of metastatic spinal cord tumors. In: Thompson R, ed. Controversies in Neurology. New York: Raven Press; 1983:57–65.
6. Sundaresan N, Krol G, Digiacinto CV, Hughes J. Metastatic tumors of the spine. In: Sundaresan B, Schiller AL, Rosenthal DL, eds. Tumors of the Spine. Philadelphia: WB Saunders; 1990:279–304.
7. Sundaresan N, Digiacinto GV, Hughes J, Cafferty M, Vallejo A. Treatment of neoplastic spinal cord compression: results of a prospective study. Neurosurgery 1991;29:645–650.
8. Lu C, Stomper PC, Drislane FW, et al. Suspected spinal cord compression in breast cancer patients: a multidisciplinary risk assessment. Breast Cancer Res Treat 1998;51:121–131.
9. Vitaz TW, Oishi M, Welch WC, Gerszten PC, Disa JJ, Bilsky MH. Rotational and transpositional flaps for the treatment of spinal wound dehiscence and infections in patient populations with degenerative and oncological disease. J Neurosurg 2004;100:46–51.
10. Loblaw DA, Laperriere NJ. Emergency treatment of malignant extradural spinal cord compression: an evidence-based guideline. J Clin Oncol 1998;16:1613–1624.
11. Ryu SI, Chang S, Kim D, et al. Image-guided hypo-fractionated stereotactic radiosurgery to spinal lesions. Neurosurgery 2001;49:838–846.
12. Shiu AS, Chang EL, Ye J-S. Near simultaneous computed tomography image-guided stereotactic spinal radiotherapy: an emerging paradigm for achieving true stereotaxy. Int J Radiat Oncol Biol Phys 2003;57:605–613
13. Amendola BE, Wolf A, Coy S, Amendola M, Bloch L. Gamma knife radiosurgery in the treatment of patients with single and multiple brain metastases from carcinoma of the breast. Cancer J 2000;6:88–92.
14. Benzil DL, Saboori M, Mogilner AY, Rochio R, Moorthy CR. Safety and efficacy of stereotactic radiosurgery for tumors of the spine. J Neurosurg 2004;101:413–418.
15. Bilsky MH, Yamada Y, Yenice KM, et al. Intensity-modulated stereotactic radiotherapy of paraspinal tumors: a preliminary report. Neurosurgery 2004;54:823–830.
16. Chang EL, Shiu AS, Lii M-F, et al. Phase I clinical evaluation of near-simultaneous computed tomographic image-guided stereotactic body radiotherapy for spinal metastases. Int J Radiat Oncol Biol Phys 2004;59:1288–1294.
17. De Salles AA, Pedroso A, Medin P, et al. Spinal lesions treated with Novalis shaped beam intensity-modulated radiosurgery and stereotactic radiotherapy. J Neurosurg 2004;101:435–440.
18. Milker-Zabel S, Zabel A, Thilmann C, et al. Clinical results of retreatment of vertebral bone metastases by stereotactic conformal radiotherapy and intensity-modulated radiotherapy. Int J Radiat Oncol Biol Phys 2003;55:162–167.
19. Ryu S, Yin FF, Rock J, et al. Image-guided and intensity-modulated radiosurgery for patients with spinal metastasis. Cancer 2003;97:2013–2018.
20. Wu JK, Wong R, Johnston M, Bezjak A, Whelan T. Meta-analysis of dose-fractionated radiotherapy trials for the palliation of painful bone metastases. Int J Radiat Oncol Biol Phys 2003;55:594–605.
21. Rades D, Fehlauer F, Stalpers L, et al. A prospective evaluation of two radiotherapy schedules with 10 versus 20 fractions for the treatment of metastatic spinal cord compression: final results of a multicenter study. Cancer 2004;101:2687–2692.
22. Rades D, Stalpers LJ, Veninga T, et al. Evaluation of five radiation schedules and prognostic factors for metastatic spinal cord compression. J Clin Oncol 2005;23:3366–3375.
23. Maranzano E, Latini P, Perrucci E, et al. Short course radiotherapy (8 Gy × 2) in metastatic spinal cord compression: An effective and feasible treatment. Int J Radiat Oncol Biol Phys 1997;38:1037–1044.
24. Rades D, Karstens JH, Alberti W. Role of radiotherapy in the treatment of motor dysfunction due to metastatic spinal cord compression: comparison of three different fractionation schedules. Int J Radiat Oncol Biol Phys 2002;54:1160–1164.
25. Hartsell WF, Scott CB, Bruner DW, et al. Randomized trial of short versus long course radiotherapy for palliation of painful bone metastases. J Natl Cancer Inst 2005;97:798–804.
26. Bruner D, Winter K, Hartsell W, et al. Prospective health related quality of life valuations (utilities) of 8 Gy in 1 fraction vs 30 Gy in 10 fractions of palliation of painful bone metastases: preliminary results of RTOG 97–14. Int J Radiat Oncol Biol Phys 2004;60:S142.
27. Auchter RM, Lamond J, Alexander E. A multi-institutional outcome and prognostic factor analysis of radiosurgery for resectable single brain metastasis. Int J Radiat Oncol Biol Phys 1996;35:27–35.
28. Chang SD, Adler J, Hancock S. The clinical use of radiosurgery. Oncology 1998;12:1181–1191.
29. Flickinger JC, Kondziolka D, Lunsford L. A multi-institutional experience with stereotactic radiosurgery for solitary brain metastasis. Int J Radiat Oncol Biol Phys 1994;28:797–802.

30. Kondziolka D, Patel A, Lunsford L. Stereotactic radiosurgery plus whole brain radiotherapy vs radiotherapy alone for patients with multiple brain metastases. Int J Radiat Oncol Biol Phys 1999;45:427–434.

31. Loeffler J, Alexander EI. Radiosurgery for the Treatment of Intracranial Metastasis. New York: McGraw-Hill; 1993.

32. Loeffler JS, Kooy HM, Wen PY, et al. The treatment of recurrent brain metastases with stereotactic radiosurgery. J Clin Oncol 1990;8:576–582.

33. Sperduto PW, Scott C, Andrews D. Stereotactic radiosurgery with whole brain radiation therapy improves survival in patients with brain metastases: report of radiation therapy oncology group phase III study 95–08. Int J Radiat Oncol Biol Phys 2002;54:3a.

34. Chang SD, Adler JR Jr. Current status and optimal use of radiosurgery. Oncology 2001;15:209–216.

35. Gerszten PC, Burton SA, Ozhasoglu C, Welch WC. Single-fraction radiosurgery for spinal metastases: clinical experience in 500 cases from a single institution. Spine 2007;32:193–199.

36. Hamilton AJ, Lulu BA, Fosmire H, Stea B, Cassady J. Preliminary clinical experience with linear accelerator-based spinal stereotactic radiosurgery. Neurosurgery 1995;36:311–319.

37. Medin PM, Solberg T, DeSalles A. Investigations of a minimally invasive method for treatment of spinal malignancies with linac stereotactic radiation therapy: accuracy and animal studies. Int J Radiat Oncol Biol Phys 2002;52:1111–1122.

38. Ryu S, Rock J, Rosenblum M, Kim JH. Patterns of failure after single-dose radiosurgery for spinal metastasis. J Neurosurg 2004;101:402–405.

39. Yin FF, Ryu S, Ajlouni M, et al. Image-guided procedures for intensity-modulated spinal radiosurgery. J Neurosurg 2004;101:419–424.

40. Colombo F, Pozza F, Chierego G. Linear accelerator radiosurgery of cerebral arteriovenous malformations: An update. Neurosurgery 1994;34:14–21.

41. Hitchcock E, Kitchen G, Dalton E, Pope B. Stereotactic linac radiosurgery. Br J Neurosurg 1989;3:305–312.

42. Pirzkall A, Lohr F, Rhein B, et al. Conformal radiotherapy of challenging paraspinal tumors using a multiple arc segment technique. Int J Radiat Oncol Biol Phys 2000;48:1197–1204.

43. Song DY, Kavanagh BD, Benedict SH, Schefter T. Stereotactic body radiation therapy rationale, techniques, applications and optimization. Oncology 2004;18:1419–1436.

44. Isacsson U. Potential advantages of protons. Radiother Oncol 1997;45:63–70.

45. Klish MD, Watson GA, Shrieve DC. Radiation and intensity-modulated radiotherapy for metastatic spine tumors. Neurosurg Clin North Am 2004;15:481–490.

46. Rock JP, Ryu S, Yin FF. Novalis radiosurgery for metastatic spine tumors. Neurosurg Clin North Am 2004;15:503–509.

47. Yamada Y, Lovelock M, Yenice KM, et al. Multifractionated image-guided and stereotactic intensity modulated radiotherapy of paraspinal tumors: a preliminary report. Int J Radiat Oncol Biol Phys 2005;62:53–61.

48. Gerszten PC, Burton SA, Ozhasoglu C, et al. Radiosurgery for the management of spinal metastases. In: Kondziolka D, ed. Radiosurgery. Basel: Karger; 2006:199–210.

49. Abbatucci JS, Delozier T, Quint R, Roussel A, Brune D. Radiation myelopathy of the central spinal cord: time, dose and volume factors. Int J Radiat Oncol Biol Phys 1978;4:239–248.

50. Boden G. Radiation myelitis of the cervical spinal cord. Br J Radiol 1948;21:464–469.

51. Hatlevoll R, Host H, Kaalhus O. Myelopathy following radiotherapy of bronchial carcinoma with large single fractions: a retrospective study. Int J Radiat Oncol Biol Phys 1983;9:41–44.

52. McCuniff AJ, Liang MJ. Radiation tolerance of the cervical spinal cord. Int J Radiat Oncol Biol Phys 1989;16:675–678.

53. Phillips TL, Buschke F. Radiation tolerance of the thoracic spinal cord. Am J Roentgenol Radium Ther Nucl Med 1969;105:659–664.

54. Wara WM, Phillips TL, Sheline GE, Schwade JG. Radiation tolerance of the spinal cord. Cancer 1975;35:1558–1562.

55. Degen JW, Gagnon GJ, Voyadzis J-M, et al. CyberKnife stereotactic radiosurgical treatment of spinal tumors for pain control and quality of life. J Neurosurg Spine 2005;2:540–549.

56. Pieters RS, Niemierko A, Fullerton BC, Munzenrider JE. Cauda equina tolerance to high dose fractionated irradiation. Int J Radiat Oncol Biol Phys 2006;64:251–257.

57. Emami B, Lyman J, Brown A, et al. Tolerance of normal tissue to therapeutic irradiation. Int J Radiat Oncol Biol Phys 1991;21:109–122.

58. Tong D, Hendrickson F. The palliation of symptomatic osseous metastases: final results of the study by the radiation therapy oncology group. Cancer 1982;50:893–899.

59. Gerszten PC, Burton S, Ozhasoglu C, et al. Stereotactic radiosurgery for spine metastases from renal cell carcinoma. J Neurosurg Spine 2005;3:288–295.

60. Gerszten PC, Burton SA, Welch WC, et al. Single fraction radiosurgery for the treatment of spinal breast metastases. Cancer 2005;104:2244–2254.

61. Gerszten PC, Burton SA, Quinn AE, Agarwala SS, Kirkwood JM. Radiosurgery for the treatment of spinal melanoma metastases. Stereotact Funct Neurosurg 2006;83(5–6):213–221.

62. Gerszten PC, Ozhasoglu C, Burton S, et al. CyberKnife frameless stereotactic radiosurgery for spinal lesions: clinical experience in 125 cases. Neurosurgery 2004;55:89–99.

63. Ryken TC, Meeks SL, Pennington EC, et al. Initial clinical experience with frameless stereotactic radiosurgery: analysis of accuracy and feasibility. Int J Radiat Oncol Biol Phys 2001;51:1152–1158.

64. Rock JP, Ryu S, Shukairy MS, et al. Postoperative radiosurgery for malignant spinal tumors. Neurosurgery 2006;58:891–898.

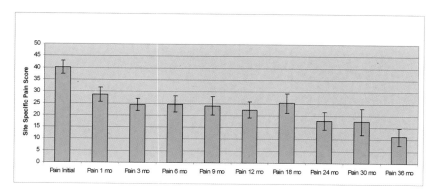

Figure 10.1 Pain scores by the Visual Analog Scale as a function of time following CyberKnife radiosurgery of the spine.

surgery were self-limited and mild in most cases. One patient developed breakdown at a surgical site, requiring surgery for débridement and reclosure of the wound, although it was not possible to assign this complication to CyberKnife radiosurgery, the patient's prior external beam radiotherapy, or two spinal surgeries. Otherwise, several patients experienced mild esophagitis or dysphagia, fatigue, and transient diarrhea. There was no evidence of myelitis or neurologic damage in any patient as a result of radiosurgery.

Pain Scores

Initial and follow-up treatment site-specific pain scores by the Visual Analog Scale (VAS) are given in **Fig. 10.1**. Initial site-specific pain scores prior to treatment ranged from 0 to 100 (mean 44). Eighty-two percent of patients reported some degree of pain prior to treatment, and 18% had asymptomatic disease. At 1 month after treatment, 39% of the evaluable patients reported that they were pain free. Paired t-test analysis was used to evaluate the change in pain scores over time compared with the starting level of pain. Pain scores were significantly decreased at 1-month follow-up (mean 29, decrease of 19, $p < .001$). Scores remained significantly decreased compared with the starting level over the entire

follow-up period (12 months: mean of 24, decrease of 11, $p = .009$; 24 months: mean of 20, decrease of 14, $p = .01$; 36 months: mean of 12, decrease of 26, $p = .05$). Pain relief appeared to be quite durable. Sixteen spinal sites received subsequent additional CyberKnife treatment.

SF-12 Scores

The PCS (**Fig. 10.2**) and MCS (**Fig. 10.3**) scores did not change significantly over the follow-up period. The mean initial PCS score was 33. Mean follow-up PCS scores were 1 month, 34; 12 months, 34; 24 months, 37; and 36 months, 40. The mean initial MCS score was 46. Mean follow-up MCS scores were 1 month, 49; 12 months, 51; 24 months, 52; and 36 months, 51. There was a trend toward improved MCS scores at 1- to 9-months follow-up. Patients did not experience a decline in their quality of life by SF-12 assessment. There appeared to be stabilization of quality of life following treatment.

It is possible to consider the different component scores of the SF-12 individually. These are presented in **Fig. 10.4.** They show, in general, a slow trend to improvement over a several-month period across all eight scales, and it is not possible to ascribe stabilization or improvement in the SF-12 scores to one scale or another. Rather, the quality of life

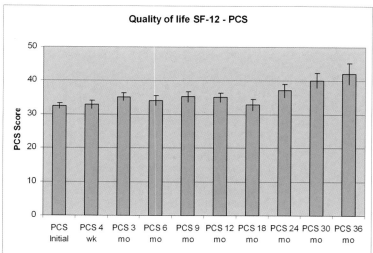

Figure 10.2 Physical component scores (PCS) from the SF-12 as a function of time following CyberKnife radiosurgery of the spine.

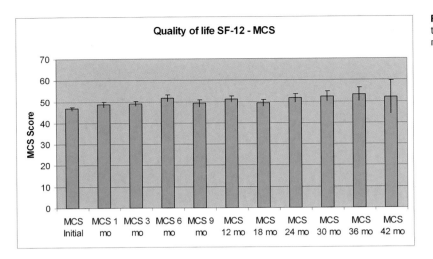

Figure 10.3 Mental component scores (MCS) from the SF-12 as a function of time following CyberKnife radiosurgery of the spine.

benefits appear to be broad, given the limitations of the instrument.

Maintenance of adequate spinal function is essential for an active lifestyle, and disturbances of this function are dramatic in their impact on activity and quality of life. Malignant involvement of the spine is a common occurrence in the natural history of many malignancies and a cause of much disturbance. Treatments for malignant spinal involvement, although successful on occasion, are often limited, often by the need to preserve the remnants of the same functions being impaired. We are interested in radiosurgery using the CyberKnife system. It is our belief that the accuracy in dose deposition, the conformity, and the homogeneity are unequaled in the radiation treatment of spinal malignancies. Outcomes data, however, are accruing and were incomplete

AQ2

at the time of this writing. For example, it is not clear if the higher doses using these techniques are associated with more durable local control, let alone a possible small survival improvement, although it is possible to report relatively mature quality of life data.

◆ Conclusion

Our measures of quality of life reveal improvements in pain scores and SF-12 scores. Whether these improvements are expected only from CyberKnife radiosurgery is also debatable; it is entirely conceivable that other radiosurgical systems, intensity-modulated radiation therapy, or other external beam techniques might be equally efficacious. What

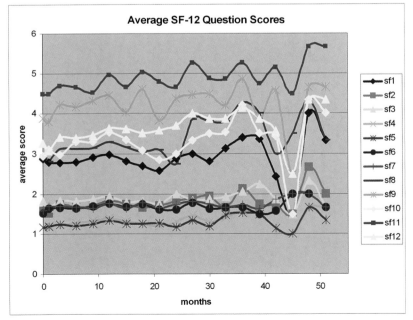

Figure 10.4 SF-12 scores after CyberKnife radiosurgery treatment for all 12 quality of life questions averaged over the study population. Potential scores depend on the question and range from 2 to 6. In general, there is a slow trend upward, indicating improved quality of life for several months. Values after 30 months are based on small sample sizes and are not expected to be reliable. *Physical functioning* is a combination of items 2 and 3 (sf2 and sf3), *role limitations from physical problems* is a combination of sf4 and sf5, and *role limitations* from emotional problems is a combination of sf6 and sf7; *bodily pain* is scored by sf8, *general health* by sf1, *vitality* by sf10, *social functioning* by sf12, and *mental health* by sf9 and sf11.

is encouraging in our studies is the extent and duration of palliative response with very few acute or long-term toxicities. We are continuing to collect outcomes data and remain impressed by the efficacy of our fractionated approach.

References

1. Campbell NA, Reece JB. Biology. 6th ed. Menlo Park, CA: Benjamin/Cummings; 2002:ch. 34.

2. Koob TJ, Long JH. The vertebrate body axis: evolution and mechanical function. Am Zool 2000;40:1–18.

3. Henderson FC, Gagnon GJ, McRae D. CyberKnife radiosurgery for spinal tumors with emphasis on tumor biology and treatment technique. In: Bucholz RD, Gagnon GJ, Gerszten PC, et al, eds. Pioneering Techniques in Robotic Radiosurgery. Vol 1. Sunnyvale, CA: CyberKnife Society Press; 2005.

4. Sherry MM, Greco FA, Johnson DH, Hainsworth JD. Metastatic breast cancer confined to the skeletal system: an indolent disease. Am J Med 1986;81:381–386.

5. Harrington KD. Orthopedic Management of Metastatic Bone Disease. St. Louis: CV Mosby; 1992:283–307.

6. Body JJ. Metastatic bone disease: clinical and therapeutic aspects. Bone 1992;13:S57–S62.

7. Markman M. Early recognition of spinal cord compression in cancer patients. Cleve Clin J Med 1999;66:629–631.

8. Stewart AL, Ware JE. Measuring Functioning and Well-Being: The Medical Outcomes Study Approach. Durham, NC: Duke University Press; 1992.

9. Ware JE, Kosinski M. SF-36 Physical and Mental Health Summary Scales: A Manual for Users of Version 1. 2nd ed. Lincoln, RI: QualityMetric Inc.; 2001.

10. Ware J Jr, Kosinski M, Keller SD. A 12-item short-form health survey: construction of scales and preliminary tests of reliability and validity. Med Care 1996;34(3):220–233.

11. Ware JE, Kosinski M, Keller SD. SF-12: How to Score the SF-12 Physical and Mental Health Summary Scales. 4th ed. Boston: QualityMetric Inc.; July 2002:67–70.

11

Treatment of Spinal Canal Compromise

Jack P. Rock, Samuel Ryu, and Ian Y. Lee

Spinal cord compression from the epidural spread of cancer is both common and debilitating. Up to 2.5% of all cancer patients have at least one admission to the hospital for epidural cord compression. At presentation, 90% have either local or radicular pain, sensory changes, or bowel and bladder incontinence, and up to 50% may have lost the ability to ambulate. As a result of complications due to decreased mobility, these patients frequently develop infection and deep vein thrombosis (DVT), complications associated with decreased life expectancy. Their medical condition and pain are difficult to manage and present a great challenge to families and society as a whole.

Before radiation therapy was contemplated as a treatment modality for the management of metastatic epidural disease, surgical decompression was the primary option. Until recently, little consideration was given to the anatomical characteristics of the lesion causing the spinal cord compression, and the primary surgical approach consisted of posterior decompressive laminectomy. However, given that most epidural disease is located anterior to the spinal cord, strategies approaching from posterior to the spinal cord frequently resulted in insufficient tumor removal and spinal instability. Surgical outcomes based on posterior strategies were thus less likely to lead to neurologic improvement.

After the establishment of radiation therapy as an effective treatment for epidural metastatic disease, laminectomy fell out of favor as subsequent clinical investigations failed to demonstrate a benefit for surgery as compared with radiation therapy alone. External beam radiotherapy has been reported to improve ambulatory function in about 30 to 40% of patients with epidural spinal cord compression.[1,2]

Unfortunately, neither posterior surgical decompression (i.e., laminectomy) nor radiation therapy represents a truly satisfactory method for treating malignant epidural spinal cord compression. Recently, advances in surgical technique for decompression and stabilization have led to more frequent use of anterior surgical approaches tailored to the anatomical characteristics of the lesion compressing the spinal cord. Although these contemporary surgical strategies have led to apparently superior clinical outcomes, presumably due to more thorough tumor removal, spinal cord decompression, and spinal stabilization, it remains unclear whether these more extensive surgical interventions will prove to be more effective than radiation alone. Patchell et al performed a randomized trial comparing the use radiation therapy alone with the use of up-to-date surgical strategies in combination with radiation therapy.[3] Patients who received surgery and radiation retained the ability to ambulate longer than those treated with radiation alone. Patients in the surgical cohort also survived longer and had less pain. It was concluded that metastatic epidural lesions were best treated by the combination of surgery, anatomically tailored to tumor location, followed by external beam radiation therapy. Presumably, the improved clinical and survival outcomes were partly influenced by the fact that greater numbers of patients were ambulatory, which, in turn, led to a decreased incidence of DVT and infection, both of which strongly influence morbidity. Given these encouraging results, one must remain aware of the general infirmity of these patients and realize that operative morbidity can be significant, even though the rate of complications in the patients in the surgical cohort of this investigation was not higher than that noted for patients in the radiation therapy alone cohort.

More recently, stereotactically delivered radiation has served as an effective alternative to surgery for many lesions located in the brain and, based in part on improvements in the technology of image guidance, has been applied for the management of lesions in and around the spine and spinal cord.[4-14] Given its focused nature, radiosurgery can treat a tumor with high doses of conformal radiation while exposing the surrounding spinal cord to relatively low doses. Radiosurgery currently stands as a treatment alternative to surgery and conventional radiation therapy and may well prove to be superior to conventional radiotherapy for neoplasms in and around the spine and spinal cord. As it becomes more apparent that radiosurgery can serve effectively in the management of certain neoplastic lesions, the question remains whether radiosurgery can be considered an alternative to surgery for tumors located within the spinal canal and, in certain instances, tumors directly compressing the spinal cord.

Currently, there is little literature that specifically addresses the role of radiosurgery in the management of neoplastic spinal canal compromise and spinal cord compression, although a considerable body of evidence supports the use of radiosurgery for spinal tumors and other spinal conditions.[15]

◆ Radiosurgery Procedure

At the Henry Ford Hospital (Detroit, Michigan), we have been conducting a phase II clinical trial addressing the use of radiosurgery in the management of spinal epidural disease and epidural spinal cord compression. Since December 2005, 75 patients with neoplastic disease within the spinal canal have been enrolled. Of these, clinical and radiographic follow-up was available for 42 lesions in 38 patients; these patients comprise the study group for this investigation.

All patients were treated with single-fraction spine radiosurgery according to previously detailed protocols used at the Henry Ford Hospital and described elsewhere.[12–14,16] The frameless image-guided Novalis system from Brain-Lab AG (Feldkirchen, Germany) and the dosimetric characteristics have been reported.[17,18] Patient positioning was achieved using the BodyFix system (Medical Intelligence Medizintechnik GmbH, Schwabmünchen, Germany) with vacuum bags or other positioning devices, as needed. Infrared reflective markers were placed on the skin. Computed tomographic (CT) simulation was performed with intravenous contrast in 2 to 3 mm slices without spacing. Using the dedicated planning system with the BrainScan planning computer (BrainLab), image fusion was routinely achieved with simulation CT and T1-weighted gadolinium contrast and T2-weighted magnetic resonance (MR) images. The radiosurgery target volume and spinal cord were delineated. Radiosurgical treatment generally consisted of multiple (usually 7–9 beams) intensity-modulated radiation beams to minimize the dose to the critical organs, and image-guided repositioning was achieved using infrared marker and image fusion of internal bony structures (i.e., vertebral bony anatomy). Prior to radiation delivery, orthogonal portal films were obtained for final verification of the isocenter.

The guidance process that brings the treatment isocenter into alignment with the preplanned isocenter uses six degrees of freedom, with rotations along three axes also considered. Because a target positioning process based solely on infrared skin fiducials is incapable of providing the high precision localization required for treating spinal lesions, the final adjustments (i.e., bringing the target isocenter to the preplanned treatment isocenter) are accomplished with an automated patient-positioning device, which represents co-ordination between the ExacTrac and Novalis Body systems (both BrainLab). The details of these systems are described in other chapters.

Definition of Tumor Volume and Spinal Cord

All patients received single-dose radiosurgery to the involved spine only, and the target volume included the involved vertebral body and pedicles. When paraspinal or epidural soft tissue tumor was present, the involved spine and the gross tumor were both included in the target volume. The spinal cord at-risk volume was consistently defined as the volume extending from 6 mm above to 6 mm below the radiosurgery target. The target tumor and the spinal cord were delineated by fusing data from contrast-enhanced simulation CT images, T1-weighted images (with and without gadolinium contrast), and T2-weighted MR images.

The radiation dose was consistently prescribed to the 90% isodose line, which encompassed the periphery of the target. Although radiosurgery doses were selected as part of a dose-escalation paradigm, the primary criteria determining dose selection were the spinal cord dose and the tumor volume coverage constraints. When the spinal cord dose constraint (< 10 Gy to < 10% of the spinal cord volume) was not met, the overall dose prescription had to be reduced. The median radiosurgery dose was 16 Gy, and the median target volume was 66.75 cc. All patients had clinical follow-up from 2 to 30 months (mean 9.2 months, median 8.0 months) and pre- and post-treatment radiographic follow-up (mean 8.46 months, median 8.10 months).

Grading of Canal Compromise and Outcome of Radiosurgery

The pretreatment grading system was based on a combination of radiographic and neurologic data (**Fig. 11.1**):

Grade 0   No visible tumor within the spinal canal
Grade I   Tumor identified within the spinal canal but not involving the dura; normal neurologic examination
Grade II   Tumor involving/distorting the dura without spinal cord involvement; normal neurologic examination
Grade III   Tumor compressing/distorting the spinal cord; normal neurologic examination
Grade IV   Tumor compressing the spinal cord; abnormal neurologic examination

Tumor was noted within the spinal canal in all cases.

Post-treatment outcomes were separately classified based on radiographic and neurologic status. Radiographic outcome grades were stable (A), partial response (B), complete resolution (C), and progression (D). Clinical outcome grades were neurologically stable (A), neurologic improvement (B), and neurologic progression (C).

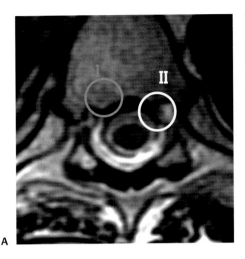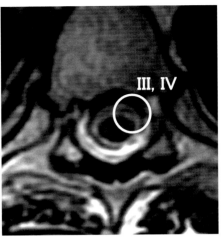

Figure 11.1 **(A,B)** Canal compromise grading system. Grade 0: no visible tumor within the spinal canal. Grade I: tumor in the spinal canal without dural involvement. Grade II: tumor involving the dura; normal neurologic examination. Grade III: tumor compressing the spinal cord; normal neurologic examination. Grade IV: tumor compressing the spinal cord; abnormal neurologic examination.

A   B

◆ Results

Patients with a neurologic deficit prior to radiosurgery were clinically stable or improved in 12 of 16 (75%) cases and clinically progressed in 4 of 16 (25%) cases. Patients without a neurologic deficit prior to radiosurgery were clinically stable or improved in 22 of 26 (84.6%) cases and clinically progressed in 4 of 26 (15.4%) cases (**Tables 11.1** and **11.2**).

Image progression was noted in 3 of 42 (7.1%) cases. Image progression was noted with colon (1), melanoma (1), and renal (1) cancers (**Table 11.3**). Clinical progression was noted with breast (1), lung (1), melanoma (1), follicular thyroid (1), colon (1), hepatocellular (1), renal (1), and papillary thyroid (1) cancers.

◆ Discussion

With more than 20,000 new cases of spinal cord compression noted yearly and controversy surrounding optimal treatment recommendations, Patchell et al performed a multi-institutional, randomized trial and found that direct (i.e., surgery tailored to the anatomical location of the tumor) decompressive surgery plus radiation therapy was superior to radiation therapy alone for the treatment of patients with metastatic spinal cord compression.[3] In the "radiation alone" arm, patients were treated with the established standard regimen consisting of 30 Gy in 10 fractions.

Radiosurgery is a relatively recent development and has been used as a treatment alternative for neoplastic lesions involving the spine, with encouraging results published.[4–14,16]

In most instances, radiosurgery has been administered as a single fraction and used for metastatic spinal disease. Although spine radiosurgery is becoming an accepted means to treat neoplastic disease within and around the vertebral column, it is unclear whether it should be considered as a primary treatment for disease within the spinal canal associated with radiographic spinal cord compression, particularly when there are neurologic deficits secondary to that spinal cord compression.

Given the functional status of many patients with metastatic spinal disease, especially those with spinal cord compression, a treatment regimen that could avoid surgery entirely would be welcomed. Bearing in mind Patchell et al's data,[3] we have used our spinal database to assess the clinical and radiographic outcomes in patients treated with single-fraction spine radiosurgery for metastatic spinal canal compromise and spinal cord compression.

In this series, the control rate for tumor growth within the target volume was 92.9%. Of the lesions treated with spine radiosurgery 34 of 42 (81%) were stable (67%) or improved (14%) at the time of follow-up, which ranged from 2 to 30 months (median 8.6 months). Additional stratification divided patients into two groups: those with canal compromise and a normal neurologic examination and those with canal compromise and an abnormal neurologic examination. Patients with a neurologic deficit prior to radiosurgery were clinically stable or improved in 12 of 16 (75%) cases and clinically progressed in 4 of 16 (25%) cases. Patients without a neurologic deficit prior to radiosurgery were clinically stable or improved in 22 of 26 (84.6%) cases and clinically progressed in 4 of 26 (15.4%) cases. Image progression was noted in 3 of 42 (7.1%) cases; colon (1), melanoma (1), and renal (1) cancers were all considered to be radioresistant. All three of these patients deteriorated clinically as well. Of the three radiographic failures, two instances were secondary to continued tumor growth within and adjacent to the radiosurgery target volume, and the third was secondary to retropulsion of vertebral bone (i.e., compression fracture) into the spinal canal after successful tumor treatment.

Table 11.1 Neurologic Outcome of Radiosurgery

	Neurologic Status before Radiosurgery		
	Overall	Intact	Deficit
Improved or stable	81%	84.6%	75%
Progressed	19%	15.4%	25%

Table 11.2 Patients with Radiographic or Neurologic Progression

Primary Diagnosis	Spine Level	Pretreatment Canal Compromise Grade	Target Volume (cc)	Radiosurgery Dose (Gy)	Cause of Failure	Post-treatment Radiologic (Target) and Clinical Grade
Imaging progression						
Adenocarcinoma (colon)**	L2	III	54.72	16	Tumor growth within and adjacent to target volume	D, C
Melanoma*	T12	IV	195.4	16	Tumor growth within and dorsal to target volume	D, C
Adenocarcinoma (kidney)***	T10	III	79.92	18	Bony retropulsion causing cord compression	D, # C
Clinical progression						
Adenocarcinoma (breast)	T4–T6	IV	66.81	16	Tumor growth adjacent and distant to target volume	B, C
Squamous carcinoma (lung)	T4	IV	88.59	16	Tumor growth within target volume	A, C
Melanoma*	T12	IV	195.4	16	See above	D, C
Follicular carcinoma (thyroid)	T6	IV	21.71	18	Tumor growth within and adjacent to target volume	A, C
Adenocarcinoma (colon)**	L2	III	54.72	16	See above	D, C
Adenocarcinoma (liver)	T12	III	162.77	14	Tumor growth adjacent to target volume	A, C
Adenocarcinoma (kidney)***	T10	III	79.92	18	See above	D, # C
Papillary carcinoma (thyroid)	T7	III	79.22	16	Tumor progression adjacent to target volume	A, C

*, **, *** represent the same patients.
Image and clinical progression secondary to compression fracture and cord compression.

Table 11.3 Results Based on Histology

Histology	Clinically Worse (8/42)			Radiologically Worse (3/42)			
	A	B	C	A	B	C	D
1 Unknown adenocarcinoma	1					1	
8 Breast	6	1	1	1	4	3	
1 Chordoma	1			1			
1 Colon	1				1		
5 Liver	4		1	3	2		
2 Lung	1		1	1		1	
1 Liposarcoma	1				1		
1 Lymphoproliferative	1				1		
2 Melanoma	1		1	1			1
5 Multiple myeloma	3	2		1	1	3	
1 Neuroendocrine	1			1			
1 Paraganglioma	1			1			
6 Prostate	5	1		3	1	2	
3 Renal	2		1	1	1		1
1 Thyroid, papillary			1	1			
1 Thyroid, follicular			1	1			
1 Thyroid, medullary	1					1	
1 Vulval		1			1		

Table 11.4 Causes of Tumor Progression

Tumor factors
    Radioresistant histology
    Tumor shape and size
    Location of tumor: paraspinal or epidural
Geometric factors
    Proximity to spinal cord
    Position of spinal cord
    Inadequate target definition
    Possible microscopic epidural extension
Inadequate radiosurgery dose

Although clinical deterioration in patients with metastatic cancer can be caused by numerous conditions, careful analysis of our outcome data provided several insights (**Tables 11.2** and **11.4**). First, an inadequate target volume definition may serve as a primary cause of failure. The use of CT in the treatment planning phase leads to images that are of inferior resolution compared with MRI, and even though an image fusion algorithm is used for final target delineation, during the contouring process the treating physician must keep this in mind so that too limited a target volume is not prescribed, which can negatively affect the outcome.

Second, consideration should be given to the potential for microscopic (i.e., nonenhancing) tumor extension beyond the gross (i.e, enhancing) tumor visible on the imaging studies. This region of possible tumor involvement will then fall outside the 90% isodose line and thereby be a source of tumor recurrence and, ultimately, adverse outcomes. **Figure 11.2** shows an instance of spinal cord compression secondary to prostate cancer. The lesion (45.07 cc) was treated with 18 Gy, and imaging at 6 months demonstrated complete resolution. Ten months later, however, the patient presented with neurologic deficit once again, and imaging revealed an apparently "new" tumor adjacent to the original target. This suggests that initially there may have been inadequate target delineation. Therefore, it may be prudent to include additional volume within the target extending superiorly, inferiorly, and laterally, but it is not clear how many additional millimeters should be added. Recent information for brain metastases indicates that microscopic deposits of tumor can extend 1 to 3 mm beyond the contrast-enhancing tumor visible on imaging studies.[19] This pathological situation undoubtedly occurs in the spine as well, underscoring the need to consider extending the high-dose field beyond the obvious target when possible. We are planning a surgicopathological study to evaluate this potential pitfall.

Third, dose selection may have compromised some outcomes. During the last 5 years, as our experience with radiosurgery has grown, we have encountered no instances of radiation-induced myelopathy, and throughout this time we have gradually escalated treatment doses. Our dose selection has ranged from 14 to 18 Gy, and it is unclear whether dose selection should be histology dependent as well as the extent to which the dose can be safely elevated. Our experience with dose escalation over the past 5 years has shown that the spinal cord can safely tolerate an exposure of 10 Gy.[20] Recently, however, we noted one case of radiation-induced spinal cord signal change in a patient who has remained asymptomatic. Although the spinal cord can most probably tolerate even higher doses, during treatment planning we attempt to limit spinal cord exposure to 10 Gy.

Finally, although clinical progression in cancer patients often relates directly to actual epidural tumor progression, other systemic conditions, comorbidities such as diabetes, vascular insufficiency, and stroke, and side effects of systemic treatments, some of which may act as radiation sensitizers, also can contribute to a patient's observed clinical deterioration. These conditions should not be mistakenly interpreted as failure of the radiosurgical treatment.

Relative to the tumor per se, the causes of progression appear to be related, in large part, to the anatomical aspects of the target, including its volume and proximity to the spinal

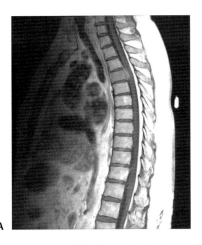 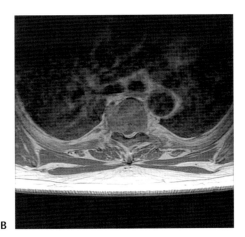 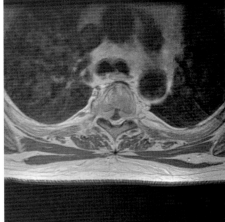

A   B   C

Figure 11.2 **(A)** The patient had a prostate metastasis. **(B)** Six months after radiosurgery, the lesion had completely resolved. **(C)** Ten months after radiosurgery, recurrence was noted slightly above the original radiosurgery target.

Table 11.5 Pretreatment Clinicoradiographic Classification of Spinal Canal Compromise

	Canal Compromise	Dura Involved/Compressed	Spinal Cord Involved/Compressed*	Neurologic Deficit
Grade 0	–	–	–	–
Grade I	+	–	–	–
Grade II	+	+	–	–
Grade III	+	+	+	–
Grade IV	+	+	+	+

* The terms *involved, distorted,* and *compressed* each relate to the imaging features (i.e., in grade I, features do not necessarily appear as distorted or compressed but simply as involved).

cord, the primary dose-limiting organ. The soft tissue tumor component in the spinal area can be divided into two regions—epidural and paraspinal. Although paraspinal tumors can be treated easily with higher doses of radiosurgery because of the relative distance between the tumor margin and the spinal cord, epidural tumors are a challenge because of their intimate anatomical relationship to the spinal cord. In this regard, intensity modulation in treatment planning may be critical. This capability allows for optimal tumor coverage with preservation of the adjacent spinal cord (i.e., treatment optimization).

In this series of patients, objective tumor response (i.e., radiological outcomes grades B + C, in-field) rate was noted in 55% (93% including those tumors that were stable and improved: grades A, B, and C) and tumor progression in 7.1%. Significantly, 41 of 42 (98%) of these lesions were associated with spinal cord compression, and 16 of 42 (38%) had spinal cord compression and neurologic deficit. Therefore, it is likely that, based on traditional treatment paradigms, surgery would have been offered to at least 16 of the patients (and possibly to 41 of 42 patients). Our data indicate that in a significant majority of these patients, surgery was avoidable without a negative impact on outcome. Additionally, although dose–response relationships have not been

definitively established, higher radiosurgery doses (16–20 Gy) seem more effective for tumor control.

These encouraging clinical outcomes have led us to consider the development of a classification system for spinal canal compromise and epidural spinal cord compression (**Figs. 11.1** and **11.3** and **Table 11.5**). There are, practically speaking, five different grades of spinal canal compromise:

Grade 0 No visible tumor within the spinal canal
Grade I Only epidural fat involvement; neurologic signs absent
Grade II Dura involved/distorted/compressed; neurologic signs absent
Grade III Spinal cord involved/distorted/compression; neurologic signs absent
Grade IV Spinal cord distorted/compressed; neurologic signs present (usually long tract signs with compromised ambulatory status)

We are also working to merge the pre- and post-treatment grading systems so that radiological and neurologic data may be more easily combined. Using this classification system for spinal canal compromise and spinal cord compression, we are continuing to accrue patients specifically to address the question of whether radiosurgery or surgery can

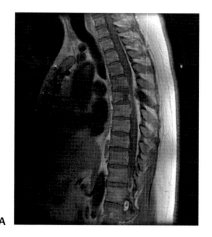
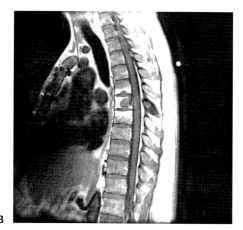
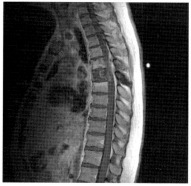

A   B   C

Figure 11.3 **(A)** The patient has multiple myeloma and was barely ambulatory but refused surgery. **(B)** Ten days after radiosurgery, there was a small but apparent decrease in the extent of spinal cord compression, and neurologically, the patient's lower extremity numbness had resolved completely. He remained ambulatory. **(C)** Three months later, the lesion was totally resolved, and the patient had normal lower extremity power.

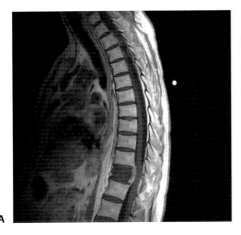

A

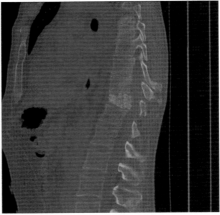

B

Figure 11.4 **(A)** Magnetic resonance imaging shows image progression in this patient with neurologic deterioration. **(B)** On computed tomography, the lesion was, in fact, a compression fracture; at the time of decompressive surgery, no tumor was found.

be considered a primary management strategy for patients with spinal cord compromise (**Table 11.6**). We currently use the patient's motor examination and ambulatory status as the primary criteria in the decision process, with histology a secondary concern. Overall, indications for surgery have not changed with decompression a primary recommendation when the patient's motor examination is significantly compromised (i.e., antigravity or worse), the neurologic deficit has progressed rapidly (< 1 week), compression is secondary to bony retropulsion, or there is overt, or the potential for, spinal instability (**Fig. 11.4**).

◆ Conclusion

Spine radiosurgery is a relatively recent development, and a considerable body of evidence now exists to support its use for the management of lesions in and around the spine and spinal cord. Clinically speaking, spinal cord compression has always carried dire implications, and surgery has always been the primary form of management based on its proven efficacy. However, many patients with metastatic spinal cord compression are either unable to tolerate or unwilling to undergo surgical intervention. Based on the literature, spine radiosurgery is now being more seriously considered in the treatment armamentarium for patients with spinal canal and spinal cord compromise. Our preliminary results lend support to the

idea that spine radiosurgery may be an effective treatment of spinal canal compromise and spinal cord compression in selected individuals. Despite these encouraging results, careful clinical follow-up and caution must be exercised.

References

1. Gilbert RW, Kim JH, Posner JB. Epidural spinal cord compression from metastatic tumor: diagnosis and treatment. Ann Neurol 1978;3:40–51.
2. Greenberg HS, Kim JH, Posner JB. Epidural spinal cord compression from metastatic tumor: results with a new treatment protocol. Ann Neurol 1980;8:361–366.
3. Patchell RA, Tibbs PA, Regine WF, et al. Direct decompressive surgical resection in the treatment of spinal cord compression caused by metastatic cancer: a randomised trial. Lancet 2005;366:643–648.
4. Bilsky MH, Yamada Y, Yenice KM, et al. Intensity-modulated stereotactic radiotherapy of paraspinal tumors: a preliminary report. Neurosurgery 2004;54:823–831.
5. Benzil DL, Saboori M, Mogilner AY, Rocchio R, Moorthy CR. Safety and efficacy of stereotactic radiosurgery for tumors of the spine. J Neurosurg 2004;101:413–418.
6. Chang SD, Main W, Martin DP, Gibbs IC, Heilbrun MP. An analysis of the accuracy of the cyberknife: a robotic frameless stereotactic radiosurgical system. Neurosurgery 2003;52:140–147.
7. De Salles AA, Pedroso AG, Medin P, et al. Spinal lesions treated with Novalis shaped beam intensity-modulated radiosurgery and stereotactic radiotherapy. J Neurosurg 2004;101:435–440.
8. Gerszten PC, Ozhasoglu C, Burton SA, et al. CyberKnife frameless single-fraction stereotactic radiosurgery for benign tumors of the spine. Neurosurg Focus 2003;14:e16.
9. Gerszten PC, Ozhasoglu C, Burton SA, et al. CyberKnife frameless stereotactic radiosurgery for spinal lesions: clinical experience in 125 cases. Neurosurgery 2004;55:89–99.
10. Gibbs IC, Chang SD, Pham C, Adler JR. Radiation tolerance of the spinal cord to staged radiosurgery. In: Konziolka D, ed. Radiosurgery. Basel, Switzerland: Karger; 2004:22–28.
11. Murphy MJ, Cox RS. The accuracy of dose localization for an image-guided frameless radiosurgery system. Med Phys 1996;23:2043–2049.
12. Ryu SI, Chang SD, Kim DH, et al. Image-guided hypofractionated stereotactic radiosurgery to spinal lesions. Neurosurgery 2001;49:838–846.
13. Ryu S, Rock R, Zhu G, et al. Image-guided radiosurgery for single spinal metastases. Proc Am Soc Clin Oncol (Abstract) 2004;8033:733.
14. Ryu S, Fang Yin F, Rock J, et al. Image-guided and intensity modulated radiosurgery for patients with spinal metastases. Cancer 2003;97:2013–2018.

Table 11.6 Working Indications for Radiosurgery versus Surgery

	Radiosurgery	Surgery
Muscle strength	Ambulatory	3* or worse
Onset of symptoms	Rapid	
Bony compression		+
Instability		+

*1, no movement of involved muscle; 2, trace movement of involved muscle; 3, antigravity movement of involved muscle; 4, moderate power of involved muscle; 5, normal muscle power.

15. Dodd RL, Ryu MR, Kamnerdsupaphon P, et al. CyberKnife radiosurgery for benign intradural extramedullary spinal tumors. Neurosurgery 2006;58:674–685.

16. Rock JP, Ryu S, Shukairy M, et al. Postoperative radiosurgery for malignant spinal tumors. Neurosurgery 2006;58:891–898.

17. Yin FF, Ryu S, Ajlouni M, et al. A technique of intensity-modulated radiosurgery (IMRS) for spinal tumors. Med Phys 2002;29:2815–2822.

18. Yin FF, Ryu S, Ajlouni M, et al. Image-guided procedures for intensity-modulated spinal radiosurgery. J Neurosurg 2004;101:419–424.

19. Baumert BG, Rutten I, Dehing-Iberije C, et al. A pathology-based substrate for target definition in radiosurgery of brain metastasis. Int J Radiat Oncol Biol Phys 2006;66:187–194.

20. Ryu S, Jin JY, Jin R, et al. Partial volume tolerance of the spinal cord and complications of single-dose radiosurgery. Cancer 2007;109:628–636.

11 Treatment of Spinal Canal Compromise

12

Treatment Failure and Complications

Samuel Ryu and Peter C. Gerszten

The clinical application of spine radiosurgery has been rapidly evolving. There is ample evidence to support integrating this modality into the treatment of spinal tumors, both malignant and benign. To maximize a successful clinical response to spine radiosurgery while maintaining a low toxicity profile, it is critical to analyze both the patterns of failure and the complications of this treatment. Because of the steep dose gradient and often small target volumes, the patterns of failure must be carefully correlated to the dosimetry profile of each case. There is currently a paucity of information regarding the patterns of failure and associated complications of spine radiosurgery, especially in clinical series with long-term follow-up. Nevertheless, the knowledge of such treatment failures and complications will help to better determine the role of radiosurgery in different clinical situations and ultimately determine the extent of the use of radiosurgery for spinal tumors. In this chapter, the patterns of clinical failures as well as the neural and non-neural complications of spine radiosurgery will be described.

◆ Patterns of Treatment Failure

Treatment failures after spine radiosurgery can be divided into three categories. *In-field failure* refers to tumor regrowth inside the treatment volume as seen on follow-up imaging studies or worsening of symptoms felt to be derived from the treated area. *Marginal failure* denotes a failure within the region of rapid dose fall-off immediately outside the target volume. Causes of marginal failure can be geographical misses due to limitations in the accuracy of treatment delivery and patient setup error or underestimation of the clinical target volume (CTV), either by limitations of imaging or underestimation of the volume at risk. *Distant failure* is progressive metastatic disease involving other untreated vertebral bodies within the spinal column. For the purpose of this discussion, distant failure may be subclassified as failure at the immediately adjacent levels or at true distant portions of the untreated spine (**Table 12.1**).

The parameters to determine treatment failures are twofold in spine radiosurgery: clinical and radiographic. Because pain is the most common symptom of spine tumors, the serial scoring of pain is a reliable, though subjective, functional end point. It is important to note that involvement of other untreated spinal pathology and nonspine metastatic sites may make pain assessment difficult and obscure the outcome assessment. Another clinical end point is the neurologic examination, especially when there was any neurologic deficit prior to treatment. This end point is an objective measurement of outcome compared with the subjective reporting of pain scores. Follow-up imaging studies (magnetic resonance imaging [MRI], computed tomography [CT], and positron emission tomography [PET]) may provide information on the anatomical extent of tumor control or possible progression.

Results of failure after radiosurgery in the initial experience of 61 treated patients with spine metastases at the Henry Ford Hospital (Detroit, Michigan) have been reported.[1] Failure of pain control from the symptomatic spine lesion was seen in 6% of the cohort. The results are illustrated in **Fig. 12.1**. There were two different categories of failure of pain control: in-field persistent pain (lack of pain response) and in-field progressive pain (symptomatic progression). In the category of persistent pain, the pain may persist without improvement, or the pain may be briefly improved but rapidly recurs.

Table 12.1 Patterns of Failure after Spine Radiosurgery

In-field persistent pain (lack of pain response)
In-field progressive pain (symptomatic progression)
Radiographic progression within the treatment volume
Marginal radiographic progression at the periphery of the target volume
Progression at the immediately adjacent spine level
Progression at remote spine levels

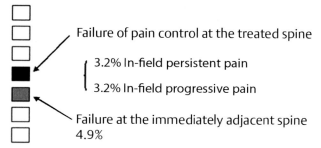

☐
☐
☐
■ ← Failure of pain control at the treated spine
■ ← { 3.2% In-field persistent pain
☐   3.2% In-field progressive pain
☐ ← Failure at the immediately adjacent spine 4.9%

Figure 12.1 Patterns of failure after radiosurgery for solitary spine metastasis.

Although the persistent or progressive pain seems to be due solely to tumor progression at the treated spine, there can be other causes of pain recurrence at the treated spine. An example of such a clinical scenario is presented here. A patient with metastatic non-small cell lung cancer developed left arm radiculopathy and upper extremity weakness with finger grip strength 3/5 of left hand. MRI revealed an enhancing epidural soft tissue mass at C7-T1 with involvement of neural foramen, more on the left side (**Fig. 12.2A**). The patient was treated with radiosurgery 16 Gy to the epidural lesion and the involved spines. After radiosurgery, muscle strength improved to 4/5 as well as radiculopathy. MRI obtained 6 months after radiosurgery showed a reduction of epidural lesion (**Fig. 12.2B**). However, 13 months after radiosurgery, the patient started having recurrent and worsening left arm pain. MRI scan showed worsening of the epidural-enhancing lesion extending longitudinally beyond the original target spines (**Fig. 12.2C**). Subsequently, the patient underwent decompressive surgery. The final pathology showed necrosis without evidence of tumor presence. This suggests that the recurrent pain was due to the tumor necrosis after radiosurgery, rather than tumor progression. Other causes are the compression fracture and spinal instability. A combined modality approach with vertebroplasty or kyphoplasty has also been shown to be effective in the treatment of pain related to compression fractures.[2]

Another type of pain failure is a progression of pain in the treated spine. This may be due to an inadequate radiosurgery dose or inadequate target definition. Some tumor histology may be more radioresistant, such as renal cell carcinoma and melanoma. A series of 60 cases of renal cell carcinoma spine

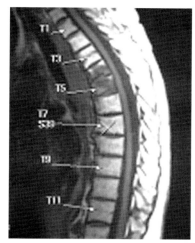

Figure 12.3 Failure at the immediately adjacent spine. This patient had a metastatic lung cancer initially involving T5 and was treated with radiosurgery. More metastases occurred at T4 after 6 months and at T3 after 8 months. These were treated with radiosurgery each time. Complete pain relief was achieved with each radiosurgery treatment. Note the thickening of the prevertebral fascia and soft tissue mass in the mediastinum extending along the vertebra.

metastases treated with radiosurgery at the same dose level used in other histologies (mean 20 Gy) demonstrated good initial pain responses in 89% of the patients. But 12% of patients underwent subsequent open surgical intervention for disease progression.[3] All failures occurred in patients receiving a lower maximum dose of 17.5 Gy. This rate of failure was not observed in other series of patients with other histologies. Dose escalation and/or the use of radiosensitizing agents may prove of benefit in some tumor histologies.

Failure at the immediately adjacent spine is an anatomical cause of failure after spine radiosurgery. It is important to identify the failure at the immediately adjacent spine because the radiosurgery targets only the involved vertebral segment. An example is illustrated in **Fig. 12.3**. This patient had a metastatic lung cancer initially involving T5 and this was treated with radiosurgery. The patient developed a T4 metastasis after 6 months, then a T3 metastasis after 8 months. These lesions were individually treated with radio-

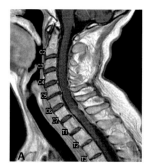 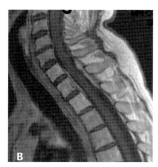 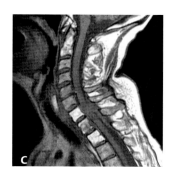

Figure 12.2 Recurrence of pain due to necrosis of epidural lesion at the treated spine. **(A)** This patient was treated for a C7-T1 metastatic lung cancer with epidural compression with a dose of 16 Gy. The patient had a arm pain relief and motor improvement. **(B)** MRI after 6 months showed stable appearance with mild reduction of the epidural lesion. **(C)** At 13 months after radiosurgery, patient had worsening pain in the arm. MRI showed progression of epidural compression. Decompressive surgery was performed. Pathology revealed necrosis with no evidence of viable tumor.

surgery. The patient had excellent symptomatic relief following each radiosurgery procedure. Note the thickening of the prevertebral fascia and soft tissue mass in the mediastinum extending along the vertebra. The patient had simultaneous tumor progression at the primary site as well as systemic metastasis. One important "limitation" of spine radiosurgery may be that it provides treatment to the targeted spinal level only. This is different from the conventional external beam radiotherapy that includes one or two spine segments both above and below the involved level. Failure rates in the immediately adjacent spine were found to be only 5%.[1] This low rate of adjacent-level failure supports the radiosurgery approach.

Failures of cases of epidural cord compressions are discussed in detail in Chapter 11, with an emphasis on the relative indications of radiosurgery versus open surgery.

◆ Neural Complications

The potential consequence of radiation-induced spinal cord injury can be severe. The classic treatment of acute and chronic radiation effects has been mainly steroid therapy and supportive care for the symptoms. Although surgical resection has been employed for focal brain radionecrosis, it cannot be readily used if a necrotic focus occurs within the spinal cord. The best way to prevent radiation myelopathy is to avoid unnecessary or excessive irradiation to the spinal cord. Therefore, it is crucial to achieve good dose conformality to the tumor volume while minimizing the dose to the spinal cord.

The nature of radiation-induced myelopathy may not be different from that of brain injury following radiosurgery or fractionated radiotherapy. The mechanism of radiation injury of the neural tissue is not well understood. A current understanding of radiation neural damage involves the existing concept of parenchymal cell loss and vascular damage and a more complex dynamic interaction with active participation of various host cells in the local tissue.[4–8] The spinal cord may have unique radiobiologic features associated with blood–spinal cord barrier disruption after radiation, in addition to the damage to long neuronal tracts.[9] Details of radiobiological consideration of spinal cord damage are described in Chapters 1 and 2. Within the spinal cord, there are several different neural tissues, and these may have varying sensitivities to radiation. It is also believed that the anterior spinal artery has the potential to be injured by high doses of radiation, leading to spinal cord ischemia. Finally, radiation-induced edema within the spinal cord can also cause acute or chronic clinical symptoms.

Neural complications may be divided into three categories based on the time of clinical manifestation after radiosurgery (**Table 12.2**). Acute complications occur in the first month after radiosurgery and are usually temporary. Subacute complications occur approximately 3 to 6 months after radiosurgery. The transient development of neurologic symptoms is thought to occur secondary to demyelination. Long-term complications occur after 6 months, and the symptoms may be either transient or permanent. The time frame of clinical

Table 12.2 Neural Complications of Spine Radiosurgery

Acute
Exacerbation of pain
Exacerbation of neurologic dysfunction
Subacute
Transient clinical deterioration
Long-term
Chronic spinal cord edema
Radiation necrosis

manifestation of complications may overlap throughout the process. In addition, there are many other tumor and host factors that predispose the patient to the development of neural complications.[10,11] Fortunately, the reported incidence of spinal cord complications seems to be very low after radiosurgery for both benign and malignant spine tumors, although long-term follow-up is still lacking.[12,16]

Acute complications after spine radiosurgery are not common. Prophylactic steroid use is not usually necessary to prevent any acute side effects, so they are not commonly administered. Indeed, a steroid taper can be started immediately after radiosurgery in patients who were already on steroids. In our patient series, there appears to be 2 to 3% of patients who developed an acute exacerbation of their existing neurologic symptoms, mostly radiculopathy (unpublished data). These symptoms occurred usually within 2 days of radiosurgery and lasted for 2 days. Steroid and anti-inflammatory treatment is advisable for the control of symptoms. A temporary exacerbation of pain after the treatment of bony metastases with standard external beam irradiation or radionuclide therapy, especially with larger dose per fraction treatment, has been known.

Long-term complications after spine radiosurgery are rare. One caveat is that the limited survival time after spine radiosurgery for metastatic disease makes the late toxicity less likely to manifest because radiation-induced cord damage may occur later than the median survival time. In this regard, longer follow-up will be necessary to better define the long-term complications of spine radiosurgery, especially radionecrosis of the spinal cord. Nevertheless, in patients with solitary spine metastasis, the overall 1- and 2-year survival rates were 49 and 39%, respectively.[17] The median survival times of patients with breast cancer, prostate cancer, and multiple myeloma were relatively long enough to manifest spinal cord toxicity. Spine radiosurgery experience with benign spine tumors will likely show the true incidence of long-term spinal cord complications.

At the University of Pittsburgh Medical Center (Pittsburgh, Pennsylvania), three patients developed radiation-induced myelitis. All three patients were treated for benign lesions (meningioma, neurofibroma, and schwannoma), and none had received prior irradiation. All three lesions were located in the cervical spinal column, and all were treated with a tumor marginal dose of 20 Gy in a single fraction. Two patients had previously undergone an attempted open surgical resection. The volume of the spinal cord receiving > 8 Gy was < 0.02 cc in all cases. In these three patients, the onset of symptoms

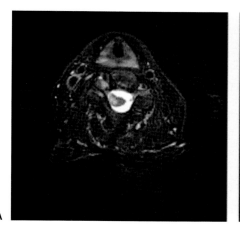

A

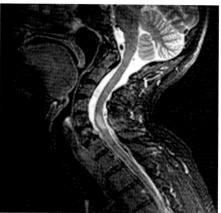

B

Figure 12.4 Brown-Séquard syndrome after radiosurgery. **(A)** Diagnosis was made based on T2-weighted magnetic resonance imaging. **(B)** The residual right C6 schwannoma is seen in the neural foramen.

consistent with a Brown-Séquard syndrome occurred within 5, 12, and 13 months after treatment. Diagnosis of radiation-induced cord damage was made based on T2-weighted signal changes seen on MRI (**Fig. 12.4**). In this case, the residual right C6 schwannoma is seen in the neural foramen on the axial image (**Fig. 12.4A**). Patients were treated with a combination of steroids, vitamin E, and gabapentin. One patient underwent a course of hyperbaric oxygen therapy.

At the Henry Ford Hospital, the constraint for the spinal cord has consistently been 10 Gy to 10% of volume at the spinal cord; hence, we defined partial volume cord tolerance.[17] The spinal cord as seen on MRI is contoured at the level of involvement and extended 6 mm cephalad and caudad to the target volume. The accumulated dose-volume histogram (DVH) of 230 consecutive procedures of dose escalation with spine radiosurgery is shown in **Fig. 12.5**. Employing this spinal cord constraint, there has been no adverse event attributable to radiation injury of the spinal cord, except for the single case of spinal cord damage as described below.

The patient had a diagnosis of invasive breast cancer. The initial treatment was mastectomy followed by chemotherapy (cyclophosphamide, methotrexate, and fluorouracil). She later developed a recurrent tumor at the chest wall,

and was treated with radiotherapy and continued hormonal therapy. After 6 years, she presented with voice change due to vocal cord paralysis and difficulty in swallowing. MRI revealed a metastatic involvement of the base of the skull, including the clivus, occipital condyle, and C1 vertebra with epidural compression (**Fig. 12.6A**). She was treated with a radiosurgery dose of 16 Gy, prescribed to the 90% isodose line encompassing the gross tumor volume (**Fig. 12.6B**). The patient had complete neurologic recovery and pain relief, as well as good radiographic response. She then received chemotherapy with carboplatin and Taxotere (docetaxel) for 6 months, and continued Herceptin (trastuzumab) as well as Zometa (zoledronic acid) and Faslodex (fulvestrant). Thirteen months after radiosurgery, however, right lower extremity weakness developed. Muscle strength was found to be four fifths. There was no sensory deficit. MRI revealed T2 signal abnormality in the cervicomedullary junction at the level of the radiosurgery target, along with contrast enhancement in the ventral aspect of the medulla and right cerebellum (**Fig. 12.6C**). These changes were consistent with radiation toxicity. The patient was treated with dexamethasone, and her symptoms improved.

Reported cases of myelopathy induced by single-dose spine radiosurgery are few. In a series of radiosurgery of benign spi-

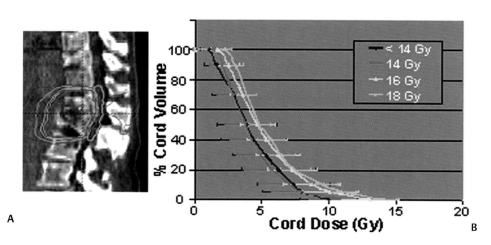

A

B

Figure 12.5 Definition of the spinal cord and dose-volume histogram (DVH) of the spinal cord. **(A)** The spinal cord was defined as 6 mm above and below the target volume (green). **(B)** The accumulated DVH of 230 procedures with spine radiosurgery shows the partial volume tolerance of the spinal cord 10 Gy to the 10% spinal cord volume.

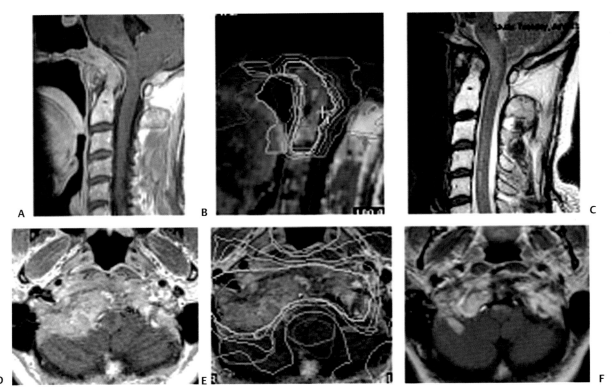

Figure 12.6 Radiation-induced cervical myelopathy. This breast cancer patient presented with vocal cord paralysis and difficulty swallowing. **(A)** Sagittal and axial magnetic resonance imaging (MRI) showed a metastatic involvement of the base of the skull, including the clivus, occipital condyle, and C1 vertebra with mild epidural compression. **(B)** The patient received a single radiosurgery dose of 16 Gy, prescribed to the 90% isodose line encompassing the gross tumor volume. The patient had complete neurologic recovery and pain relief, along with complete tumor disappearance. **(C)** She experienced a right lower extremity weakness after 13 months. Sagittal and axial MRI revealed T2 signal abnormality in the cervicomedullary junction at the level of the radiosurgery target and contrast enhancement in the ventral aspect of the medulla and right cerebellum.

nal tumors, a single patient was reported to have developed myelopathy.[18] The reported dose was 18 Gy in three fractions to a 1.73 cc volume of the spinal cord. This dose was not unusual in the researchers' experience. There were patients who received higher doses to the spinal cord but did not develop spinal cord toxicity. The authors speculated that the trauma from the previous surgical resections may have predisposed the patient to the development of the spinal cord damage.

There are many reported risk factors for radiation-induced myelopathy. These variables include total dose, fraction size, length and volume of the irradiated spinal cord, total treatment time, host factors, and other concurrent therapies.[10,11,19,20]

Radiosurgery is given to a tightly defined target, and it produces a rapid dose fall-off outside the target. It therefore leads to a significant dose gradient even within the small confines of the spinal cord. For this reason, the dose guidelines from conventional radiation tolerance using fractionated radiotherapy cannot be readily extrapolated to the practice of radiosurgery. There is currently some controversy regarding the observed versus the estimated tolerance dose.[21,22] The concept of "partial volume effect" must be carefully considered in spine radiosurgery. To define the partial volume tolerance of the spinal cord, it is necessary to consider a wide variety of variables, including the definition of spinal cord volume, the effect of the target volume in the high-dose region within the

spinal cord, the differential tolerance within the spinal cord in the cross-sectional and longitudinal planes, the functional anatomy of and within the spinal cord, the relative biologic effectiveness of different radiation dose regimens, and the combined effect with other treatment modalities.

The first consideration of partial volume effect is the consistent definition of the spinal cord contour. Because the radiosurgery is delivered to a very limited area of the spinal cord, at the Henry Ford Hospital, the spinal cord volume has been consistently defined as from 6 mm above to 6 mm below the radiosurgery target (**Fig. 12.5A**). The spinal cord proper must be contoured, not the entire spinal canal. With this definition of spinal cord volume, a DVH has been constructed for all cases (**Fig. 12.5B**). In this manner, partial volume tolerance of the spinal cord was defined to be 10 Gy to 10% of the spinal cord volume.[17] Although the maximum human spinal cord tolerance to radiosurgery has yet to be defined, in our experience there were no cases of spinal cord radionecrosis, except for the single case described above.

Second, a differential radiation sensitivity may very well exist within the spinal cord itself. A regional difference in radiosensitivity was observed within the rat cervical spinal cord. The lateral white matter was found to be more radiosensitive than the central part of the white matter.[23] Obviously, similar studies cannot be performed in humans. Nevertheless, radiosurgery creates a radiation dose gradient within

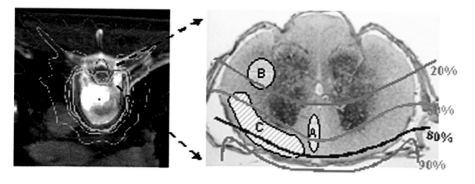

Figure 12.7 Radiation dose fall-off within the spinal cord superimposed with the functional topography of the spinal cord. (A) The anterior corticospinal tract is located within the high dose region. (B) Lateral corticospinal tracts are located in the posterolateral portion of the spinal cord. (C) The high radiation dose is located in the ventral area of the spinal cord, where mostly sensory tracts are present.

the spinal cord due to rapid dose fall-off. A diagram of radiation dose fall-off within the spinal cord is shown in **Fig. 12.7**, overlaid with the functional topography of the spinal cord. In this case (as in most cases of spine radiosurgery), the highest radiation dose is primarily deposited in the ventral portion of the spinal cord, where most sensory tracts are present (**Fig. 12.7C**). The anterior corticospinal tract (**Fig. 12.7A**) may be located within the high-dose region as well. This tract incorporates approximately 10% of the corticospinal tract that does not decussate. Injury to this tract is not likely to cause an ambulatory deficit.[24] Most of the motor function is carried by the lateral corticospinal tracts, located in the posterolateral portion of the spinal cord (**Fig. 12.7B**). Therefore, the radiation dose to the motor tract may be sufficiently lower than the actual tolerance of this portion of the spinal cord.

Patients who received these same dose constraints to the dorsal compartment of the cord similarly did not develop any neurologic abnormalities. It is not known whether the sensory tracts may be more tolerant to radiation than the motor tracts, and there also does not appear to be any difference in the spinal cord tolerance of the cervical, thoracic, or upper lumbar regions. Most radiation myelopathy cases have been reported in the cervical and thoracic regions.[25-28] The cauda equina and the spinal nerves are thought to have a higher radiation tolerance because these are actually considered peripheral nerves. Another consideration is possible long-term vascular damage to the medium-sized blood vessels, namely, the anterior spinal artery (located in the anterior sulcus) and its branches. No such clinical complication that may be attributed to this pattern of vascular damage has been described. Future studies will be required to more systematically define the cross-sectional and longitudinal differential tolerance within the spinal cord.

Third, the position of the spinal cord within the vertebral canal is of practical importance. There are significant variations in the spinal cord position between the cervical, thoracic, and lumbar regions between patients and within the same patient. There are individual variations in the position of the spinal cord at the same spine level, as well as in the diameter of the spinal cord. To overcome such individual variation, image fusion of the contrast-enhanced simulation CT with MRI (gadolinium-contrast and T2-weighted images) or myelography may help to better delineate the spinal cord.

Finally, there can be actual organ motion of the spinal cord during the radiosurgery procedure. Although the spinal cord movement by pulsation is observed intraoperatively dur-

ing surgery, this is not considered to be clinically relevant in spine radiosurgery. Other possible causes of spinal cord motion during treatment are secondary spine movement via breathing-related rib cage motion or by actual patient body movements. Patient movement issues during the radiosurgery procedure are described in Chapter 4.

◆ Non-neural Complications

Spine radiosurgery complications are not limited to the spinal cord and other neural structures. Complications may occur within any irradiated adjacent tissues depending on the targeted spine level. Complications of non-neural tissue are not different from the effect of conventional radiotherapy. Because a larger single dose is given, however, the acute effect may be more severe. These acute side effects generally resolve within 2 weeks. Similar to what has been previously discussed with the spinal cord, partial volume tolerance of other normal tissues is relevant to spine radiosurgery. Therefore, the tolerance of each individual organ needs to be redefined as a "partial volume effect" to be applicable to extracranial radiosurgery. Some of the possible non-neural complications related to spine radiosurgery are listed in **Table 12.3.** The dose–partial volume relationship of these complications has not yet been established.

Table 12.3 Non-neural Complications Reported following Spine Radiosurgery

Acute
Skin reaction
Pharyngitis
Laryngitis
Tracheitis
Transient nausea
Esophagitis
Gastritis
Enteritis
Proctitis
Long-term
Soft tissue fibrosis
Tracheoesophageal fistula
Gastrointestinal ulcer

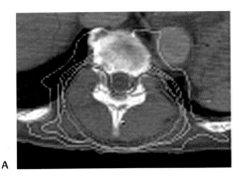
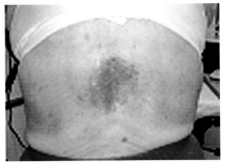

Figure 12.8 Skin reaction. **(A,B)** This patient was treated for a soft tissue tumor mass involving the spinous process. Note that the skin dose was high due to the tumor location immediately under the skin.

Skin reactions are seldom seen after radiosurgery because the radiation dose to the skin is usually minimal. The chance of skin reaction increases simply due to the location of the target, particularly when posterior elements of the spine, such as the spinous processes, are treated with radiosurgery. A case of skin reaction is shown in **Fig. 12.8** in a patient with a soft tissue mass around the spinous process. The skin dose was high in this case because the tumor extended almost to the skin. Hair loss can be seen in the irradiated field.

Mucositis of the pharynx and esophagus may occur after radiosurgery of the cervical and thoracic spines. These structures are usually within, or very close to, the range of the high-dose region or rapid dose fall-off. The clinical symptoms are usually odynophagia and dysphagia. Pharyngitis is

more frequently noted than mucositis of the larynx and trachea. The maximum dose to these structures should be kept below 10 Gy. Mucositis symptoms usually subside within 2 weeks. Transient nausea and subsequent emesis may result from treatments of lower thoracic and upper lumbar lesions posterior to the stomach. In such cases, the dose to the stomach is limited to 8 Gy in a single fraction. Patients may be treated prophylactically with antiemetics to avoid this complication.

Toxicity to the kidney has not been encountered. However, it is strongly advised to minimize the kidney dose, according to the dose-volume effect of acute and chronic renal toxicity. It should be particularly respected in patients with one kidney, transplanted kidney, and known renal disease. Renal

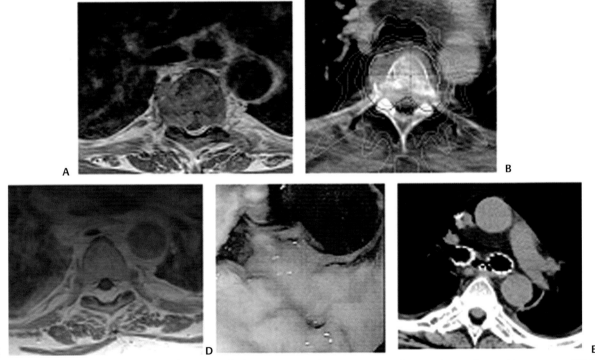

Figure 12.9 Tracheoesophageal fistula. **(A)** This patient had multiple myeloma with T4 with severe cord compression. There was a paraspinal tumor adjacent to the esophagus. **(B)** The tumor was treated with 16 Gy radiosurgery, resulting in a rapid improvement within 1 week. **(C)** Magnetic resonance imaging 6 months after radiosurgery showed a complete radiographic response. **(D)** The patient developed symptoms of cough and aspiration 13 months after radiosurgery. Esophageal endoscopy revealed a large fistula at the treated level. **(E)** Tracheal and esophageal stents were placed.

dose is of particular concern in cases of renal cell carcinoma metastases when such patients often have only a single remaining kidney; these tumors are most frequently encountered in the thoracolumbar region.

Long-term non-neural complications of spine radiosurgery are also rare. There was one case of tracheoesophageal fistula seen at the Henry Ford Hospital. This patient had multiple myeloma involving T4 with severe spinal cord compression causing paraparesis (**Fig. 12.9A**). There was paraspinal tumor adjacent to the esophagus. It was not clear whether the esophagus was involved by the tumor. The tumor volume was treated with 16 Gy single fraction (**Fig. 12.9B**). The patient had prompt clinical improvement within 1 week, and MRI obtained 6 months after radiosurgery showed a complete radiographic response (**Fig. 12.9C**). The patient had symptoms of cough and aspiration 13 months after radiosurgery. Further workup with esophageal endoscopy revealed a large fistula at the treated level (**Fig. 12.9D**). Tracheal and esophageal stents were placed (**Fig. 12.9E**). This complication was thought to be primarily the result of the radiosurgery treatment. This patient also suffered from frequent episodes of infections, however, particularly atypical mycobacterial infection as well as fungal infection, after many different courses of chemotherapy and bone marrow transplantation.

◆ Conclusion

Many factors can influence the subsequent development of radiosurgical complications. These include the proximity and/or extension of the tumor to adjacent normal tissues, concurrent systemic therapy, compounding morbidity such as acute infection, prior surgery at the treated level, and the patient's comorbidities, such as diabetes, collagen vascular disease, hypertension, and genetic predisposition to radiosensitivity. A careful assessment of the patient's clinical condition as well as the dosimetry plan and DVH is necessary to reduce the potential risk of radiation-induced tissue injury. Measures that may modify the incidence and severity of radiation damage should be incorporated in future clinical trials.

References

1. Ryu S, Rock J, Rosenblum M, Kim JH. Pattern of failure after single dose radiosurgery for single spinal metastasis. J Neurosurg 2004;101:402–405.
2. Gerszten PC, Germanwala A, Burton SA, et al. Combination kyphoplasty and spinal radiosurgery: a new treatment paradigm for pathologic fractures. J Neurosurg Spine 2005;3(4):296–301.
3. Gerszten PC, Burton SA, Ozhasoglu C, et al. Stereotactic radiosurgery for spine metastases from renal cell carcinoma. J Neurosurg Spine 2005;3(4):288–295.
4. van der Kogel AJ. Central nervous system injury in small animal models. In: Gutin RH, Leibel SA, Sheline GE, eds. Radiation Injury to the Nervous System. New York: Raven Press; 1991:91–111.
5. Hopewell JW. Radiation injury to the central nervous system. Med Pediatr Oncol 1998;1:1–9.
6. Tofilon PJ, Fike JR. The radioresponse of the central nervous system: a dynamic process. Radiat Res 2000;153:357–370.
7. Raju U, Gumin GJ, Tofilon PJ. Radiation-induced transcription factor activation in rat cerebral cortex. Int J Radiat Biol 2000;76:1045–1053.
8. Belka C, Budach W, Kortmann RD, Bamberg M. Radiation-induced CNS toxicity: molecular and cellular mechanisms. Br J Cancer 2001;85:1233–1239.
9. Tsao MN, Li YQ, Lu G, Yu X, Wong CS. Upregulation of vascular endothelial growth factor is associated with radiation-induced blood-spinal cord barrier disruption. J Neuropathol Exp Neurol 1999;58:1051–1060.
10. Rampling R, Reynolds P. Radiation myelopathy. Curr Opin Neurol 1998;11:627–632.
11. Ang KK. Radiation injury to the central nervous system: clinical features and prevention. Front Radiat Ther Oncol 1999;32:145–154.
12. Rock JP, Ryu S, Shukairy MS, et al. Postoperative stereotactic radiosurgery for malignant spinal tumors. Neurosurgery 2006;58:891–898.
13. Gerszten PC, Ozhasoglu C, Burton SA, et al. CyberKnife frameless single-fraction stereotactic radiosurgery for benign tumors of the spine. Neurosurg Focus 2003;14:e16.
14. Degen JW, Gagnon GJ, Voyadzis JM, et al. CyberKnife stereotactic radiosurgical treatment of spinal tumors for pain control and quality of life. J Neurosurg Spine 2005;2:540–549.
15. Gerszten PC, Burton SA, Welch WC, et al. Single-fraction radiosurgery for the treatment of spinal breast metastases. Cancer 2005;104:2244–2254.
16. Ryu S, Yin FF, Rock J, et al. Image-guided intensity-modulated radiosurgery for spinal metastasis. Cancer 2003;97:2013–2018.
17. Ryu S, Jin R, Jin JY, Rock J, Ajlouni M, Movsas B, Kim JH. Partial volume tolerance and complication of spinal cord to single dose radiosurgery. Cancer 2007;109:628–636.
18. Dodd RL, Ryu MR, Kamnerdsupaphon P, et al. CyberKnife radiosurgery for benign intradural extramedullary spinal tumors. Neurosurgery 2006;58:674–685.
19. Ryu S, Gorty S, Kazee AM, et al. "Full dose" re-irradiation of human cervical spinal cord. Am J Clin Oncol 2000;23:29–31.
20. Schultheiss TE, Kun LE, Ang KK, Stephens LC. Radiation response of the central nervous system. Int J Radiat Oncol Biol Phys 1995;31:1093–1112.
21. Wara WM, Phillips TL, Sheline GE, Schwade JG. Radiation tolerance of the spinal cord. Cancer 1975;35:1558–1562.
22. Emami B, Lyman J, Brown A, et al. Tolerance of normal tissue to therapeutic irradiation. Int J Radiat Oncol Biol Phys 1991;21:109–122.
23. Bijl HP, van Luijk P, Coppes RP, et al. Regional differences in radiosensitivity across the rat cervical spinal cord. Int J Radiat Oncol Biol Phys 2005;61:543–551.
24. Carpenter MB. Human Neuroanatomy. 7th ed. Baltimore: Williams & Wilkins; 1976:255–256.
25. Abbatucci JS, Delozier T, Quint R, Roussel A, Brune D. Radiation myelopathy of the cervical spinal cord: time, dose and volume factors. Int J Radiat Oncol Biol Phys 1978;4:239–248.
26. Hatlevoll R, Host H, Kaalhus O. Myelopathy following radiotherapy of bronchial carcinoma with large single fractions: a retrospective study. Int J Radiat Oncol Biol Phys 1983;9:41–44.
27. McCunniff AJ, Liang MJ. Radiation tolerance of the cervical spinal cord. Int J Radiat Oncol Biol Phys 1989;16:675–678.
28. Phillips TL, Buschke F. Radiation tolerance of the thoracic spinal cord. Am J Roentgenol Radium Ther Nucl Med 1969;105:659–664.

13

Radiosurgery for Benign Extramedullary Tumors of the Spine

Iris C. Gibbs, Steven D. Chang, Robert L. Dodd, and John R. Adler Jr.

Benign extramedullary spinal tumors represent a spectrum of tumors, including meningiomas, schwannomas, and neurofibromas. Although surgery is widely thought to be the treatment of choice for benign extramedullary spinal tumors, small case series support the use of radiation therapy as adjuvant treatment after subtotal resection or for recurrence.[1-7] Recently, the delivery of highly conformal radiosurgery of spinal tumors has been made possible by image guidance.[8,9] Extrapolating from the effectiveness of radiosurgery for intracranial meningiomas and nerve sheath tumors, where tumor control rates > 90% have been reported, radiosurgery has been explored for benign extramedullary spinal tumors.[10-15] Furthermore, the limitations of surgical options for patients with medical comorbidities, recurrent tumors, or familial phakomatoses make radiosurgery an attractive management option.

In 2001 Stanford University established the feasibility of image-guided spine radiosurgery for benign tumors when researchers there reported the first clinical experience that included two spinal schwannomas and one spinal meningioma.[8] Although larger series have reported the efficacy of radiosurgery for metastatic spinal lesions, there is a paucity of reports detailing clinical outcomes of radiosurgery for benign spinal tumors. Evaluation of radiosurgery for these lesions requires longer follow-up to confirm durable safety and efficacy, particularly because, according to surgical reports, recurrences may occur more than 5 years later.[8,16-20]

Although other commercial radiation systems designed to achieve precision radiosurgery for spinal tumors, such as Synergy (Elekta AB, Stockholm, Sweden) and TomoTherapy (TomoTherapy Inc., Madison, Wisconsin), are in early use, the available data on the clinical outcome of patients with benign extramedullary spinal tumors treated with radiosurgery come from investigators at a small number of institutions using modified linear accelerator (linac) systems, including CyberKnife (Accuray Inc., Sunnyvale, California) and Novalis (BrainLab AG, Feldkirchen, Germany) (**Table 13.1**).[1,21-24]

In their brief review of radiation for benign neurofibromas, Chopra et al reported the results of a 12-year-old child with neurofibromatosis type 1 (NF1) whose tumor was stable at 20 months.[1] Collectively, there are only six patients whose outcomes are available after treatment with the Novalis system.[21,22] Two other groups report a collective experience of 60 patients treated by CyberKnife. To date, the report by Dodd et al represents the largest single institution series of patients with extended follow-up that may help to ascertain the efficacy of this approach.[23]

Current clinical indications for benign spine tumors radiosurgery include benign spine tumors located in surgically difficult regions of the spine, recurrent benign spinal tumors after prior surgical resection, and benign spine tumors in patients who have significant medical comorbidities that preclude surgery. Relative contraindications for radiosurgery for benign spine tumors include tumors without well-defined margins, tumors with significant spinal cord compression resulting in acute neurologic symptoms, and tumors that can easily be resected with conventional surgical techniques.

◆ Technical and Dose Considerations

Geometrically accurate visualization of the target tumor on imaging is essential for radiosurgery treatment planning. Fortunately, most benign tumors of the spine enhance brightly and have well-defined margins. Magnetic resonance imaging (MRI) is the imaging modality of choice for diagnostic purposes, though issues of spatial distortion need to be considered if MRI is used directly for planning. Because signal intensities of MR images do not reflect a direct relationship with electron densities, unless attenuation coefficients are manually assigned to the regions of interest, spatial distortion limits the accuracy of using MRI directly in radiosurgery planning.[25] Because computed tomography (CT) is geometrically accurate, a common solution to improving target visu-

Table 13.1 Series of Radiosurgery for Benign Extramedullary Spinal Tumors

Series	Menin-gioma	Schwan-noma	Neuro-fibroma	Mean Age (years)	Total Patients	Indication	Dose/ Number of Fractions	Length of F/U (months)	Outcome
Dodd et al[23] (CyberKnife)	16	30	9	46	51	51% recurrent/ residual	16 to 30 Gy/ 1 to 5 fractions	25	96% stable/decreased 3 repeat surgery 1 progression 1 new myelopathy
Chopra et al[1] (linac)	0	0	1	12	1	Residual	12.5 Gy/ 1 fraction	20	NED
De Salles et al[22] (Novalis)	1	1	1	62	3		12 to 15 Gy/ 1 fraction	6	Stable
Benzil et al[21] (Novalis)	1	2	0	61	3	NR	5.0 to 50.4 Gy/ variable	NR	Rapid pain relief
Gerszten et al[24] (CyberKnife)	2	2	5	NR	9	One-third prior surgery	12 to 20 Gy/ 1 fraction	12	Pain relief

Abbreviations: F/U, follow-up; NR, not reported; NED, no evidence of disease.

alization is to co-register MRI images with CT images. The currently available commercial radiosurgery systems use CT for treatment planning and delivery. Therefore, the ability to identify tumors on CT together with the probability of generating an adequate image fusion with MRI is key to defining the radiosurgery target. Furthermore, because virtually all extramedullary spinal tumors show some degree of contrast enhancement, postcontrast CT is sometimes used directly to define the target. However, some nerve sheath tumors exhibit heterogeneous enhancement and may be identified by image fusion with MRI. Spinal image fusion of the spine can be much more complex than brain MRI-CT fusion because it is more dependent on the technical aspects of image acquisition. The quality of MR spinal image fusion often requires that the patient's imaging position closely matches the intended treatment position.

By virtue of their origin along the dura and spinal nerve roots, extramedullary spinal tumors can significantly impinge on the spinal cord to cause neurologic symptoms. The goal of radiosurgery is to provide a clinically significant radiation dose to the tumor while observing the dose tolerance to the spinal cord and surrounding soft tissue. The degree of impingement of the tumor on the spinal cord may prevent the generation of a suitable radiosurgery treatment plan. Similar to radiosurgery doses prescribed for intracranial tumors, spine radiosurgery doses generally range from 12 to 20 Gy in a single fraction; doses as high as 30 Gy have been delivered when the treatment was hypofractionated in up to five sessions (**Table 13.1**). Benzil et al also included patients treated with conventional radiation fraction doses up to 50.4 Gy.[21]

◆ Spinal Meningiomas

Meningiomas arise from cells of the meningeal coverings of the central nervous system and occur more frequently within the brain than the spinal cord, with approximately a 5:1 ratio (**Table 13.2**).[26] Spinal meningiomas show a predilection for the thoracic spine and an overwhelming female predominance of 75 to 85%.[7,27] Spinal meningiomas, in general, have a more favorable prognosis relative to their intracranial counterparts. In a study of histological and micro-array data of meningiomas, Sayaguès et al determined that spinal meningiomas were most commonly associated with lower proliferative rates and more indolent histologies (psammomatous, transitional variants), and showed characteristic genetic and genomic differences compared with intracranial meningiomas.[26] Both histology and age at presentation are important. The Mayo Clinic compared 40 patients under age 50 with spinal meningiomas with a random group of older patients having the same condition and showed that younger patients had higher mortality rates (10%) and recurred more frequently (22% vs 5%) compared with older patients.[28] These patients also had a higher number of predisposing risks, such as neurofibromatosis type 2 (NF2), trauma, and radiation exposure. Although radiosurgery for these tumors is an attractive option, longer follow-up will determine the true efficacy. In the Dodd et al series, all of the 15 of 16 meningiomas with radiographic follow-up were controlled, though one patient required surgery and another sustained the only complication reported in the series.[23] Clearly, the radiosurgery-treated patients represent a more difficult group to treat, with most being treated after subtotal surgery or

Table 13.2 Characteristic Features of Benign Extramedullary Spinal Tumors

Characteristic	Meningioma	Schwannoma	Neurofibroma
Age of presentation	5th–7th decade	5th decade	4th decade
Spinal level predominance	Thoracic (80%)	All levels evenly	Cervical (66%)
Multiplicity	1 to 2%	Rare unless NF2 associated	Common
Proportion of primary spinal tumors	25%	~33%	3.5%
Gender predominance	Female (75–85%)	None	None
Associations	More commonly psammomatous or transitional histologies	NF2, merlin/schwannomin gene on chromosome 22	NF1, neurofibromin gene on chromosome 17

Abbreviations: NF1, neurofibromatosis type 1; NF2, neurofibromatosis type 2.

recurrence. Still, 70% of the meningiomas treated in this series were symptomatically stable or improved.

Figure 13.1 shows the pretreatment sagittal T1-weighted postcontrast MRI (**Fig. 13.1A**) and the sagittal view of the radiosurgery treatment plan for a 35-year-old man who developed multiple lumbar spinal meningiomas after receiving therapeutic radiation as an adolescent 20 years prior. The CyberKnife radiosurgery treatment plan is shown for the 5.63 cm³ L4 target lesion outlined in red and the prescription isodose reflected in green (**Fig. 13.1B**). A total dose of 20 Gy was delivered in two sessions of 10 Gy each. This tumor showed nearly complete resolution at 2 years' follow-up, as seen on the sagittal MRI (**Fig. 13.1C**). Two other meningiomas developed at the level of L1 and L2–L3 and were treated successfully with radiosurgery. At 1-year follow-up, these tumors have also decreased significantly.

◆ Spinal Schwannomas

Nerve sheath tumors are comprised of schwannomas and neurofibromas. Schwannomas account for nearly one third of primary spinal tumors, whereas neurofibromas constitute only 3.5%.[29–31] Patients with nerve sheath tumors typically present with local pain, radiating pain, and/or paraparesis and a relatively long duration of symptoms varying from 6 weeks to over 5 years. Although many reports in the literature describe these tumors collectively, there are sufficient differences between the two tumor types to warrant a separate discussion of each. For example, schwannomas arise most commonly in the dorsal nerve root, are more commonly completely intradural (> 80%), and are generally amenable to complete resection.[29,30] On the contrary, neurofibromas arise more commonly in the ventral nerve root, are predisposed to multiple tumors by a strong association with NF1, and present with both intradural and extradural components in 66% of cases.[31] These tumors are also uniquely different with respect to predisposing genetic defects. The merlin/schwannomin gene on chromosome 22 is associated with schwannomas in NF2, whereas the neurofibromin gene on chromosome 17 is associated with NF1 and neurofibromas.[29–31]

NF2 is an autosomal dominant genetic disorder that predisposes patients to developing multiple central and peripheral nervous system tumors. Schwannomas are the most common spinal tumor that occurs in these patients. Though sporadic occurrences of schwannomas unrelated to NF2 are not uncommon, those tumors associated with NF2 are more aggressive and recur more often after treatment.[32,33] In a retrospective review of 87 patients with spinal nerve sheath tumors removed by surgery, 17 of whom had NF2-associated schwannomas, all NF2-related tumors recurred by 9 years compared with a 10-year recurrence rate of 28%

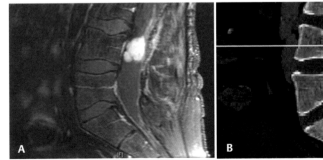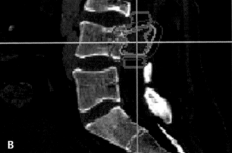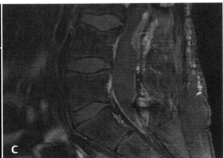

Fig. 13.1 A 35-year-old man with radiation-induced L4 meningioma. **(A)** Preradiosurgery sagittal T1-weighted postcontrast magnetic resonance imaging (MRI) with fat suppression. **(B)** Sagittal computed tomography digitally reconstructed radiograph illustrating the radiosurgery treatment plan with the L4 tumor contoured in red, a portion of the spinal canal contoured in dark green, the prescription isodose curve (79%) shown in light green, and the 50% isodose curve shown in purple. **(C)** Sagittal MRI at 2 years' follow-up showing near complete resolution of the tumor.

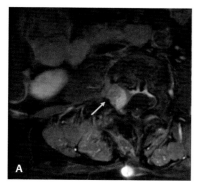 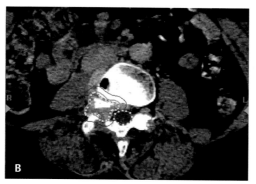 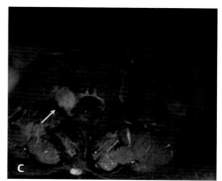

Fig. 13.2 A 72-year-old woman with recurrent L3–L4 schwannoma 3 years after resection treated by radiosurgery to 21 Gy in three sessions. **(A)** The recurrent tumor is indicated by the yellow arrow on the axial T1 postcontrast MRI. **(B)** The radiosurgery treatment plan with the tumor outlined in red with yellow dots, the prescription isodose curve in light green, the 50% isodose curve in purple, and the spinal canal outlined in dark green. **(C)** Stable tumor indicated by the yellow arrow at 2 years' follow-up on T1 postcontrast magnetic resonance image.

in tumors not associated with NF2.[33] Indeed, in this analysis, factors strongly predictive of recurrence after surgery were partial resection, prior recurrence, NF2, and advanced age. It is therefore not surprising that of the schwannomas treated by radiosurgery in the Dodd et al series, 40% of tumors were NF2 related, and 41% of these patients were treated for recurrent or residual tumor after surgery. Early follow-up of 25.4 months showed encouraging results, with 96% of tumors controlled and most patients experiencing stable to improved symptoms.[23]

Figure 13.2 illustrates the case of a 72-year-old woman with a recurrent right L3–L4 schwannoma, back pain, and right leg radicular pain 3 years after initial resection. This patient had undergone a laminectomy for a synovial cyst 7 years prior to surgery in a similar location. The schwannoma was felt to be a possible result of the previous trauma. Despite near-total resection, the tumor recurred, heralded by intractable pain. The patient was treated by CyberKnife radiosurgery in a multiple-session approach over 3 consecutive days to a total dose of 21 Gy. Two years after the procedure, the tumor is radiographically stable, and the back pain is improved, but the patient still reports radiating pain down the right leg.

◆ Spinal Neurofibromas

Neurofibromas are less common than schwannomas, constituting only 3.5% of primary spinal tumors. Peripheral and central nervous system neurofibromas are commonly associated with NF1, an autosomal dominant inherited disorder with highly variable expression. Approximately 2% of patients with NFl will develop 2% symptomatic spinal tumors. Multiple spinal tumors are not uncommon.[31] As with other nerve sheath tumors, patients present with pain and paraparesis. Two thirds of neurofibromas occur in the cervical spine. These tumors grow both intra- and extradurally. Surgical extirpation of these tumors commonly requires sectioning of the originating nerve roots to completely resect the lesion. Although asymptomatic spinal neurofibromas are common in NF1 patients, the high incidence of developing second neurofibromas warrants close clinical follow-up.

The clinical response after radiosurgery is variable. Gerszten et al detailed the outcome of one of the five neurofibromas treated with CyberKnife radiosurgery using fiducial tracking.[24] This was the case of a 32-year-old woman with NF1 and a highly symptomatic L5 neurofibroma, who was treated to a single dose of 16 Gy; at 1-year follow-up, the pain remained significantly improved. In the Dodd et al series, all of the nine neurofibromas arose in patients with NF1. After a mean follow-up of 20 months, half of the patients developed worsening pain and neurologic symptoms.[23] Given these results, the role of radiosurgery for neurofibromas remains unclear, particularly considering that a significant number of the NF1 patients were myelopathic at presentation. It is worth noting that the neurofibromas were stable radiographically in all patients. The poor clinical responses seen in this study appear to mimic the finding by Seppala et al that only 1 of 15 patients who were alive at long-term follow-up after surgery reported complete freedom from symptoms.[31] It is likely that the most realistic and attainable goal of neurofibroma treatment in myelopathic patients is tumor control without significant expectations for symptomatic improvement. Furthermore, given that many of the patients with neurofibromas had multiple lesions along their spine, it can often be difficult to determine whether symptom progression was due to the treated lesion or from any of the other neurofibroma lesions within the spine.

The clinical case presented in **Fig. 13.3** illustrates the case of a 38-year-old man with NF1 and multiple innumerable spinal and peripheral nerve neurofibromas. After presenting with progressive pain and weakness of the upper extremities, radiosurgery was offered with the goal of controlling the tumor growth of the left C2 neurofibroma. A dose of 18 Gy was delivered over two sessions. Despite the radiographic stability of the tumor at 1 year following treatment, the patient showed progressive symptoms. Patients with multiple tumors such as the one presented here represent a difficult management challenge. Here the decision was made to treat the largest tumor that approximately topographically co-localized to the patient's symptoms. The lack of symptomatic response may have correlated with the uncertainty in accurately co-localizing the offending lesion for treatment.

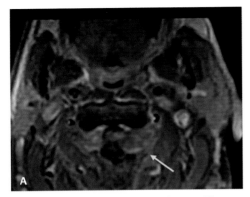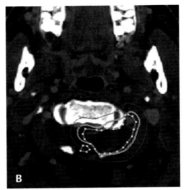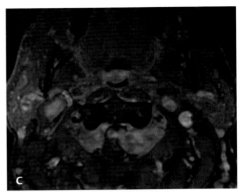

Fig. 13.3 A 38-year-old man with neurofibromatosis type 1 and multiple spinal neurofibromas presenting with progressive weakness. **(A)** Left C2 neurofibroma indicated by the yellow arrow was targeted for radiosurgery. **(B)** Radiosurgery plan of 18 Gy in two fractions shows the tumor outlined in red with yellow dots, the displaced spinal cord outlined in green, the prescription isodose curve in light green, and the 50% isodose curve in purple. **(C)** At 1-year follow-up, the tumor was radiographically stable, although not symptomatically improved.

◆ Complications of Spine Radiosurgery for Benign Spinal Tumors

Ultimately, the goals of tumor control and symptom alleviation have to be balanced with toxicity of the treatment. Because the available clinical series have short follow-up, the late effects of spine radiosurgery remain largely unknown. Transient parotitis and alopecia have been reported as mild early complications of radiosurgery.[24] More severe complications including two patients with transient radiculitis requiring intervention were reported by Benzil et al.[21] Dodd et al reported the first published case of radiation-induced myelopathy after radiosurgery for benign spinal tumors.[23] This case involved a 29-year-old woman with a cervicothoracic spinal meningioma who developed myelopathic symptoms 8 months after CyberKnife radiosurgery to a dose of 24 Gy over three sessions. It was felt that the relatively large volume of spinal cord (1.7 cm^3) irradiated above 18 Gy (over three sessions of 6 Gy) may have been the contributing factor. In their dose-volume analysis, the irradiated volume of spinal cord in this patient represented an outlier compared with other patients in the series. Although most authors who prefer to deliver radiosurgery in a single treatment attempt to limit the maximum spinal cord dose to 8 to 10 Gy, roughly based on the observed tolerance of other radiosensitive nerves, the tolerance of the spinal cord to other fractionated schedules remains unknown. Given this report, it is clear that caution is still required when considering radiosurgery for these tumors. Longer follow-up will be needed to determine the safety and efficacy of radiosurgery for benign spinal tumors.

◆ Conclusion

Radiosurgery for benign spinal tumors is feasible, safe, and in many cases effective in controlling tumor growth. The optimum dose-fraction regimens required for tumor ablation and the dose tolerance limit of the normal spinal cord remain to be determined. However, in general, meningiomas and schwannomas have high tumor control rates. Pain relief can be attained in the majority of patients with meningioma and schwannomas; improvement of weakness and sensory loss is observed in many of these patients as well. NF1 patients with neurofibromas, though demonstrating excellent tumor growth control following stereotactic radiosurgery, often do not show improvement in clinical symptoms. Longer follow-up is required to establish efficacy of spine radiosurgery for benign spinal tumors, but the clinical outcomes of the current short-term follow-up is promising.

References

1. Chopra R, Morris CG, Friedman WA, Mendenhall WM. Radiotherapy and radiosurgery for benign neurofibromas. Am J Clin Oncol 2005;28(3):317–320.
2. Gezen F, Kahraman S, Canakci Z, Beduk A. Review of 36 cases of spinal cord meningioma. Spine 2000;25(6):727–731.
3. Gottfried ON, Gluf W, Quinones-Hinojosa A, Kan P, Schmidt MH. Spinal meningiomas: surgical management and outcome. Neurosurg Focus 2003;14(6):E2.
4. Roux FX, Nataf F, Pinaudeau M, et al. Intraspinal meningiomas: review of 54 cases with discussion of poor prognosis factors and modern therapeutic management. Surg Neurol 1996;46(5):458–463, discussion 463–454.
5. Asazuma T, Toyama Y, Maruiwa H, Fujimura Y, Hirabayashi K. Surgical strategy for cervical dumbbell tumors based on a three-dimensional classification. Spine 2004;29(1):E10–E14.
6. Gambardella G, Gervasio O, Zaccone C. Approaches and surgical results in the treatment of ventral thoracic meningiomas: review of our experience with a postero-lateral combined transpedicular-transarticular approach. Acta Neurochir (Wien) 2003;145(5):385–392.
7. Parsa AT, Lee J, Parney IF, Weinstein P, McCormick PC, Ames C. Spinal cord and intradural-extraparenchymal spinal tumors: current best care practices and strategies. J Neurooncol 2004;69(1–3):291–318.
8. Ryu SI, Chang SD, Kim DH, et al. Image-guided hypo-fractionated stereotactic radiosurgery to spinal lesions. Neurosurgery 2001;49(4):838–846.
9. Yin FF, Ryu S, Ajlouni M, et al. A technique of intensity-modulated radiosurgery (IMRS) for spinal tumors. Med Phys 2002;29(12):2815–2822.

10. Chang SD, Adler JR Jr, Hancock SL. Clinical uses of radiosurgery. Oncology 1998;12(8):1181–1188, 1191.

11. Chen HJ, Liang CL, Lu K, Lin JW, Cho CL. Implication of telomerase activity and alternations of telomere length in the histologic characteristics of intracranial meningiomas. Cancer 2000;89(10):2092–2098.

12. Flickinger JC, Kondziolka D, Lunsford LD. Radiosurgery of benign lesions. Semin Radiat Oncol 1995;5(3):220–224.

13. Kondziolka D, Nathoo N, Flickinger JC, et al. Long-term results after radiosurgery for benign intracranial tumors. Neurosurgery 2003;53(4):815–821.

14. Lunsford LD, Kondziolka D, Flickinger JC. Stereotactic radiosurgery for benign intracranial tumors. Clin Neurosurg 1993;40:475–497.

15. Pan HC, Chung WY, Guo WY, et al. Effects of gamma knife radiosurgery for brain tumors: clinical evaluation. Zhonghua Yi Xue Za Zhi (Taipei) 1998;61(7):397–407.

16. Gerszten PC, Ozhasoglu C, Burton SA, Kalnicki S, Welch WC. Feasibility of frameless single-fraction stereotactic radiosurgery for spinal lesions. Neurosurg Focus 2002;13(4):E2.

17. Gerszten PC, Ozhasoglu C, Burton SA, et al. CyberKnife frameless stereotactic radiosurgery for spinal lesions: clinical experience in 125 cases. Neurosurgery 2004;55(1):89–98.

18. Degen JW, Gagnon GJ, Voyadzis JM, et al. CyberKnife stereotactic radiosurgical treatment of spinal tumors for pain control and quality of life. J Neurosurg Spine 2005;2(5):540–549.

19. Gerszten PC, Burton SA, Ozhasoglu C, et al. Radiosurgery for the management of spinal metastases. Radiosurgery 2006;6:199–210.

20. Schick U, Marquardt G, Lorenz R. Recurrence of benign spinal neoplasms. Neurosurg Rev 2001;24(1):20–25.

21. Benzil DL, Saboori M, Mogilner AY, Rocchio R, Moorthy CR. Safety and efficacy of stereotactic radiosurgery for tumors of the spine. J Neurosurg 2004;101(Suppl 3):413–418.

22. De Salles AA, Pedroso AG, Medin P, et al. Spinal lesions treated with Novalis shaped beam intensity-modulated radiosurgery and stereotactic radiotherapy. J Neurosurg 2004;101(Suppl 3):435–440.

23. Dodd RL, Ryu MR, Kamnerdsupaphon P, et al. CyberKnife radiosurgery for benign intradural extramedullary spinal tumors. Neurosurgery 2006;58(4):674–685.

24. Gerszten PC, Ozhasoglu C, Burton SA, et al. CyberKnife frameless single-fraction stereotactic radiosurgery for benign tumors of the spine. Neurosurg Focus 2003;14(5):E16.

25. Khoo VS, Joon DL. New developments in MRI for target volume delineation in radiotherapy. Br J Radiol 2006;79(Spec No 1):S2–S15.

26. Sayaguès JM, Tabernero MD, Maillo A, et al. Microarray-based analysis of spinal versus intracranial meningiomas: different clinical, biological, and genetic characteristics associated with distinct patterns of gene expression. J Neuropathol Exp Neurol 2006;65(5):445–454.

27. King AT, Sharr MM, Gullan RW, Bartlett JR. Spinal meningiomas: a 20-year review. Br J Neurosurg 1998;12(6):521–526.

28. Cohen-Gadol AA, Zikel OM, Koch CA, Scheithauer BW, Krauss WE. Spinal meningiomas in patients younger than 50 years of age: a 21-year experience. J Neurosurg 2003; 98(3, Suppl)258–263.

29. Conti P, Pansini G, Mouchaty H, Capuano C, Conti R. Spinal neurinomas: retrospective analysis and long-term outcome of 179 consecutively operated cases and review of the literature. Surg Neurol 2004;61(1):34–43.

30. Seppala MT, Haltia MJ, Sankila RJ, Jaaskelainen JE, Heiskanen O. Long-term outcome after removal of spinal schwannoma: a clinicopathological study of 187 cases. J Neurosurg 1995;83(4):621–626.

31. Seppala MT, Haltia MJ, Sankila RJ, Jaaskelainen JE, Heiskanen O. Long-term outcome after removal of spinal neurofibroma. J Neurosurg 1995;82(4):572–577.

32. Halliday AL, Sobel RA, Martuza RL. Benign spinal nerve sheath tumors: their occurrence sporadically and in neurofibromatosis types 1 and 2. J Neurosurg 1991;74(2):248–253.

33. Klekamp J, Samii M. Surgery of spinal nerve sheath tumors with special reference to neurofibromatosis. Neurosurgery 1998;42(2):279–289.

14

Treatment of Primary Spine Tumors

Mark H. Bilsky and Yoshiya Yamada

Primary malignant bone tumors of the spine present significant treatment challenges with regard to achieving local tumor control while preserving neurologic function. The most common primary tumors involving the spinal column are chordoma, chondrosarcoma, and osteogenic sarcoma. Significant advances in both surgery and radiation are redefining their roles in the treatment of these lesions. Advanced surgical techniques for en bloc resection of primary spine tumors improves the ability to achieve marginal or wide curative resections;[1-3] however, many tumors are not amenable to en bloc resection. Conventional external beam radiation is not an effective adjuvant for many primary spine tumors. Poor outcomes with conventional radiation therapy are likely related to the relatively low dose of radiation that can be given near the spinal cord. Concern for spinal cord tolerance has typically limited radiation doses to < 5400 cGy in standard fractions.[4,5] Low-dose areas within the irradiated field are the most likely to result in disease recurrence.[6] Three radiation techniques are currently being used to increase the dose to the tumor while sparing normal tissue tolerance in an attempt to treat primary spine tumors: particle beam treatment, such as proton beam therapy; brachytherapy; and high-dose conformal photon therapy, such as image-guided intensity-modulated radiation therapy (IGRT) and Cyber-Knife. Although no class 1 evidence exists to demonstrate the contribution of high-dose radiation in achieving local tumor control for spine sarcomas, several studies have lent support to this hypothesis. The ability to deliver stereotactic radiosurgery using IGRT may also be useful in the neoadjuvant or postoperative setting.

◆ Surgery

The role of en bloc resection to achieve a marginal or wide resection is well established for extremity sarcomas.[7-9] Over the past 10 years, spine surgeons have developed techniques for en bloc resection of primary spine tumors that improve cure rates compared with piecemeal, curettage techniques.

These techniques are safe for patients with isolated vertebral body or posterior element disease. Boriani et al published a surgical series regarding en bloc spondylectomy for low-grade chondrosarcoma of the mobile spine in 22 patients.[10] Of the 12 patients who underwent en bloc excision, 9 (75%) maintained local control at a median follow-up of 81 months (range 2–236 months). Of the three recurrences, two had contaminated margins at surgery from epidural disease. The remaining 10 patients underwent curettage resection and by definition had intralesional resections with positive histologic margins. At a median follow-up of 36 months, the recurrence rate was 100%, and 80% died of disease.[10] Of note, in this group, three patients received conventional-dose external beam radiation, and no patients received high-dose conformal radiation with proton beams or IGRT.

Although curative resections are feasible in some patients, many present with factors that may preclude en bloc resection that achieves negative histologic margins. En bloc resection of the isolated vertebral body or posterior elements is technically feasible. However, according to the classification by Boriani et al,[11] patients who present with epidural tumor, multilevel large paraspinal masses, or circumferential bone disease are not candidates for marginal or wide excisions (i.e., en bloc with negative margins). The feasibility of achieving a wide or marginal excision is limited by the risk of neurologic or adjacent structure injury. For example, resecting the dura en bloc with a specimen will possibly provide a margin on epidural tumor. Unfortunately, the loss of spinal fluid buffering the spinal cord increases the probability of injury to the spinal cord and complications of cerebrospinal fluid (CSF) leak. If tumor is spilled during resection, there seems to be a higher probability of intradural seeding as well.[12] In a series of 59 spine sarcomas reviewed using the radiographic criteria established by Boriani et al's classification, about 15% of patients were candidates for en bloc excisions that could achieve a wide or marginal margins. As noted in extremity sarcomas, once the tumor is violated, the risk of recurrence significantly increases.[13] However, the treatment of sarcomas at other sites has demonstrated the utility of adjuvant high-dose radiation in the setting of microscopic or gross residual disease postresection.[14]

◆ Radiation Therapy

Radiation therapy is an extremely important modality in the treatment of primary spine tumors. However, the relative radioresistance of these tumors requires doses well above spinal cord tolerance for potential local tumor control. From the paradigm of extremity sarcomas, radiation doses > 60 Gy in 2 Gy per fraction are required for the control of positive microscopic margins and > 70 Gy for gross residual disease.[15] Traditional concepts of spinal cord tolerance using conventional radiation techniques establishes the TD 5/5 (the dose at which there is a 5% probability of myelitis necrosis at 5 years from treatment) at 50 Gy in 1.2 to 2.0 Gy per fraction, above which there appears to be a significantly increased risk of developing radiation myelitis.[16] Toxicity to the spinal cord may also be associated with the length of cord irradiated. In addition to the spinal cord, additional toxicities to paraspinal structures, such as bowel, kidneys, and the esophagus, need to be considered. Three radiation techniques are currently being used to increase the dose to the spinal cord while sparing normal tissue tolerance: proton beam therapy, brachytherapy, and high-dose conformal photon therapy, such as image-guided IGRT.

Proton Beam

The rationale for using proton beams is the excellent dose distribution at the tumor target and virtually no exit dose beyond the target volume. The Bragg peak phenomenon characteristic of proton beam radiation results in an extremely steep dose fall-off that can be measured over a course of millimeters. A relatively large experience exists in the treatment of neuraxis tumors using proton beams to deliver fractionated therapy. Proton beam radiotherapy's main limitation is the extreme expense of building and maintaining such facilities. The cost–benefit ratio of proton beam treatment is controversial. Excellent results for uveal melanoma have been reported using proton beam therapy in a hypofractionated manner (median dose 70 cobalt gray equivalent [CGE] in five fractions),[17] but there are no data reporting the use of single-fraction radiation with proton beam therapy for the management of tumors of the neuraxis.

Hug reported radiation results from 47 patients treated for primary or recurrent osteogenic and chondrogenic tumors treated with combined proton/photon therapy.[18] In this series, 23 patients received postoperative doses of 73.9 CGE, 17 pre- and postoperative therapy patients received 69.8 CGE, and 7 received 61.8 CGE as sole treatment at 1.8 to 2.0 CGE per fraction once daily. Preoperative radiation, 20 to 50 Gy, was delivered using photons in conventional fractions. In the group including chondrosarcoma, chordoma, and osteogenic sarcoma, surgical treatment consisted of two biopsies, eight subtotal resections, and four gross total resections. The 5-year local control rates were 53% for chordoma, 50% for osteogenic sarcoma, and 100% for chondrosarcoma.[18] Of the six failures, five were in-field recurrences, and one was out of field. A trend was noted toward improved local tumor control in pa-

tients receiving > 77 CGE. The failures were seen primarily in patients with < 77 CGE delivered to the tumor volume. Of the failures, 2 of 10 recurred following radiation after the initial resection, but 2 of 4 were treated for recurrent disease.

Austin-Seymour et al reported a case series of 141 patients treated for chordoma and chondrosarcoma of the skull base and cervical spine, using mixed proton/photon beam therapy at a median of 69 CGE.[17] Twenty-six failures were noted. Of these failures, 23% received the prescribed tumoral dose. However, 77% of failures occurred in areas that received less than the prescribed tumoral dose, most of which were in regions constrained by normal tissue tolerance. Other failures were outside the field, either in the surgical approach or marginal recurrences, underscoring the importance of radiation dose in ultimately successful treatment.

Intensity-Modulated Radiation Therapy

At the Memorial Sloan-Kettering Cancer Center in New York, we have reported the use of high-dose IMRT for the management of primary malignancies of the mobile spine. The actuarial local control was found to be 75%, with follow-up extending to a maximum of 40 months. No patient experienced myelitis. The median dose was 66 Gy (54–72 Gy) in 2 Gy fractions.[19] We treated seven chordomas and five chondrosarcomas, two of which were high grade and the remaining intermediate or low grade. At median follow-up of 18 months, the local control rate for chordomas was 86% and for chondrosarcomas 80%, with the single failure occurring in a high-grade patient. The follow-up is too short to draw meaningful conclusions, but fractionated therapy using IGRT is possible at doses similar to those reported for proton beam therapy.[20]

Brachytherapy

Brachytherapy has also been used to treat primary tumors. [125]Iodine has commonly been used to treat positive microscopic disease or minimal residual gross disease following tumor resection. Good results have been reported in the treatment of paraspinal tumors and epidural disease.[21,22] Rogers et al reported a series of 25 patients who were implanted intraoperatively with [125]iodine seeds.[22] Twenty-two (88%) failed prior external beam radiotherapy. At a mean follow-up of 19.2 months, four patients demonstrated local failure, and the 3-year actuarial control rate was 72.9%. No radiation toxicity was seen in this study. However, radiation myelitis has been reported 34 months following the routine administration of [125]iodine for metastatic thyroid cancer. The level of myelitis corresponded to a level at which significant epidural disease was nearly circumferential, likely resulting in a high surface dose to the spinal cord over a short period of time.[23]

Delaney et al developed applicators for the delivery of high-dose radiation using [92]iridium and [90]yttrium.[24] [90]Yttrium is a pure B-emitter and ideal for delivering high-dose radiation (i.e., 7.5–15Gy) to the dura without toxicity to the spinal cord. The [90]yttrium dose penetrance is 29% at 2 mm and 9% at 4 mm. This provides an adequate margin on the spinal cord, if the gross tumor has been resected in the absence of a spinal fluid leak. In this series, seven of eight patients were treated for sarcoma, six of which were controlled at a

Table 14.1 Comparison of the Biologically Effective Dose with the Fraction Size as the Variable for Acute and Late Effects

Effect	Dose/Number of Fractions					
	24 Gy/12	24 Gy/8	24 Gy/6	24 Gy/4	24 Gy/2	24 Gy/1
Late (α/β = 2)	48 Gy	72 Gy	96 Gy	120 Gy	168 Gy	312 Gy
Acute (α/β = 10)	29 Gy	31 Gy	34 Gy	38 Gy	53 Gy	81.6 Gy

median of 24 months. No radiation myelitis has been seen to date. [90]Yttrium may ultimately prove to be excellent as an adjuvant therapy for radioresistant tumors with epidural disease when combined with IGRT or proton beam therapy. IGRT uses dose painting to lessen the dose at the spinal cord margin to spare spinal cord tolerance, potentially underdosing this area. [90]Yttrium may improve the dose distribution for epidural disease and facilitate treatment planning and delivery of IGRT. The limitations of [90]yttrium are that the applicators are custom made for each patient and the isotope has a very short half-life. If the epidural tumor resection is more extensive than predicted by the MRI or the case is delayed several days, the plaque may be wasted.

◆ Stereotactic Radiosurgery

The role of stereotactic radiosurgery in the treatment of primary tumors has yet to be determined, and experience is limited compared with proton beam therapy. Theoretically, high-dose single-fraction therapy may improve local tumor control compared with standard-fraction therapy. From a biologic standpoint, tumor histologies with low alpha/beta (α/β) ratios, such as sarcomas, respond better to larger frac-

tion sizes. Evidence suggests that single-fraction therapy > 15 Gy results in apoptosis of tumor cells based on the acid sphingomyelinase pathway.[23] Microvascular damage in the tumor from high-dose fractions likely contributes to cell death.

The radiobiologic benefit may be most pronounced in tumor types traditionally considered resistant to standard fractionated radiation therapy. A construct called the biologically effective dose (BED) has become a widely accepted way to compare the potency of different radiation dose schedules.[25] Although the assumptions made for BED calculations based on linear quadratic formalism are not likely to be accurate at high doses per fraction, such as radiosurgery,[26] a comparison of different dose schedules demonstrates the significant advantage of increasing the dose of radiation per fraction for radioresistant tumors (α/β = 2) compared with relatively sensitive tumors (α/β = 10). Thus, increasing the fraction size is a form of biologic dose escalation. Based on this simplified analysis, a course of proton beam radiotherapy giving 76 Gy in 2 Gy fractions would give the BED of 152 Gy for radioresistant tumors, whereas a single dose of 24 Gy would give a BED more than double the value calculated for the former dose schedule (**Table 14.1**). Although the true utility of applying linear quadratic formalism in the setting of single fraction radiotherapy is controversial, the increased

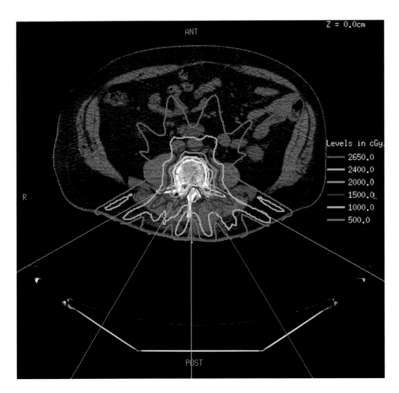

Fig. 14.1 Dose distribution for 24 Gy prescribed to the 100% isodose line for an L3 chordoma.

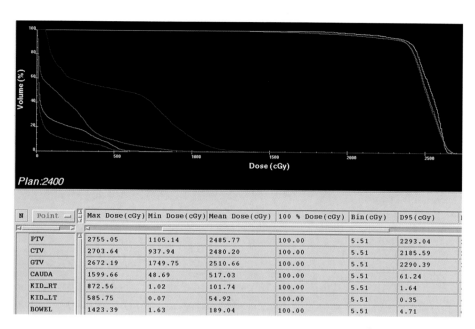

Fig. 14.2 Dose-volume histogram for the L3 target.

Plan:2400

N	Point		Max Dose(cGy)	Min Dose(cGy)	Mean Dose(cGy)	100 % Dose(cGy)	Bin(cGy)	D95(cGy)	
	PTV		2755.05	1105.14	2485.77	100.00	5.51	2293.04	
	CTV		2703.64	937.94	2480.20	100.00	5.51	2185.59	
	GTV		2672.19	1749.75	2510.66	100.00	5.51	2290.39	
	CAUDA		1599.66	48.69	517.03	100.00	5.51	61.24	
	KID_RT		872.56	1.02	101.74	100.00	5.51	1.64	
	KID_LT		585.75	0.07	54.92	100.00	5.51	0.35	
	BOWEL		1423.39	1.63	189.04	100.00	5.51	4.71	

biologic effect of very high dose single fraction radiation is a tantalizing in the setting of primary spine tumors.

In order for such high biologic doses of radiation to be administered safely, it is critical that radiation be delivered in a very conformal manner with high accuracy and precision, to prevent the exposure of dose sensitive normal tissues to high doses. Image-guided techniques[27] coupled with IMRT have provided the avenue for such treatment. The extremely high local control rates and very low toxicity associated with radioresistant histologies such as metastatic renal cell carcinoma spine lesions treated with high-dose single-fraction radiosurgery appears to support this paradigm.[28] **Figure 14.1** represents the axial dose distribution for a chordoma involving L3, treated to 24 Gy in a single fraction. The dose-volume histogram for this treatment is shown in **Fig. 14.2.** The cauda equina was identified on a myelogram and constrained to a maximum dose of 16 Gy. **Figure 14.3** is the 8-week post-treatment MR image suggesting central necrosis. Although

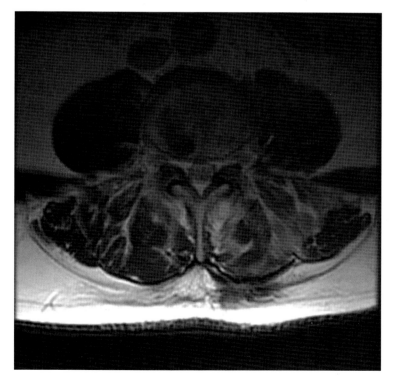

Fig. 14.3 Magnetic resonance image suggesting central necrosis 8 weeks post-treatment.

anecdotal and without sufficient follow-up, these findings are suggestive that very high dose single-fraction radiation (and extremely high BED) may represent an alternative treatment paradigm to the use of conventional fraction sizes for the management of these traditionally highly radioresistant lesions.

Stereotactic radiosurgery is currently being used as neoadjuvant therapy in our center. For tumors such as chordoma, chondrosarcoma, and liposarcoma, neoadjuvant radiation may decrease the possibility of tumor dissemination from intralesional resection. This may also benefit patients who ultimately undergo en bloc resection with negative histologic resections in which tumor dissemination is sometimes found. Although it is feasible to use IMRT to give high-dose radiation in standard fractionation, many primary tumors of the spine may respond best to high-dose hypofractionated or single-fraction radiation. However, when administering such high-dose therapy, extreme care and caution are mandatory to minimize complications. From a surgical perspective, the advantage of using highly conformal delivery of radiation is the decreased soft tissue damage and consequent decreased risk of wound complications. Patients may be safely operated within 2 weeks of IGRT.

◆ Conclusion

From available data, en bloc resection achieving negative histologic margins may have a good rate of local tumor control. For patients who are not candidates for marginal or wide resections, adjuvant radiation adds a measure of tumor control. Proton beam, intraoperative radioactive implants, and high-dose conformal photon therapy all play a role in local tumor control and possibly cure.

References

1. Boriani S, Bandiera S, Biagini R, et al. Chordoma of the mobile spine: fifty years of experience. Spine 2006;31(4):493–503.
2. Tomita K, Kawahara N, Baba H, et al. Total en bloc spondylectomy: a new surgical technique for primary malignant vertebral tumors. Spine 1997;22(3):324–333.
3. Yao KC, Boriani S, Gokaslan ZL, et al. En bloc spondylectomy for spinal metastases: a review of techniques. Neurosurg Focus 2003;15(5):e6.
4. Fuller DB, Bloom JG. Radiotherapy for chordoma. Int J Radiat Oncol Biol Phys 1988;15(2):331–339.
5. Krochak R, Harwood AR, Cummings BJ, Quirt IC. Results of radical radiation for chondrosarcoma of bone. Radiother Oncol 1983;1(2):109–115.
6. Austin JP, Urie MM, Cardenosa G, et al. Probable causes of recurrence in patients with chordoma and chondrosarcoma of the base of skull and cervical spine. Int J Radiat Oncol Biol Phys 1993;25(3):439–444.
7. Bell RS, O'Sullivan B, Liu FF, et al. The surgical margin in soft-tissue sarcoma. J Bone Joint Surg Am 1989;71(3):370–375.
8. Pisters PW, Leung DH, Woodruff J, et al. Analysis of prognostic factors in 1,041 patients with localized soft tissue sarcomas of the extremities. J Clin Oncol 1996;14(5):1679–1689.
9. Tanabe KK, Pollock RE, Ellis LM, et al. Influence of surgical margins on outcome in patients with preoperatively irradiated extremity soft tissue sarcomas. Cancer 1994;73(6):1652–1659.
10. Boriani S, De Iure F, Bandiera S, et al. Chondrosarcoma of the mobile spine: report on 22 cases. Spine 2000;25(7):804–812.
11. Boriani S, Weinstein JN, Biagini R. Primary bone tumors of the spine: terminology and surgical staging. Spine 1997;22(9):1036–1044.
12. Bilsky MH, Boland PJ, Panageas KS, et al. Intralesional resection of primary and metastatic sarcoma involving the spine: outcome analysis of 59 patients. Neurosurgery 2001;49(6):1277–1286.
13. Bell RS, O'Sullivan B, Liu FF, et al. The surgical margin in soft tissue sarcoma. Chir Organi Mov 1990;75(1, Suppl)126–130.
14. O'Sullivan B, Davis AM, Turcotte R, et al. Preoperative versus postoperative radiotherapy in soft-tissue sarcoma of the limbs: a randomised trial. Lancet 2002;359(9325):2235–2241.
15. DeLaney TF, Trofimov AV, Engelsman M, Suit HD. Advanced-technology radiation therapy in the management of bone and soft tissue sarcomas. Cancer Control 2005;12(1):27–35.
16. Emami B, Lyman J, Brown A, et al. Tolerance of normal tissue to therapeutic irradiation. Int J Radiat Oncol Biol Phys 1991;21(1):109–122.
17. Austin-Seymour M, Munzenrider JE, Goitein M, et al. Progress in low-LET heavy particle therapy: intracranial and paracranial tumors and uveal melanomas. Radiat Res Suppl 1985;8:S219–S226.
18. Hug EB. Review of skull base chordomas: prognostic factors and long-term results of proton-beam radiotherapy. Neurosurg Focus 2001;10(3):e11.
19. Yamada Y, Lovelock DM, Yenice KM, et al. Multifractionated image-guided and stereotactic intensity-modulated radiotherapy of paraspinal tumors: a preliminary report. Int J Radiat Oncol Biol Phys 2005;62(1):53–61.
20. Terezakis S, Lovelock M, Bilsky M, et al. Image-guided and stereotactic intensity-modulated photon radiotherapy using a multifractionated regimen to paraspinal chordomas and rare sarcomas. Int J Radiat Oncol Biol Phys 2007;69(5):1502–1508.
21. Cheng EY, Ozerdemoglu RA, Transfeldt EE, et al. Lumbosacral chordoma: prognostic factors and treatment. Spine 1999;24(16):1639–1645.
22. Rogers CL, Theodore N, Dickman CA, et al. Surgery and permanent 125I seed paraspinal brachytherapy for malignant tumors with spinal cord compression. Int J Radiat Oncol Biol Phys 2002;54(2):505–513.
23. Garcia-Barros M, Paris F, Cordon-Cardo C, et al. Tumor response to radiotherapy regulated by endothelial cell apoptosis. Science 2003;300(5622):1155–1159.
24. Delaney TF, Chen GT, Mauceri TC, et al. Intraoperative dural irradiation by customized ^{192}iridium and ^{90}yttrium brachytherapy plaques. Int J Radiat Oncol Biol Phys 2003;57(1):239–245.
25. Hall EJ, GA. Radiobiology for the Radiologist. 6th ed. New York: Lippincott Williams & Wilkins; 2006:521.
26. Flickinger JC, Kondziolka D, Lundsford LD. Radiobiologic analysis of tissue responses following radiosurgery. Technol Cancer Res Treat 2003;2(2):87–92.
27. Lovelock DM, Hua C, Wang P, et al. Accurate setup of paraspinal patients using a noninvasive patient immobilization cradle and portal imaging. Med Phys 2005;32(8):2606–2614.
28. Gerszten PC, Burton SA, Ozhasoglu C, et al. Stereotactic radiosurgery for spinal metastases from renal cell carcinoma. J Neurosurg Spine 2005;3(4):288–295.

15

Spinal Cord Arteriovenous Malformation Radiosurgery

Steven D. Chang, Steven L. Hancock, Iris C. Gibbs, and John R. Adler, Jr.

Stereotactic radiosurgery has emerged over the past three decades as an alternative to microsurgical resection and embolization for cerebral arteriovenous malformations (AVMs). Since this technique was first described by Steiner et al in 1972,[1] over 5000 patients worldwide were successfully treated with this modality through December 2006. Radiosurgery causes gradual hyperplasia of the endothelial tissue within the arteries of the nidus of the AVM, which leads to vessel occlusion.[2] Numerous reports show that cerebral AVMs have an 80 to 85% obliteration rate for vascular malformations < 2.5 cm.[3-9]

With the success of radiosurgery in the management of brain AVMs, the treatment of spinal cord AVMs with radiosurgery would be a logical next step. Given the various subtypes of spinal cord AVMs, those with a relatively compact nidus would represent the optimal targets. Spinal cord AVMs are typically classified into four distinct pathologic groups based on the location of the arteriovenous connections. Types I and IV are dural and perimedullary arteriovenous fistulas, and are often optimally treated with endovascular embolization and/or microsurgical resection. Type III, also called juvenile-type spinal AVMs, are characterized by large and diffuse intramedullary nidi, which can also extend into the extramedullary space. They are less well defined and do not represent optimal radiosurgical targets. Type II, also called glomus AVMs, represent a compact vascular nidus and are often suitable radiosurgery targets. These are also difficult if not impossible to treat with embolization and microsurgery alone and often were not treated prior to the development of spine radiosurgery.

The ability to treat spinal cord AVMs with radiosurgery was not feasible prior to the development of image-guided spine radiosurgery.[10] As with brain radiosurgery, spine radiosurgery relies on the delivery of a large number of cross-fired radiation beams to deliver an effective dose of radiation to a specific target within the spine. Much of radiosurgery to spinal AVMs was based on prior experience of radiosurgery for spinal tumors.[10-12] Despite the success with tumors, there remained a concern that high doses of radiation to focal areas within the spinal cord itself would represent a potentially

significant risk to patients. The ability of frameless image-guided radiosurgery to deliver multiple sessions of radiosurgery to intramedullary vascular malformations played a role in reducing this risk.

Our experience to date in the treatment of patients with spinal cord radiosurgery is based on a series of 23 patients treated between 1997 and 2006 with the CyberKnife. The following chapter represents the details of this 10-year experience.

◆ Patient Selection

It has been our practice to offer CyberKnife (Accuray Inc., Sunnyvale, California) radiosurgery to those patients with type II spinal cord AVMs who are not candidates for either microsurgical or endovascular embolization. In addition, a small subset of type III spinal cord AVMs are considered candidates for radiosurgery if the vascular nidus is a reasonable target based on size. Currently, we do not feel that type I and type IV spinal cord AVMs are optimally treated with radiosurgery. At Stanford, these types of spinal cord AVMs typically are treated successfully with either open microsurgery or embolization. Low-flow spinal cord and vascular malformations, such as cavernous malformations, are not considered candidates for spinal cord radiosurgery.

◆ Pretreatment Preparation

All potential candidates for radiosurgery of spinal cord AVMs undergo formal review by our multidisciplinary cerebrovascular and radiosurgery team. Team members include neurosurgeons and interventional radiologists experienced in spinal cord AVMs, as well as radiation oncologists. All patients who are considered candidates for radiosurgery undergo formal radiographic evaluation. This consists of spine magnetic resonance imaging (MRI) scans and conventional spinal angiography to identify the size, shape, and location of the vascular malformation.[13] Feeding arteries and draining veins are identified to exclude them from the target volume. More recently, the use of three-dimensional (3D) angiography has improved our ability to visualize these vascular lesions.[13–16] Although we have not utilized fusions between 3D angiography and computed tomography (CT) or MRI, we typically use 3D angiography to assist with our treatment planning.

In some cases, patients with spinal cord AVMs undergo preradiosurgery embolization if it is felt that the AVM volume could be significantly reduced before radiosurgery. We have found, however, that the embolization glue can cause significant artifact on treatment planning CT and MRI scans; thus, we typically do not perform preradiosurgical embolization for smaller spinal cord AVMs.

Once a candidate is approved for radiosurgery, informed consent is obtained. Our early experience in treating spinal cord AVMs relied on the placement of percutaneous fiducials into the bony anatomy of the spine to assist with target localization. More recently, advances in the CyberKnife treatment planning software have allowed the treatment of these spinal cord AVMs without fiducials, thereby eliminating one step in the treatment process.

As with spinal cord tumors, the first step in preparation includes treatment setup. This typically involves obtaining thin-slice postcontrast axial CT images (using 1.25 mm slice thickness). It is also common to perform postcontrast axial stereotactic MRI to produce a CT-MRI fusion to assist with outlining the target volume. All patients have undergone prior two-dimensional (2D) spinal angiography prior to treatment; more recently, 3D angiography was obtained prior to treatment in certain patients.

Treatment planning consists of outlining the nidus of the vascular malformation. Although the spinal cord is considered the primary normal critical structure, it was often difficult to outline the spinal cord independent of the AVM if the nidus was localized within the center of the cord or if the nidus occupied the entire cross-sectional volume of the cord on axial CT and MRI slices. In certain patients, the nidus was located eccentrically on one side; this allowed us to demarcate the spinal cord on the other side of the canal as the

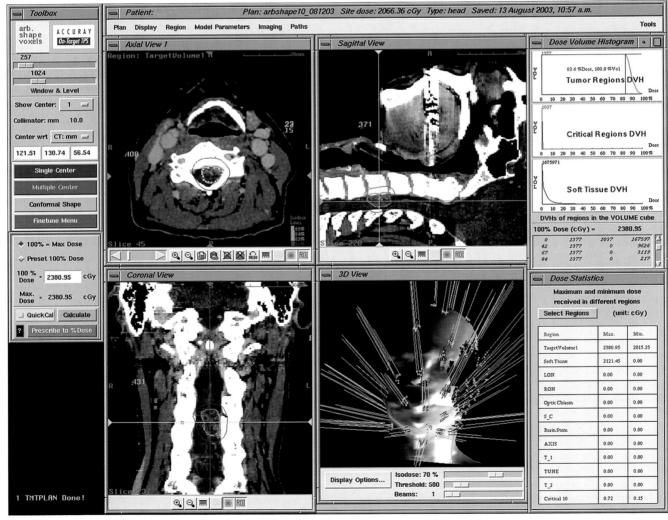

Fig. 15.1 A typical CyberKnife treatment plan for a cervical spinal cord arteriovenous malformation. (From Sinclair J, Chang SD, Gibbs IC, Adler JR Jr. Multisession CyberKnife radiosurgery for intramedullary spinal cord arteriovenous malformations. Neurosurgery 2006;58[6]:1081–1089, with permission.)

critical structure. Inverse treatment planning was then used to generate a treatment plan for the patient (**Fig. 15.1**).

◆ Radiosurgical Dosing for Spinal Cord AVMs

Our initial choice of radiosurgical dosing was quite conservative based on the lack of any experience within the medical literature on the treatment of spinal cord AVMs with radiosurgery. Early patients were treated with 20 Gy delivered in four sessions. Based on the lack of morbidity noted in this group of patients, we progressed to a dose of 21 Gy delivered in three sessions. Our recent experience has been to treat spinal cord AVMs with 20 Gy in two sessions. This, by definition, delivers a dose of 10 Gy to the surrounding spinal cord, which we feel is reasonably tolerated in most patients. Two of our patients with very small spine AVMs located within the conus region were treated with a single session of radiosurgery because we felt the risk of spinal cord injury was small based on the target volume.

◆ Radiographic and Clinical Follow-up

Following radiosurgical treatment, patients underwent MRI of the spine at 6-month intervals. This imaging allowed us to assess the extent of AVM obliteration and to observe for the possible development of any spinal cord radiation edema. Clinical exams were also performed on patients at 6-month intervals. This allowed us to assess for changes in motor and sensory function, and possibly bowel or bladder dysfunction. Once MRI indicated probable AVM obliteration, patients underwent formal spine angiography to confirm AVM obliteration. Those patients who were > 3 years following their spinal cord radiosurgery also underwent spine angiography to assess the extent of residual AVM and to determine what proportion of the AVM had been obliterated.

◆ Results of the Stanford Experience

We have previously published our earlier experience in the treatment of the first 15 patients undergoing spinal cord radiosurgery for their AVMs.[17] As of December 2006, 23 patients with spinal cord AVMs have been treated using CyberKnife radiosurgery. Twenty-two of these patients had glomus spine and AVMs, and 1 had a type III juvenile spinal cord AVM. Spinal AVM locations included the cervical spine (12 patients), thoracic spine (8 patients), and conus region (3 patients). Thirteen of the 23 patients (57%) presented with hemorrhage, which was multiple in 6 of the patients. In the remaining 10 patients, progressive neurologic dysfunction was the presenting symptom. Ten of the 23 patients (43%) underwent prior embolization to their AVMs. A median of three treatment sessions was performed. Mean target volume was 2.8 cm³, with a range of 0.26 to 15.0 cm³. The mean marginal dose used was 20.3 Gy, with a range of 16 to 21 Gy. A median of two sessions was used in this patient population, with a range of one to four treatments. The mean maximal internidal dose was 25.8 Gy and ranged from 22.5 to 30.0 Gy. As mentioned above, the radiosurgical dose was gradually escalated over the course of this study as we gained experience.

Clinical follow-up ranged from 4 to 83 months, with a mean of 35 months. Radiographic follow-up averaged 25.3 months, with a range of 0 to 72 months. Although postoperative MRI demonstrated noticeable reduction in the volume of all AVMs over the course of follow-up, only 8 of the 23 patients underwent formal spine angiography. Of these eight patients, three had complete angiographic obliteration (**Figs. 15.2** and **15.3**). As of December 2006, no patients have suffered a rebleed after spine radiosurgery, and the clinical outcome was improved

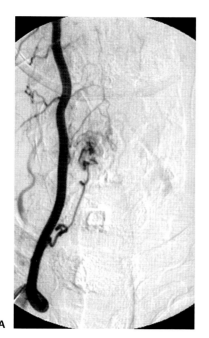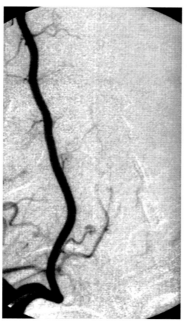

Fig. 15.2 **(A)** Preradiosurgery lateral cervical spine angiogram demonstrates a C5 type II spinal cord arteriovenous malformation (AVM). **(B)** Three years after CyberKnife radiosurgery, a lateral cervical spinal cord angiogram demonstrates obliteration of the AVM nidus. (From Sinclair J, Chang SD, Gibbs IC, Adler JR Jr. Multisession CyberKnife radiosurgery for intramedullary spinal cord arteriovenous malformations. Neurosurgery 2006;58[6]:1081–1089, with permission.)

A   B

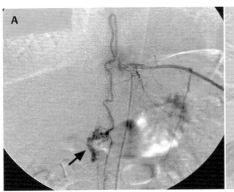
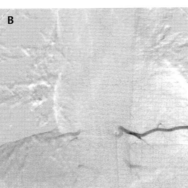

Fig. 15.3 Preradiosurgery (**A**) and postradiosurgery (**B**) angiograms demonstrating angiographic obliteration of a conus type II spinal cord arteriovenous malformation. (From Sinclair J, Chang SD, Gibbs IC, Adler JR Jr. Multisession CyberKnife radiosurgery for intramedullary spinal cord arteriovenous malformations. Neurosurgery 2006;58[6]:1081–1089, with permission.)

or unchanged in 96% of patients. A single patient who was neurologically severely impaired prior to radiosurgery deteriorated further at 9 months following radiosurgery. MRI demonstrated a significant decrease in flow voice as well as high signal in the adjacent spinal cord on T2 imaging. Although this patient is < 3 years following radiosurgical treatment, and thus AVM obliteration may still occur, it appears that the patient has developed a case of radiation myelopathy. One other patient experienced significant onset of radiation edema (for a conus AVM), but this AVM obliterated rapidly over 9 months, and the patient was one of three who proceeded to have complete obliteration of his AVM.

◆ Future Directions for CyberKnife AVM Radiosurgery

The use of CyberKnife radiosurgery to treat spinal cord AVMs is continually evolving. Over time, improvements in imaging have allowed us to more accurately define the AVM nidus for treatment. One of the more recent advances in radiographic imaging consists of high-quality 3D angiography (**Fig. 15.4**). These 3D images provide a potentially improved view of many spinal AVMs compared with standard 2D angiography or MRI and CT imaging. Algorithms that allow fusion of 3D

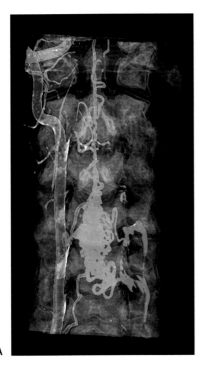
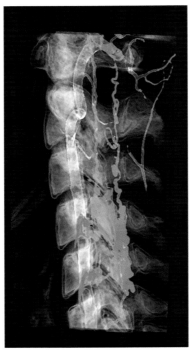

Fig. 15.4 Three-dimensional angiography shows a cervical spinal cord arteriovenous malformation in the anteroposterior (**A**) and lateral (**B**) views.

angiography images to either CT or MR images represent a potential advance in radiosurgical treatment by allowing more accurate targeting of spinal AVMs.

Additional work needs to be done in terms of our understanding of the tolerance of the spinal cord tolerance to radiosurgery. Our current obliteration rate for spinal AVMs is lower than that existing in the neurosurgical literature for intracerebral AVMs of comparable size, likely due to conservative dosing. If further studies show a greater tolerance of the spinal cord to certain radiosurgical doses, one could then either escalate the dose of spinal cord AVM radiosurgery when performing multisession radiosurgical treatment or increase the number of spinal cord AVMs treated in a single session in an attempt to achieve greater obliteration rates while maintaining an acceptable risk.

◆ Conclusion

CyberKnife radiosurgery appears to be an effective treatment for spinal cord AVMs. The CyberKnife allows the flexibility of multisession radiosurgery for these AVMs, which may reduce the risk of treatment. Additional challenges remain with respect to obtaining a better understanding of the tolerance of the spinal cord to radiosurgery. The development of 3D angiography and the possibility of incorporating this imaging into AVM radiosurgery treatment planning may further reduce risk.

References

1. Steiner L, Leksell L, Greitz T, Forster DM, Backlund EO. Stereotaxic radiosurgery for cerebral arteriovenous malformations: report of a case. Acta Chir Scand 1972;138:459–464.
2. Chang SD, Shuster DL, Steinberg GK, Levy RP, Frankel K. Stereotactic radiosurgery of arteriovenous malformations: pathologic changes in resected tissue. Clin Neuropathol 1997;16:111–116.
3. Betti OO, Munari C, Rosler R. Stereotactic radiosurgery with the linear accelerator: treatment of arteriovenous malformations. Neurosurgery 1989;24:311–321.
4. Coffey RJ, Lunsford LD, Bissonette D, Flickinger JC. Stereotactic gamma radiosurgery for intracranial vascular malformations and tumors: report of the initial North American experience in 331 patients. Stereotact Funct Neurosurg 1990;54:535–540.
5. Colombo F, Benedetti A, Pozza F, Marchetti C, Chierego G. Linear accelerator radiosurgery of cerebral arteriovenous malformations. Neurosurgery 1989;24:833–840.
6. Colombo F, Pozza F, Chierego G, et al. Linear accelerator radiosurgery of cerebral arteriovenous malformations: an update. Neurosurgery 1994;34:14–20.
7. Friedman WA, Bova FJ. Linear accelerator radiosurgery for arteriovenous malformations. J Neurosurg 1992;77:832–841.
8. Steinberg GK, Fabrikant JI, Marks MP, et al. Stereotactic heavy-charged-particle Bragg-peak radiation for intracranial arteriovenous malformations. N Engl J Med 1990;323:96–101.
9. Steiner L. Radiosurgery in cerebral arteriovenous. In: Fein JM, Flamm ES, eds. Cerebrovascular Surgery. New York: Springer-Verlag; 1985:1161–1215.
10. Ryu SI, Chang SD, Kim DH, et al. Image-guided hypo-fractionated stereotactic radiosurgery to spinal lesions. Neurosurgery 2001;49:838–846.
11. Dodd RL, Ryu MR, Kamnerdsupaphon P, et al. CyberKnife radiosurgery for benign intradural extramedullary spinal tumors. Neurosurgery 2006;58:674–685.
12. Ryu SI, Kim DH, Chang SD. Stereotactic radiosurgery for hemangiomas and ependymomas of the spinal cord. Neurosurg Focus 2003;15:e10.
13. Prestigiacomo CJ, Niimi Y, Setton A, Berenstein A. Three-dimensional rotational spinal angiography in the evaluation and treatment of vascular malformations. AJNR Am J Neuroradiol 2003;24:1429–1435.
14. Cavedon C. Three-dimensional rotational angiography (3DRA) adds substantial information to radiosurgery treatment planning of AVM's compared to angio-CT and angio-MR. Med Phys 2004;31:2181–2182.
15. Kakizawa Y, Nagashima H, Oya F, et al. Compartments in arteriovenous malformation nidi demonstrated with rotational three-dimensional digital subtraction angiography by using selective microcatheterization: report of three cases. J Neurosurg 2002;96:770–774.
16. Stancanello J, Cavedon C, Francescon P, et al. Development and validation of a CT-3D rotational angiography registration method for AVM radiosurgery. Med Phys 2004;31:1363–1371.
17. Sinclair J, Chang SD, Gibbs IC, Adler JR Jr. Multisession CyberKnife radiosurgery for intramedullary spinal cord arteriovenous malformations. Neurosurgery 2006;58:1081–1089.

16

Biomechanical Assessment of Spinal Instability and Stabilization

Boyle C. Cheng and William C. Welch

Traditionally, the study of spinal biomechanics and stability has been heavily influenced by congenital, traumatic, developmental, and degenerative conditions such as scoliotic deformities, degenerative disks, and burst fractures. Although it has been recognized that spinal lesions due to metastases can cause clinical instability, basic biomechanical testing in metastatic disease states has been limited. This may be due to the inherent limitations in acquiring diseased specimens for testing, or there may be other reasons for the paucity of scientific literature in this highly specialized field.

From a clinical oncological standpoint, spinal metastases are common. The prevalence of bony metastases involving the spine has been estimated as high as one in three of all cancer patients[1] and one in two elderly patients diagnosed with cancer.[2] Many patients who harbor metastatic disease will have systemic issues that take treatment precedence over the spinal diseases. However, because of advances in systemic therapies, patients are living longer, and their spine disease may ultimately require treatment.

Spinal metastases can directly afflict one or multiple vertebral bodies and, in specific cases, compromise the structural integrity of the spine segment. Subsequent instability and neurologic complications may result. Thus, spinal metastases have the potential to become a biomechanical issue and require surgical intervention.

The proliferation of metastatic disease in the bony anatomy of the spine has been shown to be indiscriminate; consequently, if structural components, including the posterior wall, pedicles, facets, and other osteoligamentous elements of a functional spinal unit (FSU; two vertebral bodies and the disk space), are damaged, the potential for instability, including burst fracture, is highly probable.[3] Challenges in anticipating such events, including the inability to visualize the early onset of vertebral body involvement on plain film radiograph, have made diagnostic predictions of structural failure more difficult. Researchers have estimated that 30 to 50% of the vertebrae by volumetric measurements must be involved before a spinal tumor may be radiographically identifiable.[4]

Different methods of classifying spinal metastases have been proposed with the intent of rationalizing surgical indications. Currently, there is little consensus on an objective criterion in the estimation of the risk of burst fracture and neurologic compromise. It has been suggested that with the many treatment options and combinations available, including irradiation, chemotherapy, steroids, diphosphonates, and surgery, the complete management of a patient's condition would require that both symptomatic and prophylactic issues be taken into consideration.[2] Should the patient still warrant surgery, biomechanical aspects of the metastases, along with the treatment, should be considered.

◆ Introduction to Biomechanics

Clinically relevant biomechanical studies involving the spine have been available for more than 5 decades. These studies have not addressed metastatic disease per se, but they have covered several topics from anulus fibril orientation to vertebral bone strength to the effects of instrumented procedures. An early study by Virgin described various biomechanical aspects of the intervertebral disk, including the effects of compressive loading and the observation of hysteresis during loading and unloading.[5] Likewise, Hirsch and Nachemson reported on the influence of spine motion and the associated disk pressures.[6] The study of FSUs under controlled loading provides biomechanical insight into clinically relevant issues, including instability related to the spine. Moreover, the instrumentation and the ability to achieve FSU stability can potentially be important in the clinical decision-making process for the adjuvant treatment of spinal tumors.

Instability has various definitions, and as it relates to degenerative biomechanics of the spine, a kinematic response for an FSU under a given physiologic load in excess of the normal healthy condition (e.g., excessive range of motion [ROM] in a lumbar FSU) can be used to characterize the instability of a motion segment. Clinically, multiple factors have been used to describe instability for symptomatic patients. Surgical intervention has the potential to treat certain aspects of metastatic conditions afflicting the spine, including instability. Such outcomes are of interest to both clinicians and biomechanicians. Should the clinical conditions be appropriate for a surgical intervention, a repeatable kinematic response of the FSU should be predictable and well described. Instability in the spine that harbors metastatic disease may more closely mimic osteoporotic disease, as the metastases most commonly affect the vertebral bodies, as opposed to the soft tissue structures (e.g., ligaments or disks).

Biomechanical loading and displacement protocols on test frames have been developed for spinal treatment comparisons. In conjunction, precision measuring devices have been necessary to measure the relative motion between vertebral bodies. Subsequent interpretation of the data becomes more significant if there are clinical conclusions that can be derived from in vitro biomechanical testing. For example, in a cadaveric calf corpectomy model, Heller et al determined that restoration of stability is dependent upon instrumentation constructs.[7] Results from other studies have since corroborated the fact that the type of instrumentation significantly alters the ROM, as well as the type of surgical procedure performed. Kanayama et al concluded that anteroposterior instrumentation is more effective in cases involving total spondylectomies, whereas anterior instrumentation may not be significantly more stable than circumferential fixation in subtotal spondylectomies.[8] The in vitro biomechanical description of stability in a human cadaveric FSU provides a guideline for in vivo clinical techniques.

The clinical relevance of biomechanical testing is difficult to correlate perfectly in any disease state. The variables associated with testing—the test apparatus, the representative spine segment model, and the difficulty in patient assessment—cause difficulty in repeating studies in either the clinical or laboratory setting. Regardless of biologic variability, patient compliance, and artifacts of biomechanical studies, the fundamental basis of measurement parameters should be understood and taken into consideration to fully appreciate a patient's condition and the ramifications of surgical intervention.

◆ Biomechanics of Instrumented FSU in the Treatment of Spinal Tumors

Surgical treatment for the neoplastic spine is designed to decompress neural elements, restore neurologic function, and reduce pain by providing increased support. Because instrumentation has the potential to improve the quality of life through stabilization, surgical intervention can, to some extent, be evaluated based on in vitro biomechanical performance. The surgical techniques may be anterior or posterior, or both. Choices in implant materials include metal and polymer technologies. Polymer technologies, including polymethyl methacrylate (PMMA), fiber-reinforced composites, and poly(etheretherketone) (PEEK), provide solutions to spinal stability not achievable with traditional fixation hardware. However, metal constructs, including posterior pedicle screw fixation, vertebral body replacements, and anterior rods and plates, are still essential to the reduction of motion

and the stiffness of the treated FSU. Regardless of approach, the ability to maximize tumor decompression and restore a viable spinal unit construct is the criterion used to compare techniques and devices.

In a study by Oda et al, a series of different metal reconstructive devices were biomechanically compared in human cadaveric spines.[9] Pedicle screws were found to be most effective when used in combination with anterior instrumentation. Additionally, effectiveness was measured in the three major modes of loading and was determined to have significant multiplanar reduction in motion compared with the intact state.[9] In a similar study, Shannon et al were interested in the use of a PMMA cement, in lieu of rigid metal instrumentation.[10] One purported advantage is the ability to implant the material in a liquid state and to cure in situ.[10] Subsequently, the implant conforms and fills the void volume and provides an excellent implant bone interface. Additionally, the anterior column support provided by the PMMA can be implanted from a posterior technique. In the study by Shannon et al, the results suggest biomechanical stability can be achieved through a polymer-based implant following a spondylectomy.

Vahldiek and Panjabi compared the stability of various constructs in stabilizing a spine following a spondylectomy treatment.[11] In that study, the anterior column support was based on a carbon fiber cage measuring 35 mm in diameter, which occupied the space created by the vertebral resection. Various combinations of metal posterior and anterior instrumentation supplemented this construct. From a biomechanical stabilization aspect, the study concluded that carbon fiber vertebral body replacement in conjunction with posterior screws or carbon fiber vertebral body replacement with both anterior and posterior hardware provided sufficient rigidity for vertebral body replacement surgery. In contrast, the anterior instrumentation used with the same carbon fiber vertebral body replacement did not provide sufficient stabilization.[11]

Evidence of translational application of research (i.e., biomechanical human cadaveric testing to the clinical setting) has been documented in the treatment of metastatic disease. The stabilization effects of implants and approaches found effective have been considered based on a host of factors. Clinical validation of Vahldiek and Panjabi's biomechanical cadaveric study was in part confirmed in a case study reported by Samartzis et al, in which a patient was diagnosed with Ewing sarcoma of T8 and T9.[12] The authors reported an en bloc spondylectomy of T8 and T9 followed by reconstructive surgery with a stackable carbon fiber cage vertebral replacement in conjunction with anterior and posterior instrumentation. The patient was tumor free and maintained normal neurologic function with a reduction in pain. The stability determined by the in vitro testing to be biomechanically stable coupled with other patient host factors resulted in a successful outcome and eliminated even the need for radiation therapy.

◆ Methods of Spine Testing in Experimental Designs

Spine biomechanical research has evolved, including in the area of testing FSU stabilization techniques. Biomechanical test outcome should be independent of location and laboratory and repeatable from experiment to experiment. Ultimately, the goal is to build consensus among researchers as to the effects of a given technique. Several authors have defined the necessary components in standardization, including Panjabi's conceptual framework, which establishes the necessity for uniform test methods and has been widely implemented since inception.[13] More recently, the criteria have been modernized to accommodate new concepts beyond fixation.[14] The need to carefully apply and measure both load and displacement is essential for spine stability testing.

Six independent motions can completely describe the kinematic motion for a given vertebral body (i.e., three translations and three rotations). These must be defined according to three orthogonal axes and are commonly defined relative to adjacent vertebrae. This will be referred to as FSU motion. A clear understanding of the clinical biomechanics of the spine is based on the three-dimensional kinematic response of the FSU. There are several testing paradigms used for spinal evaluation. These include evaluation of FSU motion, end plate assessment for strength, and destructive loading to bone failure in assessments of degenerative conditions. FSU assessments for metastatic disease may require destructive testing, as short-term stability may be more important than long-term outcomes necessary for other spine ailments.

Ideally, a physiologic load applied to an FSU needs to respond with an ROM limited in magnitude by the intact osteoligamentous structures and the stabilizing surgical treatment. As illustrated in **Fig. 16.1**, treatments need to be compared, and many metrics, including reductions in ROM and the neutral zone, have been used to evaluate the stability of the spine following instrumentation.[7,9,14,15] Instant fixation devices provide excellent rigidity, but long-term survivability and positive patient outcome depend to some degree on arthrodesis. It should be noted that between fixation and the normal healthy condition, a continuum with a trade-off between rigidity and mobility exists. The region closest to

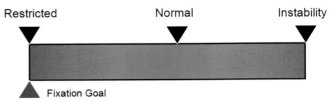

Fig. 16.2 Continuous spectrum of stability.

rigid fixation in **Fig. 16.2** should be established as a stability target following surgical intervention of metastatic tumors involving the spine.

◆ Spine Test Configurations

Spine testers are designed to apply a load in a physiologic manner to anatomically correct models from which questions of stability and treatments of instability may be measured and compared. Many methods have been documented for FSU testing. They range from reporting the kinematic response of a single axis test, to validation of finite element models, to sophisticated axial loading routines.[1,8,10,16] Because of the biologic variability that exists in biologic specimens, however, data are most useful for comparison testing, and absolute parameters have been difficult to validate clinically.

Single-axis materials testers require certain features for biologic testing. Sophisticated automated computer controls, high-grade bearing seals, and axial torsion capabilities are some of the features provided on standard spine-testing equipment. Additionally, standard spine fixtures capable of applying flexion/extension bending moments, and lateral bending moments are readily available. **Figure 16.3** represents a commercially available standard spine tester with automated follower load capability.

Flexion Extension Bending

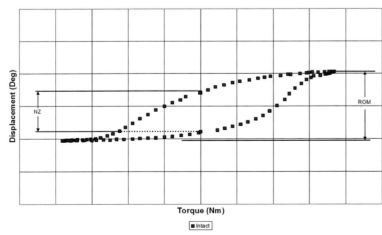

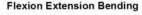

Fig. 16.1 Representative load displacement graph for a complete bending cycle. Note the hysteresis within the specimen.

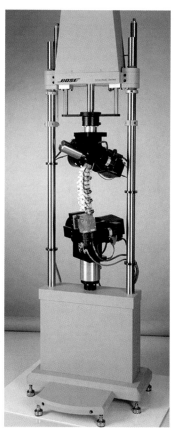

Fig. 16.3 Spine tester with automated follower load capability. (Courtesy of Welch Research Laboratory, Department of Neurological Surgery, University of Pittsburgh, Pittsburgh, PA.)

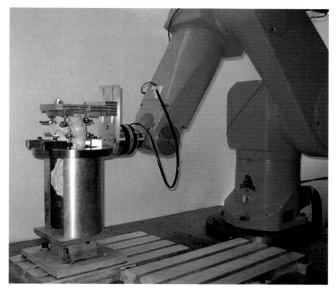

Fig. 16.4 Robotics-based spine-testing system programmed with a hybrid control algorithm that uses an iterative load control loop embedded within a displacement control loop. (Courtesy of Ferguson Laboratory, Department of Orthopaedic Surgery, University of Pittsburgh, Pittsburgh, PA.)

Generally, spine testers apply a controlled load, and a measured response is recorded. Alternatively, displacements can be controlled, and the corresponding load can be recorded. A third algorithm incorporating both load and displacement control at various stages in the protocol is possible. This is often referred to as a hybrid control algorithm; **Fig. 16.4** is one example of a robotic arm using this type of control. Test configurations are important to understand, as each comes with a set of underlying assumptions and rationales on the method in which the load is applied. The assumptions are important in understanding artifacts from testing as opposed to the effects on an FSU. Primary flexibility comparison tests depend on the application of a pure moment being applied to the test setup. An example of a moment being applied to a spinal segment through weights and pulleys is shown in **Fig. 16.5.**

One of the first automated flexion/extension/bending systems that applied pure moments was described in the literature.[17] Mounted on a materials tester capable of axial compression and axial torsion, the system was retrofitted for a matched set of stepper motors applying counteracting torques or displacements at each end. This method of pure moment application has been well documented. Cunningham et al described a similar custom-designed six degree

of freedom spine simulator (6DOF-SS), which has been the source of many studies and cited in refereed journals.[8,9,18,19] Three independent stepper motors, harmonic drives, and electromagnetic clutches provide controllable loads in several independent degrees of freedom for a given spine test specimen. Additionally, artificial shear forces can be negated in this test arrangement through the use of linear-bearing guide rails. The primary actuator provides an axial compressive capability to the system, which gives an additional degree of freedom.

Many spine test configurations have been documented for stability testing. Each of these configurations can replicate standardized load protocols for compression, torsion, and bending. As for physiologic loading, there has been an ever increasing demand, and the relationship between applied moments and physiologic loading must be further established and ultimately correlated to clinical implications.

◆ Standard Fixation Measurement Parameters

Descriptions of stability are important for several reasons. As has been suggested, instability due to neoplasm of the spine is one of many factors that may require patients to be subjected to surgical intervention. The many methods of performing ex vivo testing on constructs have provided insight into the nature of the performance. Each system has demonstrated carefully controlled loading methods. Whether the load is applied through weights and pulleys or as a pure

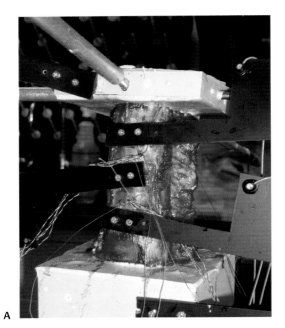

A

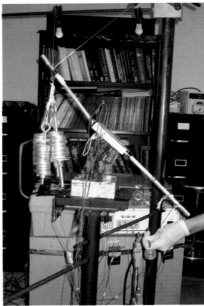

B

Fig. 16.5 *Spine tester using weights and pulleys to apply bending moments.* **(A)** Cadaveric specimen instrumented with optical tracking markers. **(B)** Spine test setup with specimen in load frame.

moment or through the end effector of a robotic arm, the response of the spine can be accurately measured.

The FSU response is most often described in a load deflection curve, as shown in **Fig. 16.1.** For any given FSU testing, there are six different types of individual loads that can be applied and six degrees of freedom that can be measured. The resulting 36 potential outcomes are important depending on the type of information that is necessary in understanding spinal instability. For example, a common parameter for surgeon measurement is flexion/extension stability. Fusion treatments require a stable environment for arthrodesis, and it has been shown that the stiffer systems promote better clinical outcomes. Thus, a reduction in normalized ROM has often been linked to stability that promotes better clinical outcomes[20] and can potentially alleviate pain in metastatic disease of the spine. Another example is load sharing, in which axial compression numbers are the important axial direction necessary to deduce the amount of load transferred through the anterior and midcolumn versus the load transferred through the posterior column. The mode of loading is most often used to determine the hardware characteristics in axial compression.[21,22] Load displacement data have been used to identify load percentages by interbody spacers and that of the fixation hardware.

Regardless of the method of testing and the attempts at standardizing FSU test configurations, the results for stability measurements can be reported and discussed with the proper reporting methods.[13,23,24] Methods and results have been published and continue to evolve.[14] As new test methods evolve and surgical paradigms change, consistent reporting of the test configurations, along with standardized results, will allow quick adaptation of sophisticated test algorithms.

Reporting of several important biomechanical parameters for implanted FSUs, including the following, are often discussed in the literature[24]:

- Neutral zone
- Range of motion
- Elastic zone
- Neutral zone stiffness
- Elastic zone stiffness

The parameters are essential to the understanding of the native intact condition, as well as the various treatments of the spinal column for most test configurations. Until recently, the methods of reporting have been independent of the method of testing. ROM can be reported whether load is applied through pure moments, with a follower load, or in a translational/pinned fixed (TPF) condition.

The resulting kinematic motion is a response for a vertebral body relative to the adjacent vertebrae and therefore a measure of the kinematic FSU response. Such results are the basis for comparison and the foundation for understanding of the biomechanical effects on the clinical FSU.

The data most often generated and reported for biomechanical FSU testing are the resultant FSU ROM. For fixation studies, the criteria are relatively simple when evaluating the biomechanical data that include ROM; that is, the smaller the ROM, the better the fixation result. Although ROM alone is not sufficient to describe the biomechanical parameters associated with an FSU, it has been a key biomechanical parameter in assessing and predicting stability. Therefore, it can be extrapolated to the clinical decision-making process. However, for newer technologies and implants, additional parameters may become more important but currently remain unclear.

◆ Conclusion

Spinal stability based on the described measurement methodologies is important for several reasons. Primarily for the metastatic involved spine, stabilization through surgical intervention can relieve pain and restore function. Moreover, it can improve the quality of life for the patient. It has also been shown in certain circumstances that radiation treatment can be avoided provided proper tumor resection and subsequent decompression and stabilization can be performed. As devices are developed that allow greater versatility and stability, clinicians still require a means to evaluate their potential. Biomechanical stability testing may help in the decision-making process for the clinical management of metastatic tumors involving the spine.

References

1. Tschirhart CE, Finkelstein J, Whyne C. Metastatic burst fracture risk assessment based on complex loading of the thoracic spine. Ann Biomed Eng 2006;34:494–505.
2. Aebi M. Spinal metastasis in the elderly. Eur Spine J 2003;12:S202–S13.
3. Ebihara H, Ito M, Abumi K, et al. A biomechanical analysis of metastatic vertebral collapse of the thoracic spine: a sheep model study. Spine 2004;29:994–999.
4. Krishnaney AA, Steinmetz MP, Benzel EC. Biomechanics of metastatic spine cancer. Neurosurg Clin N Am 2004;15:375–380.
5. Virgin WJ. Experimental investigations into the physical properties of the intervertebral disc. J Bone Joint Surg Br 1951;33-B:607–611.
6. Hirsch C, Nachemson A. New observations on the mechanical behavior of lumbar discs. Acta Orthop Scand 1954;23:254–283.
7. Heller JG, Zdeblick TA, Kunz DA, et al. Spinal instrumentation for metastatic disease: in vitro biomechanical analysis. J Spinal Disord 1993;6:17–22.
8. Kanayama M, Ng JT, Cunningham BW, et al. Biomechanical analysis of anterior versus circumferential spinal reconstruction for various anatomic stages of tumor lesions. Spine 1999;24:445–450.
9. Oda I, Cunningham BW, Abumi K, et al. The stability of reconstruction methods after thoracolumbar total spondylectomy: an in vitro investigation. Spine 1999;24:1634–1638.
10. Shannon FJ, DiResta GR, Ottaviano D, et al. Biomechanical analysis of anterior poly-methyl-methacrylate reconstruction following total spondylectomy for metastatic disease. Spine 2004;29:2096–2112.
11. Vahldiek MJ, Panjabi MM. Stability potential of spinal instrumentations in tumor vertebral body replacement surgery. Spine 1998;23:543–550.
12. Samartzis D, Marco RA, Benjamin R, et al. Multilevel en bloc spondylectomy and chest wall excision via a simultaneous anterior and posterior approach for Ewing sarcoma. Spine 2005;30:831–837.
13. Panjabi MM. Biomechanical evaluation of spinal fixation devices: 1. A conceptual framework. Spine 1988;13:1129–1134.
14. Goel VK, Panjabi MM, Patwardhan AG, et al. Test protocols for evaluation of spinal implants. J Bone Joint Surg Am 2006;88(Suppl 2):103–109.
15. Akamaru T, Kawahara N, Sakamoto J, et al. The transmission of stress to grafted bone inside a titanium mesh cage used in anterior column reconstruction after total spondylectomy: a finite-element analysis. Spine 2005;30:2783–2787.
16. Dimar JRII, Voor MJ, Zhang YM, et al. A human cadaver model for determination of pathologic fracture threshold resulting from tumorous destruction of the vertebral body. Spine 1998;23:1209–1214.
17. Kunz DN, McCabe RP, Zdeblick TA, et al. A multi-degree of freedom system for biomechanical testing. J Biomech Eng 1994;116:371–373.
18. Cunningham BW, Gordon JD, Dmitriev AE, et al. Biomechanical evaluation of total disc replacement arthroplasty: an in vitro human cadaveric model. Spine 2003;28:S110–S117.
19. Cunningham BW, Kotani Y, McNulty PS, et al. The effect of spinal destabilization and instrumentation on lumbar intradiscal pressure: an in vitro biomechanical analysis. Spine 1997;22:2655–2663.
20. Zdeblick TA. A prospective, randomized study of lumbar fusion: preliminary results. Spine 1993;18:983–991.
21. Rapoff AJ, Conrad BP, Johnson WM, et al. Load sharing in Premier and Zephir anterior cervical plates. Spine 2003;28:2648–2650.
22. Rapoff AJ, O'Brien TJ, Ghanayem AJ, et al. Anterior cervical graft and plate load sharing. J Spinal Disord 1999;12:45–49.
23. Goel VK, Goyal S, Clark C, et al. Kinematics of the whole lumbar spine: effect of discectomy. Spine 1985;10:543–554.
24. Wilke HJ, Wenger K, Claes L. Testing criteria for spinal implants: recommendations for the standardization of in vitro stability testing of spinal implants. Eur Spine J 1998;7:148–154.

17

Functional Spine Radiosurgery

Antonio A. F. De Salles and Paul M. Medin

The idea of concentrating an extremely high dose of radiation with highly collimated beams to cause changes in brain function, mostly in the treatment of medically refractory pain, gave birth to radiosurgery.[1] The evolution of medical therapy for chronic and cancer pain, as well as the relatively short-lived pain relief afforded by destruction of nuclei or pain pathways in the brain, led to the application of radiosurgery to morphological diseases of the brain, such as benign tumors,[2] vascular lesions,[3] and malignances.[4] The imaging revolution during the last quarter of the 20th century established stereotactic radiosurgery (SRS) as a viable and robust minimally invasive technique to manage extremely difficult benign and malignant pathologies of the brain.[3,5–7] It also established SRS as an important form of treatment for essential trigeminal neuralgia,[8–11] a unique recurrent and frequently medically refractory facial pain syndrome. Treatment of other dermatomal pain syndromes with SRS became a natural evolution of the technique that met substantial barriers due to the technical challenges of targeting precisely outside the skull.

Several factors have delayed the progress of SRS for the treatment of spinal cord–related pain, although the effectiveness of SRS to abate pain related to spinal metastases compressing neural elements is well known. Because the spinal cord is packed with highly eloquent pathways, imprecision in dose delivery cannot be tolerated. Methods of stereotactic localization and exquisite visualization of the spinal cord and spinal nerves were developed during the past decade; however, methods of fixation and tracking of target movement in relation to the isocenter of the SRS device are still in development. The potential of SRS to manage dermatomal pain syndromes is still to be explored.

Authors working on spinal SRS technical development have given the prevalence of metastases to the spinal column and their consequence on a patient's quality of life as an explanation for the importance of the technique.[12–14] Compromised ambulation, lack of sphincter control, and medically refractory pain are the symptoms that mostly impair the patient's quality of life. Stabilization and regression of spinal lesions with SRS are already a reality.[15–19] Because the treatment of patients with cancer has improved substantially as a result of developments in systemic chemotherapy, immunotherapy, and radiotherapy, as well as SRS, long-term survivors face the difficult problem of effective pain control during the advanced phase of their disease. Similar difficulties confront patients with chronic pain secondary to benign disease. The application of spinal SRS in the treatment of medically refractory pain requires an understanding of the scope of the problem that one is facing, as well as the limitations of this focal technique.

◆ Refractory Pain Syndromes

There are disagreements among specialists on how to manage persistent pain. These disagreements intensify when opioids and destructive procedures in the nervous system become necessary. Opioids are more acceptable when cancer pain is involved.[20] Opioid treatment for persistent pain of benign origin requires careful consideration. Primary care physicians and rheumatologists who prescribe opioids for chronic pain may not consider their long-term use to be a major problem. However, pain specialists, including neurologists, anesthesiologists, neurosurgeons, psychologists, and psychiatrists, are particularly opposed to the extended use of opioids by patients who do not have a limited life span. Complications of long-term use of opioids include intolerance (64%), physical tolerance (34%), withdrawal (17%), and abuse (13%). Psychiatrists are less likely to endorse the long-term use of opioids and are less likely to prescribe them than are anesthesiologists or neurologists.[21] Frequently, neurosurgical procedures for pain are not even thought of by a large percentage of practitioners.[22] Spinal SRS can be introduced in several instances of pain limited to few dermatomes because it is a noninvasive procedure.

Understanding and diagnosing persistent pain are the first steps in indicating SRS in its context. Medically and surgically persistent pain (MSPP) is defined here as persistent pain when all medical and curative surgical measures have been exhausted. Invasive palliative procedures in the nervous sys-

Table 17.1 Pain Categories When Considering Neurosurgical Procedures

Category	Description
Acute pain	Usually nociceptive; considered tractable by common analgesics, short course of opioids, or a curative surgical procedure
Persistent noncancer pain (chronic pain)	Usually neuropathic or mixed*
Persistent cancer pain	Usually nociceptive; lack of opioid response because of neuropathic component or opioid tolerance*

* Spinal stereotactic radiosurgery may have limited application in cases of well-defined dermatomal pain.

Table 17.2 Neurosurgical Procedures Applied to Chronic Pain Syndromes*

Peripheral nerve injury
  Chronic nerve stimulation
  Rhizotomy†
  Ganglionectomy†
  Spinal dorsal rhizotomy†
  Dorsal root entry zone lesion
Trigeminal neuralgia
  Microvascular decompression
  Radiosurgery
  Radiofrequency rhizotomy
  Glycerol retrogasserian rhizolysis
  Percutaneous balloon compression
Atypical facial pain
  Rhizotomy
  Trigeminal nerve stimulation
  Radiofrequency sphenopalatine
  Ganglinectomy
Brachial plexus avulsion
  Dorsal root entry zone lesion
Phantom limb pain
  Dorsal column stimulation
  Deep brain stimulation
  Dorsal root entry zone lesion
Failed back syndrome and whiplash syndrome
  Dorsal column stimulation
  Facet denervation†
  Deep brain stimulation
Sympathetic dystrophy†
  Radiofrequency sympathectomy
  Endoscopic sympathectomy
  Open sympathectomy
Central pain
  Cortical stimulation
  Deep brain stimulation
  Mesencephalotomy
  Thalamomtomy
  Cingulotomy

* These are the most common neurosurgical procedures for chronic pain.
† Situations in which spinal stereotactic radiosurgery may be applied.

tem become necessary to control pain when MSPP is present. In this chapter, the term *chronic pain* stands for MSPP noncancer pain; the term *cancer pain* refers to pain from cancer not responding to opioid therapy, or for cases where the side effects of opioid therapy are unbearable to the patient (**Table 17.1**). Neurosurgical procedures for these two categories of persistent pain are listed in **Table 17.2**. Critical evaluation of the neurosurgical procedure for pain leads to the realization of the limitation of spinal SRS in this complex field. However, spinal SRS may be well suited to situations where the current techniques fail or are too invasive to be applied to the frail and medically infirm patient with dermatomal pain.

◆ Chronic Pain

Chronic pain is at least of 6 months' duration and is often associated with disability, secondary gain, psychosocial dysfunction, and litigation. The most common example is the failed back syndrome. This complex syndrome has nociceptive and neuropathy components aggravated by the factors given above. These factors are important and must be considered when evaluating patients for neurosurgical procedures for pain, especially spinal SRS.

Application of spinal SRS to chronic pain syndromes has to be in the context of a multidisciplinary approach to pain management. Collaboration of pain specialists, as happens in modern pain clinics, is indispensable for the proper application of palliative invasive procedures in chronic pain patients. These patients frequently have unrealistic expectations of neurosurgical pain procedures. A succession of failed procedures increases frustration and complicates their management. There is a paucity of methods designed to measure success of surgery for pain.[21] Results that are considered excellent by some surgeons are not accepted by others. Several variables contribute to the investigators' disagreement; these include follow-up length, differences in technique applied, patient selection, and the subjectivity of pain. The evaluation becomes more difficult when drug dependence and secondary gains are at play.

◆ Technical Aspects of Stereotactic Radiosurgery for the Spine

The progress of computed image fusion has allowed the development of stereotactic techniques that no longer depend on rigid fixation,[23] as did the initial surgically invasive attempts of spinal SRS.[24] The Stanford group pioneered the frameless approach that uses image matching of pretreatment computed tomography (CT) and oblique x-rays obtained at the time of treatment.[18] Several groups have adopted this technique for spine SRS. Further development of patient positioning has relied on reflective markers attached to a patient's surface and registration by infrared-emitting cameras, similar to the prevalent image-guided systems in neurosurgery operating rooms (ExacTrac Xray 6D, BrainLab, AG, Feldkirchen, Germany). The marriage of stereotactic triangulation technique with powerful fusion of images obtained in the radiosurgical suite supported the treatment of spinal lesions.[15] Now this same technique can be developed for the treatment of carefully selected refractory pain syndromes.

Instrumentation

The Novalis Body (BrainLab) is one commercial system used for SRS. It consists of several stereotactic components. Infrared passive reflectors attached noninvasively to the patient's surface are used for positioning of the target close to the isocenter of a linear accelerator (linac). Radiographic image guidance is used for fine positioning adjustments based on internal anatomy (the spine). The infrared guidance is also used to monitor external patient motion during treatment. The infrared positioning system consists of a pair of cameras in the radiosurgery room that emit and detect infrared radiation reflected from markers placed on a patient's skin. Data are disseminated to give real-time positional information about the patient; translation and rotation in all three major axes are displayed on multiple monitors. The treatment couch is driven automatically to position the patient near the isocenter based on information from the infrared positioning system. The infrared cameras have a very high effective resolution and can determine the position of individual reflectors with a standard deviation of 0.1 to 0.2 mm.

The radiographic image guidance system consists of a pair of kilovoltage x-ray tubes suspended from the ceiling and an amorphous silicon detector mounted to the linac couch. A pair of radiographs is exposed following infrared positioning to determine the position of the spine relative to the isocenter. The radiographs are digitally transferred to a computer, where they are compared with digitally reconstructed radiographs (DRRs) generated from a pretreatment CT. DRRs represent the position of a perfectly aligned patient. Radiographs and DRRs are fused automatically to determine if any patient positioning adjustments are necessary, and the treatment couch is moved to reposition the patient appropriately. After shifts have been applied, anterior and lateral port films are exposed to confirm patient positioning. The infrared positioning system is used to monitor external patient motion throughout the treatment process. A vacuum immobilization bag and plastic wrap restraining system minimize patient movement during treatment.

◆ Feasibility of Functional Spine Radiosurgery

A feasibility animal experiment in Yucatan minipigs was performed at the UCLA School of Medicine to investigate the effects of a 90 Gy single dose of radiation on a small volume of spinal nerve. The study specifically aimed to (1) determine the most effective 1.5 T magnetic resonance imaging (MRI)

sequence for visualization of the spinal nerve and dorsal root ganglia (DRG), (2) determine if the Novalis image-guidance process (described above) is capable of accurately targeting the spinal nerve using a 5 mm circular collimator, and (3) evaluate morbidity during an 8-month follow-up period after radiosurgery. The Yucatan minipig was selected as a model, and the study implemented the timeline shown in **Fig. 17.1**.

Imaging for Visualization and Localization

For all imaging studies, animals were positioned supine on a body-length vacuum cushion (BodyFIX, Medical Intelligence Medizintechnik GmbH, Schwabmünchen, Germany). A vacuum cushion was custom shaped around each animal and was subsequently used during image-guided radiosurgery (IGRS) to promote consistent positioning. Infrared reflector spheres (ExacTrac) were distributed on the belly at a rostral/caudal level corresponding to the lumbar spine. Positions of the infrared reflector spheres were permanently recorded on the skin with black India tattoos. A CT scan of the entire lumbar spine was acquired with 1.0 mm-thick contiguous slices and a 350 mm field of view (FOV), resulting in a voxel size of $0.68 \times 0.68 \times 1.0$ mm. The FOV was wide enough to include the entire axial anatomy plus infrared guidance reflectors. No imaging contrast was used pre-IGRS.

MR images were acquired in a 1.5 T scanner (Magnetom Symphony, Siemens Medical Solutions, Malvern, Pennsylvania) using tabletop phase array coils. Many image sequences were acquired pre- and post-IGRS, including constructive interference steady state (CISS), T1 spin echo (SE), T2 SE, T2 turbo spin echo (TSE), and true three-dimensional (3D) fast imaging with steady-state precession (FISP). Gadolinium MR contrast (Omniscan, GE Healthcare, 0.1 cc per pound) was injected for the post-IGRS imaging session of one animal only.

Treatment Planning and Delivery

CT/MR image fusion and treatment planning were performed using BrainScan version 5.2 software (BrainLab). Image series were fused using a combination of the automatic and manual fusion functions of the software. The left-sided proximal spinal nerves at two consecutive levels of the lumbar spine (L1–L2 for pig 1, L2–L3 for pig 2) were identified. Each nerve was targeted at the intervertebral foramen 7 to 8 mm lateral to the spinal cord. Of the preradiosurgery MRI sequences acquired, only the 0.5 mm thick axial CISS and the 1.0 mm thick coronal T2 TSE were useful for treatment planning. The CISS image set was used exclusively for target contouring, and the coronal image set was used for verification of target location.

A treatment plan was generated to deliver a maximum dose of 90 Gy to each target using a 5.0 mm diameter (at

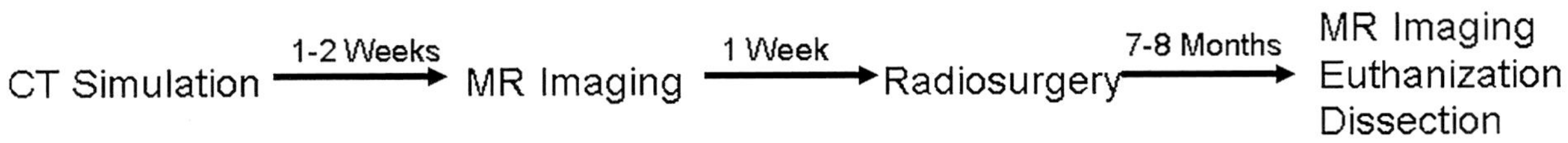

CT Simulation →(1-2 Weeks)→ MR Imaging →(1 Week)→ Radiosurgery →(7-8 Months)→ MR Imaging / Euthanization / Dissection

Fig. 17.1 Timeline for study design.

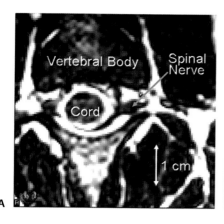
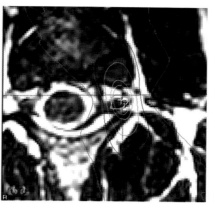

Fig. 17.2 Axial constructive interference steady state (CISS) magnetic resonance image with **(A)** and without **(B)** isodose distribution. The 90%, 80%, 50%, 30%, and 10% isodose lines are displayed.

isocenter) collimator directed in a series of eight noncoplanar arcs with a total 250 arc degrees. Arc orientations and weighting were chosen to keep the maximum spinal cord dose < 9 Gy (10% isodose line) and to minimize the dose to all other tissue outside the target volume. The 0.5 mm thick CISS axial slice displaying the isocenter is shown with and without the dose distribution in **Fig. 17.2**. Isodose distributions are all normalized to the global maximum dose point. The volumes encompassed by the 90, 50, 30, and 10% isodose lines were 0.02, 0.22, 0.61, and 6.66 cc, respectively. Typical doses calculated to the proximal edge, center, and distal edge of the spinal cord were 7, 2, and 1 Gy, respectively. Monitor units were calculated using a simple Clarkson algorithm without tissue heterogeneity corrections.

Target positioning was performed with ExacTrac 2.0 software. Radiation was delivered per plan with a Novalis 6 MV linac at a nominal dose rate of 800 monitor units per minute (8.0 Gy per minute to isocenter at a depth of 1.5 cm water in a 10 × 10 cm field). Each animal underwent one IGRS session in which both targeted spinal nerves were irradiated. The average treatment time (time from first "beam on" until conclusion) to irradiate one target was 58 minutes.

Proof of Principle and Feasibility

Animals were followed for 7 to 8 months (as described above) as planned. The lumbar segments of the spinal cord were removed with 1 to 2 cm sections of the corresponding spinal nerves. The spinal nerve from the L1 level of pig 1 was damaged during dissection and discarded. Contralateral tissues were used as normal controls. The typical dose received by contralateral spinal nerves and DRG was < 0.7 Gy. The spinal cord, ganglia, and spinal nerve were fixed in 10% buffered formalin or 2.5% glutaraldehyde. Postfixation specimens were processed as follows: (1) longitudinal sections of peripheral nerve, cross sections of DRG, and cross sections of spinal cord were embedded in paraffin, then 6 μm thick sections were cut and stained with hematoxylin and eosin; (2) cross sections of peripheral nerve were also embedded in epoxy resin, cut at 1 μm thickness and stained with toluidine blue; and (3) teased nerve fiber preparations stained with osmium tetroxide were performed on pig 1 right and left lumbar spinal nerve 2.

Both animals remained healthy throughout the study. Both animals maintained normal behavior and gait following IGRS. Pig 1 showed a marked decline in response to pinch testing over its left hind quarter 4 months post-IGRS, as evidenced by an absence of vocalization and withdrawal, but pig 2 maintained a normal response to pinch testing throughout the course of the study.

Marked signal changes were clearly visible in the bone surrounding the irradiated targets in all post-IGRS MR scans. A sagittal T2 image through the isocenter 8 months post-IGRS is shown in **Fig. 17.3**; signal enhancement is clear in the vertebral bodies of L2–L3 (irradiated) compared with L4 (not irradiated). Signal enhancement emanates from the treatment isocenter and is probably due to fatty marrow replacement. Signal changes were not as profound in the soft tissue, but signal decrease was evident in CISS images in the high dose regions (approximately ≥ 50% isodose) normally occupied by epidural fat.

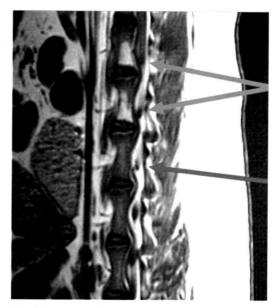

Fig. 17.3 Sagittal T2 magnetic resonance image of the Yucatan lumbar spine 8 months postradiosurgery. Green arrows, irradiated; red arrow, unirradiated.

Histopathological Observations

Spinal cords of pigs 1 and 2 were grossly unremarkable; however, there appeared to be tough, white fibrous adhesions between the dura mater surrounding the rootlets of pig 1 left DRG within the intervertebral foramina and adjacent periosteum. No other soft tissue fibrosis was noted, and the adjacent skeletal muscle appeared normal. The spinal nerves measured 1.8 mm in diameter where targeted. Plastic sections of pig 2 left L3 spinal nerve revealed focal loss of about 65% of both large and small myelinated fibers and unmyelinated fibers associated with focal collagen deposition (**Fig. 17.4**). This was not noted in the corresponding spinal nerve of the contralateral side or in the spinal nerve evaluated from L2. Plastic sections from the L2 spinal nerve of pig 1 did not demonstrate focal loss of nerve fibers on either side; however, a teased fiber preparation of the nerve distal to the left DRG showed evidence of osmiophilic ovoids due to axonal degeneration in 12 out of 96 (12.5%) myelinated fibers examined (**Fig. 17.5**). In contrast, the spinal nerve from the contralateral side showed no axonal degeneration in any of the 82 myelinated fibers examined. The findings show focal nerve damage to at least one of two spinal nerves targeted in both pigs just distal to the DRG. One small artery in the epineurium of the left spinal nerve near DRG 3 (pig 2) revealed approximately 50% luminal stenosis due to intimal hyperplasia (**Fig. 17.6**). The segmental myelinated nerve fiber loss within the fascicle in pig 2 and focal intimal hyperplasia in a small artery together with evidence of axonal (wallerian-type) degeneration in pig 1 suggest an ischemic neuropathy induced by irradiation.

Paraffin and plastic sections of the DRG demonstrated intact ganglia, satellite cells, and myelinated and unmyelinated nerve fibers leading into and out of the ganglia. Paraffin sections of the spinal cord at all levels examined from pigs 1 and

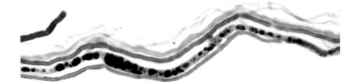

Fig. 17.5 Teased nerve fiber preparation stained with osmium tetroxide.

2 demonstrated unremarkable white and gray matter; specifically, the dorsal, lateral, and anterior columns, rootlets, and motor neurons appeared intact.

◆ Considerations of Functional Spine Radiosurgery

It is possible to irradiate spinal nerves causing partial nerve fiber degeneration, possibly decreasing conductibility through the nerve but not completely abolishing function. Further studies are necessary to establish SRS for patients with refractory dermatomal pain. These include the dose and volume of the nerve irradiated, the long-term side effects, and the effectiveness of this procedure on controlling pain. The two initial unknowns, dose and volume, can be partially understood in this animal model.

◆ Radiology and Accuracy

IGRS of nerves or ganglia demands the highest level of visualization and targeting accuracy. The small diameter of the spinal nerve and DRG, coupled with the absence of a rigidly attached frame (as is used in trigeminal SRS), presents a challenge that has been conquered using current technol-

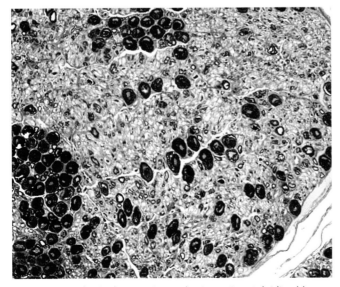

Fig. 17.4 Axial spinal nerve, 1 μm plastic section, toluidine blue (×100).

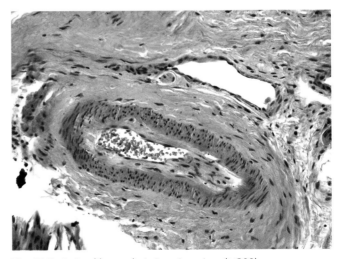

Fig. 17.6 Intimal hyperplasia in epineurium (×200).

ogy. The technical aspects of this study were to (1) determine the most effective 1.5 T MRI sequence for visualization of the spinal nerve and DRG and (2) determine if the Novalis image-guidance process is capable of accurately targeting the spinal nerve using a 5 mm circular collimator. It was apparent after dissection that, although the proximal spinal nerve can be seen in some MR images, the DRG were not distinguished from the spinal nerve in any of the image sequences acquired. The spinal nerve was viewed most clearly in the epidural space with 0.5 mm axial CISS images. Gadolinium contrast was not used in preradiosurgery MR images and was not considered useful in postradiosurgery images. Visualization was somewhat problematic for this study, but MR imaging continues to improve with changes in MRI protocols such as inclusion of additional coils and increase in magnetic field strength. Additional imaging procedures may be valuable. CT myelography could obviate the need for MRI if the DRG or spinal nerves are adequately visualized. Although myelography increases the level of patient invasion, it may increase the procedure accuracy by removing the need for CT/MRI fusion.

The localization accuracy of the radiograph/DRR fusion mode of the Novalis Body system has been reported.[19,26] Thin-slice (1 mm) CT images played an important role in this study, both to minimize errors introduced by DRR quality and to improve the resolution available for CT/MRI fusion. The spine is arguably the most amenable site to radiographic image guidance because the positional stability of the spine has been shown to be relatively independent of respiratory motion in supine pigs and humans,[27,28] and the distinct shape and high-density composition of the spine can be exploited to attain positioning information.

The accuracy of the Novalis Body system is very high by most standards. Medin et al[27] and others[15,26,28] have shown that the current accuracy of IGRS using image fusion, as in this study, and/or implanted markers is comparable to that described for frame-based cranial SRS. For perspective, Maciunas et al[29] evaluated the application accuracy of four commercially available frame-based intracranial radiosurgery systems and reported a mean accuracy of 1.2 to 1.9 mm with 0.6 to 1.0 mm standard deviation. Murphy et al[28] reported a total root-mean-square targeting accuracy of approximately 1.5 mm when using implanted markers and a CT slice thickness of 1.25 mm for targeting of spinal lesions using the CyberKnife system (Accuray Inc., Sunnyvale, California).

Collimators

Based purely on the accuracy results presented, the wisdom of using a 5 mm diameter collimator to treat functional targets in the spine is debatable. For example, assuming the isocenter is centered on a 2 mm diameter target, a positioning error of 1.5 mm in the right/left or rostral/caudal directions would result in half the target being outside the 90% isodose volume, and part of the target would be covered only by the 50% isodose volume. The same argument applies to SRS of the trigeminal root entry zone, yet 4 and 5 mm collimators remain common, and favorable results have been shown.[9,10,30–32]

It is possible that geometric misses of 1.5 mm are common in trigeminal SRS, yet the resulting dose to the nerve is suf-

ficient to produce pain relief.[9,10] Alternatively, trigeminal SRS results may be better if targeting accuracy were increased. The possibility of missing the target has to be balanced with the potential for morbidity. In the case of trigeminal nerve SRS, the risks of excessive radiation to the brainstem are well understood. The potential for morbidity when irradiating the spinal nerve or DRG is less clear, but it should be lower than the former, allowing the use of larger collimators when targeting the spinal nerves. The animals in this UCLA study showed no evidence of morbidity other than numbness, which is a potential outcome of trigeminal nerve SRS that is well tolerated by patients. It is hypothesized that only partial numbness is observed following SRS because not all fibers are demyelinated.[33]

Targeting spinal nerves or ganglia with larger collimators would lead to increased dose to the spinal cord. The radiation tolerance of the cord under the conditions of functional radiosurgery is not well known, but several previous studies in animals suggest that the cord can tolerate much higher doses than used in this UCLA swine project. Irradiated volume,[34,35] dose distribution,[36,37] dose rate,[38] previous irradiation,[39] and age[40] have all been shown to affect the tolerance of the cord but, the first two are probably the most significant to functional spine radiosurgery. The dose to the spinal cord from functional radiosurgery is unique in radiation therapy because (1) it is delivered in a single treatment, (2) a short length (2–10 mm) is irradiated, (3) only a fraction of the cross section of the cord receives a high dose, and (4) there is a steep dose gradient in all planes across the cord. Further experimental studies characterizing the tolerance of the spinal cord to radiosurgical doses and volumes need to be carried out before this technique becomes ready to treat patients with benign dermatomal pain. The 7- to 8-month postradiosurgery observation period of this study far exceeded the time frame in which radiation-induced paralysis is expected to occur. The latency period for paralysis in pigs following a single dose of radiation to the spinal cord has been reported to be 7.5 to 16.5 weeks.[40,41]

Dosimetry

The radiation tolerance of the DRG is unknown, but De Salles et al[42] reported no damage to the trigeminal ganglion from doses < 37 Gy delivered by SRS. It is unclear why one of three spinal nerves evaluated did not show significant radiation damage, but this is potentially due to poor visualization of the nerve, errors introduced in image fusion, positioning error, or a combination thereof. Vujaskovic et al[43] reported a significant decrease in nerve fiber density in the canine sciatic nerve 12 months after 28 Gy was delivered to a 5 cm length by intraoperative radiotherapy (IORT), but no damage was seen following doses of 12 or 20 Gy. Vujaskovic has also noted that the tolerance of peripheral nerves depends on the volume of irradiated nerve and surrounding tissues.[44] In a similar study with 24 month follow-up, Vujaskovic et al[45] noted mild fibrosis and nerve fiber loss in one of five dogs treated with 24 Gy. In another large IORT study, the right lumbrosacral plexus (L3–L7 plus three sacral nerves) of foxhounds was exposed surgically and given a single dose of electron radiation through a 9 cm diameter circular cone.

Groups of four dogs received doses of 10, 15, or 20 Gy at a dose rate of 2.5 Gy per minute.[46] With follow-up of ≥ 42 months, it was reported that dogs in the 10 and 15 Gy groups continued to have normal function of the right hind limb, whereas all dogs in the 20 Gy group developed clinical signs of paresis beginning 8 to 12 months postirradiation that progressed to paralysis and flexion contractures in two dogs.[46] After prolonged follow-up of 60 months, Johnstone et al[47] reported one dog in the 15 Gy group had developed paralysis (51 months), whereas dogs in the 10 Gy group remained free of neuropathy. Histological review of the paralyzed animal revealed an acute spinal hemorrhage in the milieu of chronic inflammatory change. It is suggested that the hemorrhage may have been contributed to by late damage in the fine vasculature.

◆ Conclusion

In view of imaging and targeting improvements implemented in spine radiosurgery since this project was completed, there is no longer a question of whether functional SRS is technically possible, but most aspects of this procedure remain unanswered. Among the unknown parameters are the most effective imaging modality/protocol, the lowest effective dose, the most effective target, the most appropriate collimator/lesion size, the potential for long-term morbidity, and the time course for morbidity. Most importantly, it is still not known if this procedure will provide any measure of pain relief. Matters of procedural safety and a better understanding of the response of spinal nerves to small-volume, high-dose radiation is warranted to guide this procedure to a trial in humans.

References

1. Leksell L. The stereotaxic method and radiosurgery of the brain. Acta Chir Scand 1951;102:316–319.
2. De Salles A, Bajada CL, Goetsch S, et al. Radiosurgery of cavernous sinus tumors. Acta Neurochir Suppl (Wien) 1993;58:101–103.
3. Friedman WA, Bova FJ. Radiosurgery for arteriovenous malformations. Clin Neurosurg 1993;40:446–464.
4. Mehta MP, Masciopinto J, Rozental J, et al. Stereotactic radiosurgery for glioblastoma multiforme: report of a prospective study evaluating prognostic factors and analyzing long-term survival advantage. Int J Radiat Oncol Biol Phys 1994;30:541–549.
5. Kondziolka D, Niranjan A, Lunsford LD, et al. Stereotactic radiosurgery for meningiomas. Neurosurg Clin North Am 1999;10:317.325.
6. Lunsford LD. Stereotactic radiosurgery: at the threshold or at the crossroads? Neurosurgery 1993;32:799–804.
7. Steiner L, ed. Radiosurgery: Baseline and Trends. New York: Raven Press; 1992.
8. Frighetto L, De Salles AA, Smith ZA, et al. Noninvasive linear accelerator radiosurgery as the primary treatment for trigeminal neuralgia. Neurology 2004;62:660–662.
9. Goss BW, Frighetto L, DeSalles AA, et al. Linear accelerator radiosurgery using 90 gray for essential trigeminal neuralgia: results and dose volume histogram analysis. Neurosurgery 2003;53:823–828.
10. Kondziolka D, Lunsford LD, Flickinger JC, et al. Stereotactic radiosurgery for trigeminal neuralgia: a multiinstitutional study using the gamma unit. J Neurosurg 1996;84:940–945.
11. Smith ZA, De Salles AA, Frighetto L, et al. Dedicated linear accelerator radiosurgery for the treatment of trigeminal neuralgia. J Neurosurg 2003;99:511–516.
12. Hamilton RJ, Kuchnir FT, Pelizzari CA, et al. Repositioning accuracy of a noninvasive head fixation system for stereotactic radiotherapy. Med Phys 1996;23:1909–1917.
13. Medin PM, Solberg TD, De Salles AA, et al. Investigations of a minimally invasive method for treatment of spinal malignancies with LINAC stereotactic radiation therapy: accuracy and animal studies. Int J Radiat Oncol Biol Phys 2002;52:1111–1122.
14. Zhu G, Ryu S. Efficacy of image-guided radiosurgery for spinal metastases. Int J Radiat Oncol Biol Phys 2003;57:S374–S375.
15. De Salles AA, Pedroso AG, Medin P, et al. Spinal lesions treated with Novalis shaped beam intensity-modulated radiosurgery and stereotactic radiotherapy. J Neurosurg 2004;101(Suppl 3):435–440.
16. Gerszten PC, Burton SA, Welch WC, et al. Single-fraction radiosurgery for the treatment of spinal breast metastases. Cancer 2005;104:2244–2254.
17. Gerszten PC, Ozhasoglu C, Burton SA, et al. CyberKnife frameless single-fraction stereotactic radiosurgery for benign tumors of the spine. Neurosurg Focus 2003;14:e16.
18. Ryu SI, Chang SD, Kim DH, et al. Image-guided hypo-fractionated stereotactic radiosurgery to spinal lesions. Neurosurgery 2001;49:838–846.
19. Yin FF, Ryu S, Ajlouni M, et al. A technique of intensity-modulated radiosurgery (IMRS) for spinal tumors. Med Phys 2002;29:2815–2822.
20. Cleeland CS, Gonin R, Hatfield AK, et al. Pain and its treatment in outpatients with metastatic cancer. N Engl J Med 1994;330:592–596.
21. Turk DC, Brody MC, Okifuji EA. Physicians' attitudes and practices regarding the long-term prescribing of opioids for non-cancer pain. Pain 1994;59:201–208.
22. De Salles AA, Johnson JP. More on the treatment of pain. N Engl J Med 1994;331:1528.
23. Murphy MJ, Chang SD, Gibbs IC, et al. Patterns of patient movement during frameless image-guided radiosurgery. Int J Radiat Oncol Biol Phys 2003;55:1400–1408.
24. Hamilton AJ, Lulu BA, Fosmire H, et al. LINAC-based spinal stereotactic radiosurgery. Stereotact Funct Neurosurg 1996;66:1–9.
25. Medin P, Goss B, Chute D, et al. Image guided radiosurgery of proximal lumbar spinal nerves: a technical and histopathological study. Unpublished.
26. Verellen D, Soete G, Linthout N, et al. Quality assurance of a system for improved target localization and patient set-up that combines real-time infrared tracking and stereoscopic X-ray imaging. Radiother Oncol 2003;67:129–141.
27. Medin PM, Solberg TD, De Salles AA, et al. Investigations of a minimally invasive method for treatment of spinal malignancies with LINAC stereotactic radiation therapy: accuracy and animal studies. Int J Radiat Oncol Biol Phys 2002;52:1111–1122.
28. Murphy MJ, Chang S, Gibbs I, et al. Image-guided radiosurgery in the treatment of spinal metastases. Neurosurg Focus 2001;11:e6.
29. Maciunas RJ, Galloway RL Jr, Latimer JW. The application accuracy of stereotactic frames. Neurosurgery 1994;35:682–694.
30. Maesawa S, Salame C, Flickinger JC, et al. Clinical outcomes after stereotactic radiosurgery for idiopathic trigeminal neuralgia. J Neurosurg 2001;94:14–20.
31. Pollock BE, Phuong LK, Gorman DA, et al. Stereotactic radiosurgery for idiopathic trigeminal neuralgia. J Neurosurg 2002;97:347–353.
32. Young RF, Vermeulen SS, Grimm P, et al. GammaKnife radiosurgery for treatment of trigeminal neuralgia: idiopathic and tumor related. Neurology 1997;48:608–614.
33. Kondziolka D, Lacomis D, Niranjan A, et al. Histological effects of trigeminal nerve radiosurgery in a primate model: implications for trigeminal neuralgia radiosurgery. Neurosurgery 2000;46:971–976.
34. Bijl HP, van Luijk P, Coppes RP, et al. Dose-volume effects in the rat cervical spinal cord after proton irradiation. Int J Radiat Oncol Biol Phys 2002;52:205–211.
35. Hopewell JW, Morris AD, Dixon-Brown A. The influence of field size on the late tolerance of the rat spinal cord to single doses of X rays. Br J Radiol 1987;60:1099–1108.
36. Bijl HP, van Luijk P, Coppes RP, et al. Unexpected changes of rat cervical spinal cord tolerance caused by inhomogeneous dose distributions. Int J Radiat Oncol Biol Phys 2003;57:274–281.
37. van Luijk P, Bijl HP, Coppes RP, et al. Techniques for precision irradiation of the lateral half of the rat cervical spinal cord using 150 MeV protons [corrected]. Phys Med Biol 2001;46:2857–2871.
38. Scalliet P, Landuyt W, Van der SE. Repair kinetics as a determining factor for late tolerance of central nervous system to low dose rate irradiation. Radiother Oncol 1989;14:345–353.

39. Ang KK, Jiang GL, Feng Y, et al. Extent and kinetics of recovery of occult spinal cord injury. Int J Radiat Oncol Biol Phys 2001;50:1013–1020

40. van den Aardweg GJ, Hopewell JW, Whitehouse EM, et al. A new model of radiation-induced myelopathy: a comparison of the response of mature and immature pigs. Int J Radiat Oncol Biol Phys 1994;29:763–770.

41. van den Aardweg GJ, Hopewell JW, Whitehouse EM. The radiation response of the cervical spinal cord of the pig: effects of changing the irradiated volume. Int J Radiat Oncol Biol Phys 1995;31:51–55.

42. De Salles AA, Solberg TD, Mischel P, et al. Arteriovenous malformation animal model for radiosurgery: the rete mirabile. AJNR Am J Neuroradiol 1996;17:1451–1458.

43. Vujaskovic Z, Gillette SM, Powers BE, et al. Ultrastructural morphometric analysis of peripheral nerves after intraoperative irradiation. Int J Radiat Biol 1995;68:71–76.

44. Vujaskovic Z. Structural and physiological properties of peripheral nerves after intraoperative irradiation. J Peripher Nerv Syst 1997;2:343–349.

45. Vujaskovic Z, Powers BE, Paardekoper G, et al. Effects of intraoperative irradiation (IORT) and intraoperative hyperthermia (IOHT) on canine sciatic nerve: histopathological and morphometric studies. Int J Radiat Oncol Biol Phys 1999;43:1103–1109.

46. Kinsella TJ, DeLuca AM, Barnes M, et al. Threshold dose for peripheral neuropathy following intraoperative radiotherapy (IORT) in a large animal model. Int J Radiat Oncol Biol Phys 1991;20:697–701.

47. Johnstone PA, DeLuca AM, Bacher JD, et al. Clinical toxicity of peripheral nerve to intraoperative radiotherapy in a canine model. Int J Radiat Oncol Biol Phys 1995;32:1031–1034.

18

Multidisciplinary Combined Modality Approach for Cancer of the Spinal Cord

Joseph Anderson, Marilyn J. G. Gates, Laura A. Massanisso, Kathleen M. Faber, and Samuel Ryu

Optimal management of patients with spinal cord neoplasm requires collaboration between several disciplines: medical oncology, neurology, neurosurgery, radiation oncology, and radiology. The patients are a diverse group, but there are several guiding principles that aid in their assessment and management. Goals of care for the multidisciplinary team include early and accurate diagnosis, effective treatment, prevention and management of complications and comorbidities, functional improvement, and enhanced quality of life. This chapter will focus on some of the multidisciplinary aspects of caring for these patients.

◆ Diagnosis

Most of our patients already have an established cancer diagnosis, and new patients may have an obvious primary neoplasm elsewhere, away from the spine. Occasionally, a patient presents with spinal metastases with an uncertain primary, or there may have been a time interval between a prior neoplasm and later metastases, making the tissue diagnosis uncertain. In such cases, a biopsy may be necessary. Prior to making this decision, it is useful to consider a complete workup to screen for malignancy elsewhere. For instance, an ambiguous solitary vertebral metastasis is more likely to be a metastatic focus if the workup reveals additional metastases elsewhere. Serum tumor markers can be used in this determination, such as prostate-specific antigen for prostate cancer, CA-15.3, CA-27, and CA-29 for breast cancer, and immunoglobulins for myeloma.

◆ Patient Presentation

There are three main ways that spinal tumors may present: incidental lesions in asymptomatic patients, those presenting with pain, and those presenting with neurologic symptoms.

Most spine tumors are bone metastases to vertebral bodies. A variety of cancers metastasize to bone; the most frequently seen are breast, lung, and prostate cancers.[1] We have observed that with newer and more effective systemic therapy, the natural history and metastatic pattern for certain cancers may be evolving; for instance, we have seen several cases of colorectal cancer with apparent hematogenous metastases to the spine, which previously was a rare occurrence.

When surveillance studies indicate the incidental finding of an asymptomatic spinal metastasis, a decision needs to be made on whether further diagnostic study or lesion-specific treatment is necessary. Many asymptomatic lesions detected on a bone scan can have clinical follow-up. Solitary metastases may be considered for definitive treatment on an individualized basis.

The common presenting pattern is pain. The typical picture is that of crescendo pain localized at the site of the radiographic abnormality over the spine, often with associated radicular pain or tenderness. For classic symptoms and a consistent magnetic resonance imaging (MRI) appearance, a decision may easily be made to treat. Unfortunately, the diagnosis is not always so straightforward. Back pain is a common diagnosis, even in patients without metastatic cancer. According to the results of a national survey, at least 2.5% of all medical visits in Ontario were because of malignant spinal cord compression pain.[2] In a similar survey in Saskatchewan, the prevalence of back pain in adults was 28%.[3] Patients may have pain from degenerative disease, muscular strain, or other conditions. Even in patients with definite metastases on imaging studies, their pain may not always be from the tumor. For example, vertebral compression fracture can cause pain generated by periosteal and soft tissue inflammation from the fracture. In such cases, MRI evaluation and multidisciplinary assessment will help determine the optimal management.

The next common presenting pattern is with neurologic symptoms, including weakness, paresthesia, and incontinence.[4] Making a diagnosis is usually straightforward in cases with rapid onset of classic symptoms. Typically, though, the symptoms are more subtle and can be confounded by concurrent neurologic conditions, such as peripheral sensory neuropathy from chemotherapy weakness from steroids or deconditioning.[5] The most common chemotherapeutic agents that may cause neuropathy include the platinum compounds, taxanes, vinca alkaloids, thalidomide, methotrexate, and fluorouracil.[6] Because clinical outcomes are improved with early treatment of symptomatic spinal cord compression, primary physicians need to remain vigilant. Multidisciplinary evaluation may be helpful in making the diagnosis of patients with overlapping neurologic symptoms.

◆ Treatment

Multidisciplinary management can include several treatment modalities: surgery, fractionated radiotherapy, radiosurgery, systemic chemotherapy, steroids, physiotherapy, and attention to concurrent medical conditions. Many of these are addressed in other chapters.

Systemic Chemotherapy

Most intramedullary spinal tumors are treated primarily with radiotherapy. In select cases we have also incorporated systemic chemotherapy. Patients with spinal cord gliomas can be treated with concurrent radiotherapy and Temodar (tomozolomide), in a fashion similar to brain gliomas.[7] Patients with primary central nervous system (CNS) lymphoma with spine involvement may be treated primarily with chemotherapy, high-dose methotrexate, and/or rituximab.[8]

Patients may develop leptomeningeal metastases from a variety of tumors. About 5% of patients with advanced cancer may have clinical leptomeningeal metastases, but autopsy studies indicate that the prevalence may be considerably higher.[9,10] Although cerebral or cranial nerve symptoms are typical presentations, many patients present with spinal symptoms. Presymptomatic patients may have the diagnosis suggested by MRI. Cerebrospinal fluid (CSF) cytology is helpful in confirming the diagnosis, but it may not always be positive. If there is clinical suspicion, high-volume or repeat CSF cytology should be performed.[11] If intrathecal chemotherapy is planned, a nuclear cisternogram should be considered to verify adequate CSF flow.[12] If there is a block or bulky intraspinal or paraspinal tumor, then focal radiotherapy or radiosurgery may be considered to facilitate the distribution of the intrathecal medication. Chemotherapeutic agents for intrathecal administration include methotrexate, Ara C (cytarabine), and thiotepa. The spectrum of activity of these agents is limited, with predictable responses with leukemias and lymphomas, occasional responses with breast cancer, and rare responses with other solid tumors.[13] Systemic chemotherapy agents can also be considered on an individualized basis, for example, Xeloda (capecitabine) in patients with breast cancer or high-dose methotrexate for leptomeningeal lymphoma.

The majority of cases discussed at the spine tumor board at Heny Ford Hospital, Detroit, Michigan, have extra-axial systemic metastases to bone or paraspinal regions. In patients without spinal cord compression who have responsive tumors, such as lymphoma, multiple myeloma, and receptor-positive breast cancers, chemotherapy can be the primary treatment modality. A common dilemma is whether to treat with surgery or radiotherapy before systemic agents

are used. For isolated metastases, nonresponsive tumors to chemotherapy such as renal cell carcinoma, or if there is encroachment into the canal, radiosurgery may be considered. There may be several vertebral levels that would need to be targeted. In such cases, multidisciplinary planning may be helpful to minimize the radiotherapy field and preserve marrow function to allow for later systemic therapy.

Hormone therapy can achieve a rapid response in a subset of patients who present with pain and have advanced potentially hormone-responsive tumors, such as receptor-positive breast cancers and prostate cancer. We have seen dramatic responses within 1 or 2 days in prostate cancer patients treated with ketoconazole, or in breast cancer patients treated with an aromatase inhibitors. A patient with prostate cancer with spinal cord compression at T6 and T10–T11 causing lower extremity weakness is shown in **Fig. 18.1.** The T6 lesion was treated with ketoconazole alone, and the more severe T10–T11 lesion was treated with radiosurgery. A follow-up MRI scan showed significant tumor response to these treatments. However, special care must be taken because of the risk of tumor flair from luteinizing hormone-releasing hormone (LHRH) analogues or antiestrogens. Short-term follow-up with MRI and ancillary studies such as serum tumor markers should be performed in conjunction with clinical assessment. Patients responding to hormone therapy may have other modalities of treatment held, whereas those without early response may be considered for radiation.

Bisphosphonates

Bisphosphonates decrease osteoclastic activity, necessary for the lysis of bony cortex by skeletal metastases. They may also change the marrow microenvironment, with effects on

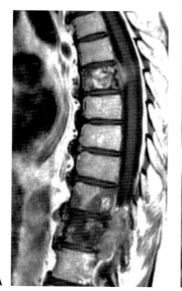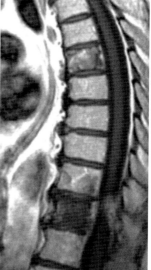

A   B

Figure 18.1 Ketoconazole effect for prostate spinal cord compression. This patient presented with T6 and T10–T11 spinal cord compression with neurologic symptoms. The T6 compression was treated with ketoconazole alone, and the more severe T10–T11 compression was treated with 18 Gy radiosurgery. **(A)** Before treatment. **(B)** Two months after treatment.

the initiation and growth of metastases. Studies have documented reduction of pain and skeletal events in appropriately selected patients who are treated with these agents.[14-16] The clinical benefits include a reduction in the rate of pathologic fractures, vertebral compression fractures in the spine tumor board population. Pain control may be enhanced with Zometa in patients with skeletal metastases.[17] Patients with solitary or isolated metastases without apparent pathology in surrounding bone may not need systemic diphosphonates therapy. Most patients with diffuse disease, especially with a lytic component on plain film or CT, should be considered for treatment.

Bisphosphonates can also be used in patients with long-term steroid usage, those with ongoing treatment with aromatase inhibitors, and others at risk for osteoporosis. Bone density assessment can aid in determining which patients are candidates.[18,19]

Bisphosphonates can be used for prevention of compression fracture because the drugs can prevent bone loss.[20] We have used Zometa after radiosurgery for spine metastasis. We observed osteoblastic change of the treated spine after radiosurgery and Zometa treatment. One example case is described here. This patient presented with widespread painful bone metastasis with squamous cell carcinoma of unknown primary. The patient was treated with spine radiosurgery 16 Gy to T11 spine, with excellent pain relief. The patient continued with intravenous Zometa 4 mg every other month. Follow-up imaging studies showed gradual osteoblastic change with time, as shown in **Fig. 18.2.** It is not known whether this change is from the combined effect of radiosurgery or Zometa. This case shows the potential of radiosurgery and Zometa for bone reshaping and strengthening, ultimately to prevent compression fracture.

Pain Management

In many patients with advanced cancer, appropriate multimodality antineoplastic therapy will adequately control their pain. Other patients, unfortunately, have ongoing pain syndromes and may require treatment primarily with analgesics. It is important that the multidisciplinary team include individuals with expertise in using narcotic analgesics and other adjuvant medications. We also collaborate regularly with Henry Ford Hospital's palliative medicine team.[21]

Radiosurgery with Vertebroplasty or Kyphoplasty

Pain is the primary presenting complaint of patients with metastatic disease to the spine. This may be related to spinal cord compression, nerve root compression, periosteal stretching, mechanical failure, and/or compression fracture of involved vertebral bodies. Radiosurgery can relieve pain in these areas within as little as 1 day and lasting up to 6 months or more in 75% of cases.[22-26] The pain of pathologic compression fracture may require additional intervention, however, in the form of vertebroplasty or kyphoplasty or even surgical stabilization.

Vertebroplasty is a percutaneous procedure that allows for injection of polymethyl methacrylate (PMMA) into the fractured vertebral body. The procedure requires placement of a larger bore needle, under fluoroscopic guidance, into the fractured vertebral body and injection, under pressure, of PMMA. Vertebroplasty was originally applied to painful vertebral hemangiomas and osteoporotic compression fractures and was used to stabilize metastatic osteolytic lesions. PMMA stabilizes and reinforces the inner vertebral body and the superior end plate, which has been shown to have a marked positive effect on pain experienced by the patient. Multiple studies have shown this to be an effective and safe procedure.[27-29]

Kyphoplasty involves the application of an intravertebral balloon that is inflated under pressure (KyphX, Kyphon, Inc., Sunnyvale, California). The inflation, done under fluoroscopic guidance, provides a space for application of the PMMA, an indication of the volume required, and may increase the height of the fractured vertebral body. PMMA is injected anterior to posterior, again, with fluoroscopic guidance. Pain relief may be almost immediate in some patients. Patients are treated as ambulatory or kept in the hospital overnight for observation and local pain management at the sites of the needle placement.

Patients who may be candidates for kyphoplasty should have T2-weighted images available that demonstrate edema within the fractured bone.[30] These individuals are likely to have had pathological fracture within the past 3 to 6 months and would likely have bone that would respond. Patients will need to be off all anticoagulation, antiplatelet, nonsteroidal anti-inflammatory, and related medications that can prolong clotting for 7 to 10 days. The complication rate of vertebro-

RS 16 Gy   2 mon   4 mon   7 mon

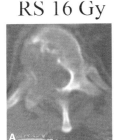 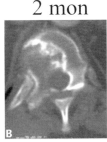 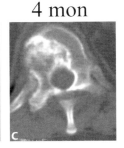 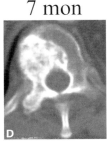

Figure 18.2 A case of bone reshaping by radiosurgery and Zometa treatment for painful spine metastasis. **(A)** A T11 compression was treated with radiosurgery (16 Gy). The patient had complete pain relief. The patient then continued treatment with Zometa every month. **(B–D)** Follow-up imaging studies showed evidence of gradual osteoblastic change.

plasty and kyphoplasty is 2 to 3% in most studies. There is a 1% incidence of spinal cord compression. Other complications include injection of PMMA into the pleural cavity or vascular spaces and extravasation into the adjacent disk. Any change in the neurologic examination should prompt immediate evaluation and, if necessary, may require emergency decompression.

Combined use of radiosurgery and vertebroplasty or kyphoplasty is not yet fully explored. Gerszten et al[22] reported their experience in combining these modalities in patients with compression fracture. Radiosurgery with 16 Gy was delivered at a mean time of 12 days after kyphoplasty. The combined procedures were well tolerated with excellent results of pain control. In our institution, these procedures are done in interventional radiology and coordinated through the spine tumor board so that these modalities can be used ideally to control the symptoms and improve spine stability. Organized literature does not reflect studies with regard to the ideal timing of vertebroplasty and kyphoplasty with radiosurgery. The literature and our experience suggest, however, that it is safe to combine these procedures for maximum pain relief. It also seems reasonable that these procedures can be used in a planned manner or according to the clinical symptoms.

Radiosurgery Combined with Open Surgery

Operative intervention is often required for extirpation of the tumor, reduction of tumor volume, and surgical stabilization. Surgical intervention usually stops with laminectomy, but, with the evolution of technologies, surgical stabilization is possible. In autopsy series, up to 36% of patients with metastatic disease demonstrated observable metastatic disease to the spine.[31,32] Spinal cord compression occurs in 10 to 20% of those with metastases to the bone.[33,34] Most of the metastases occur in the thoracic spine, 20% in the lumbar spine, and 10% in the cervical spine.[35] Most surgeons would consider surgical stabilization in patients who have a life expectancy > 3 months. However, accurate determination of survival and, more importantly, quality of life in the peri- and postoperative period is much more difficult to assess. For this reason, appropriate discussions between the oncologic and surgical teams are necessary. An excellent channel in our institution has been the spine tumor board. Determination of the clinical appropriateness of the surgery (in light of neurologic decline, duration of decline, and status prior to treatment), in addition to the anticipated outcome, general health, and life expectancy, is necessary. Several individuals have proposed prognostic scoring systems that may be of use in determining candidacy for surgery.[36–38] Indeed, we are in the process of developing a grading system of epidural spinal cord compression with radiographic and neurologic scoring criteria.

Several studies have been published that indicate successful surgical stabilization. Sundaresan et al studied 80 patients with 60% ambulatory prior to surgery and 55% with significant pain.[39] Following surgery, 98% of patients were ambulatory, including 94% who were not preoperatively, and stability was improved in 95% of patients. Other studies showed about 85% success when defined as the percentage of patients who continued to be ambulatory following surgery or who regained function.[40-44] A randomized controlled study of radiation alone versus surgical intervention and postoperative radiotherapy demonstrated that 56% of those who were not ambulatory prior to surgery were able to regain that ability as compared with 19% in the group receiving radiation only.[45]

Experience with the combined use of surgical resection and radiosurgery is scant. Postoperative radiosurgery has been tested following open surgical resection in 18 patients with spine metastasis with or without epidural compression.[23] Radiosurgery with a marginal dose of 6 to 16 Gy was delivered to the level of spine involvement usually 1 to 2 weeks after surgery. Ninety-two percent of the patients remained neurologically stable or improved. Only one patient became neurologically worse because of tumor progression. These results suggest that radiosurgery as prescribed in this series of postoperative patients with residual spinal tumor is well tolerated and associated with little or no significant morbidity. One caveat is the difficulty in delineating the tumor and spinal cord due to a poor image quality secondary to interference of hardware used for spine stabilization, even with the use of MRI fusion.

Multidisciplinary Spine Tumor Board

Tumors involving the spinal column are complex. They manifest not only the symptoms of pain or neurologic deficits but also other general medical and oncologic problems, even with socioeconomic issues. In addition, any symptoms arising from the weight-bearing central skeleton directly affect the function and quality of life. More complicating clinical dilemmas include intercurrent degenerative changes, osteoporosis and associated spine bone changes, and spine instability problems, particularly in elderly patients. There also can be many different treatment approaches for the issues occurring from the spine. In our institution, these issues were considered important for patient care and warranted the formation of a multidisciplinary spine tumor board. The spine tumor board/clinic is a forum of a true spine oncology program with medical, radiation, and surgical spine oncology, as well as radiology and pathology. Support programs are provided by spine nurses, a pain management team, physical therapists, social workers, and a coordinator. The purpose of the spine tumor board is to coordinate comprehensive total care of spine tumor patients using a multimodality approach.

◆ Patient Care and Education for Spine Radiosurgery

Patient education and orientation begins at the time of consultation. It is natural for patients and their families to experience a variety of emotions, with fear being the most common. Once they understand the process of radiosurgery and what they are going to experience, their fears and hesitations are dramatically reduced. It is reassuring for patients and their families to learn that radiosurgery is noninvasive and does not require an incision or hospital admission, as typical surgery does. It is also helpful to show them the radiosurgery treatment room and equipment so they can see the actual table and setup. We explain the actual radiosurgery procedures in five steps:

1. Preparation for positioning and immobilization. This includes the planning process, also known as simulation. The patient's vital signs are monitored, and the intravenous line is set up for contrast media to help image-guided localization and hydration with medications, if needed. It is also explained that a special body-molding device or a head frame is used. The body is kept still with the aid of a vacuum pump or other positioning devices.

2. Imaging acquisition. With the immobilization device, CT and/or MRI scans are taken with intravenous contrast for the area where the target tumor is located. It is explained to the patient that some stereotactic frames and tools can be used to help precise localization of tumor and normal tissues. After the imaging is complete, the immobilization device is removed, and the patient is free to get dressed.

3. Treatment planning. The images are sent to the radiosurgery planning computer to develop precise treatment and dosage. State-of-the-art methods are used to achieve the optimal treatment plan. The patient is allowed to relax in a comfortable position. If desired, the patient is sent home, and the actual treatment is done the next day.

4. Repositioning and radiosurgery. Patient education in the treatment room is important. When the patient is ready, the therapist and the nurse escort the patient to the treatment room. We try to alleviate the patient's anxiety and fears by explaining to the patient what is going to happen and when. If a patient is experiencing pain and discomfort, he or she is asked to take prescribed pain medication before the treatment. Having the patient comfortable on the table ensures a smoother and less time-consuming treatment. The patient is reassured that there will be no pain, that nothing will touch him or her, that the treatment equipment may be robotically turned around the patient's body, and that he or she will be carefully monitored. If anything happens that is not planned, the treatment will stop automatically. Validation of alignment is done using the image-guided and other positioning systems. The actual treatment takes about 30 minutes.

5. Removal of positioning device and discharge with instructions of post-treatment care. Once the treatment is over, the patient is taken off the treatment table. There is a brief observation period, including checking vital signs. Discharge instructions including for medication are reviewed with the patient, along with follow-up instructions. We call the patient within 24 hours and in 1 week to check his or her general and clinical status. At the 4-week follow-up, the patient is asked to fill out a survey regarding the experience. Surveys have revealed that the extra time spent with patients explaining the process greatly reduces their fears and apprehension. Patients and family members also appreciate the fact that our team is multidisciplinary and that their cases have been discussed at the spine tumor board prior to radiosurgery treatment.

References

1. Loblaw DA, Laperriere NJ, Mackillop WJ. A population-based study of malignant spinal cord compression in Ontario. Clin Oncol (R Coll Radiol) 2003;15:211–217.
2. Hart LG, Deyo RA, Cherkin DC. Physician office visits for low back pain: frequency, clinical evaluation, and treatment patterns from a U.S. national survey. Spine 1995;20(1):11–19.
3. Cassidy JD. Saskatchewan health and back pain survey. Spine 1998;23(17):1923.
4. Boogerd W, van der Sande JJ. Diagnosis and treatment of spinal cord compression in malignant disease. Cancer Treat Rev 1993;19:129–150.
5. Batchelor TT, Taylor LP, Thaler HT, et al. Steroid myopathy in cancer patients. Neurology 1997;48(5):1234–1238.
6. Keime-Guibert F, Napolitano M, Delattre JY. Neurological complications of radiotherapy and chemotherapy. J Neurol 1998;245(11):695–708.
7. Stupp R, Mason WP, van den Bent MJ. Radiotherapy plus concomitant and adjuvant temozolomide for glioblastoma. N Engl J Med 2005;352:987–996.
8. Batchelor T. Treatment of primary CNS lymphoma with methotrexate and deferred radiotherapy: a report of NABTT 96–07. J Clin Oncol 2003;21(6):1044–1049.
9. Kaplan JG, DeSouza TG, Farkash A, et al. Leptomeningeal metastases: comparison of clinical features and laboratory data of solid tumors, lymphomas and leukemias. Neuro-oncology 1990;9(3):225–229.
10. Wasserstrom WR. Diagnosis and treatment of leptomeningeal metastases from solid tumors: experience with 90 patients. Cancer 1982;49(4):759–772.
11. Glantz MJ, Cole BF, Glantz LK, et al. Cerebrospinal fluid cytology in patients with cancer: minimizing false-negative results. Cancer 1998;82:733–739.
12. Grossman SA. Cerebrospinal fluid flow abnormalities in patients with neoplastic meningitis: an evaluation using 111indium-DTPA ventriculography. Am J Med 1982;73(5):641–647.
13. DeAngelis LM. Current diagnosis and treatment of leptomeningeal metastasis. Neuro-oncol 1998;38(2–3):245–252.
14. Hortobagyi GN, Theriault RL, Porter L, et al. Efficacy of pamidronate in reducing skeletal complications in patients with breast cancer and lytic bone metastases: Protocol 19 Aredia Breast Cancer Study Group. N Engl J Med 1996;335(24):1785–1791.
15. Hillner BE. American Society of Clinical Oncology 2003 update on the role of bisphosphonates and bone health issues in women with breast cancer. J Clin Oncol 2003;21(21):4042–4057.
16. Berenson JR. Zoledronic acid reduces skeletal-related events in patients with osteolytic metastases. Cancer 2001;91(7):1191–1200.
17. Ross JR, Saunders Y, Edmonds PM, et al. Systematic review of role of bisphosphonates on skeletal morbidity in metastatic cancer. BMJ 2003;327(7413):469.
18. NIH Consensus Development Panel on Osteoporosis Prevention, Diagnosis, and Therapy: Osteoporosis prevention, diagnosis, and therapy. JAMA 2001;285(6):785–795.
19. American College of Rheumatology Ad Hoc Committee on Glucocorticoid-Induced Osteoporosis. Recommendations for the prevention and treatment of glucocorticoid-induced osteoporosis: 2001 update. Arthritis Rheum 2001;44(7):1496–1503.
20. Ahmad K. Zoledronic acid prevents bone loss. Lancet Oncol 2007;8:375.
21. Lieberman IH. Initial outcome and efficacy of "kyphoplasty" in the treatment of painful osteoporotic vertebral compression fractures. Spine 2001;26(14):1631–1638.
22. Gerszten PC, Germanwala A, Burton SA, Welch WC, Ozhasoglu C, Vogel WJ. Combination kyphoplasty and spinal radiosurgery: a new treatment paradigm for pathological fractures. J Neurosurg Spine 2005;3:296–301.
23. Rock JP, Ryu S, Shukairy MS, et al. Postoperative radiosurgery for malignant spinal tumors. Neurosurgery 2006;58:891–897.

24. Ryu S, Fang Yin FF, Rock J, et al. Image-age-guided and Intensity-modulated radiosurgery for patients with spinal metastasis. Cancer 2003;97:2013–2018.
25. Schachar NS. Specific strategies for nonoperative treatment of patients with tumor-induced osteolysis from metastatic bone disease. Clin Orthop Relat Res 2001;382:75–81.
26. Cortet B, Cotton A, Boutry N, et al. Percutaneous vertebroplasty in the treatment of osteoporotic vertebral compression fractures: an open prospective study. J Rheumatol 1999;26:2222–2228.
27. Deramond H, Depriester C, Galibert P, Le Gars D. Percutaneous vertebroplasty with polymethylmetharylate: technique,indications and results. Radiol Clin North Am 1998;36:533–546.
28. Jensen ME, Evans AJ, Mathis JM, et al. Percutaneous polymethylmethacrylate vertebroplasty in the treatment of osteoporotic VB compression fractures: technical aspects. AJNR Am J Neuroradiol 1997;18:1897–1904.
29. Peters KR, Guiot BH, Martin PA, Fessler RG. Vertebroplasty for osteoporotic compression fractures: current practice and evolving techniques. Neurosurgery 2002;51:S96–S103.
30. Stallmeyer MJ, Zoarski GH, Obuchowski AM. Optimizing patient selection in percutaneous vertebroplasty. J Vasc Interv Radiol 2003;14:683–696.
31. Wong DA, Fornasier VL, MacNab I. Spinal metastases: the obvious, the occult, and the impostors. Spine 1990;15:1–4.
32. Klimo P, Schmidt MH. Surgical management of spinal metastases. Oncologist 2004;9(2):188–196.
33. Gerszten PC, Welch WC. Current surgical management of metastatic spinal disease. Oncology 2000;14:1013–1024.
34. Lada R, Kaminski HJ, Ruff R. Metastatic spinal cord compression. In: Vecht C, ed. Neuro-oncology. Part 3: Neurological Disorders in Systemic Cancer. Neurooncology 1997:167–189.
35. Byrne TN. Spinal cord compression from epidural metastases. N Engl J Med 1992;327:614–619.
36. Gilbert RW, Kim JH, Posner JB. Epidural spinal cord compression from metastatic tumor: diagnosis and treatment. Ann Neurol 1978;3:40–51.
37. Tokuhashi Y, Matsuzaki H, Toriyama S, et al. Scoring system for the preoperative evaluation of metastatic spine tumor prognosis. Spine 1990;15:1110–1113.
38. Sundaresan N, Steinberger AA, Moore F, et al. Indications and results of combined anterior-posterior approaches for spine tumor surgery. J Neurosurg 1996;85:438–446.
39. Sundaresan N, Digiacinto GV, Hughes JE, et al. Treatment of neoplastic spinal cord compression: results of a prospective study. Neurosurgery 1991;29:645–650.
40. Cooper PR, Errico TJ, Martin R, et al. A systematic approach to spinal reconstruction after anterior decompression for neoplastic disease of the thoracic and lumbar spine. Neurosurgery 1993;32:1–8.
41. Hammerberg KW. Surgical treatment of metastatic spine disease. Spine 1992;17:1148–1153.
42. Sundaresan N, Rothman A, Manhart K, et al. Surgery for solitary metastases of the spine: rationale and results of treatment. Spine 2002;27:1802–1806.
43. Gokaslan ZL, York JE, Walsh GL, et al. Transthoracic vertebrectomy for metastatic spinal tumors. J Neurosurg 1998;89:599–609.
44. Wise JJ, Fischgrund JS, Herkowitz HN, et al. Complication, survival rates, and risk factors of surgery for metastatic disease of the spine. Spine 1999;24:1943–1951.
45. Patchell RA, Tibbs PA, Regine WF, et al. Direct decompressive surgical resection in the treatment of spinal cord compression caused by metastatic cancer: a randomized trial. Lancet 2005;366:643–648.

INDEX

Index

Index